"We have long needed a book like this to deal with the challenges of work. But I didn't know what form that perfect book would take. *The Performance Edge* is it. It is shockingly appropriate for our times. Dr. Cooper is a national treasure. He masterfully combines science, philosophy, and common sense to guide us toward real success in our lives. Having this book is like having a brilliant friend with inside information who is willing to tailor a program for you not only to deal with job stress, but to turn your challenges into victories for everyone involved. The reward for reading and using this book will be a continual full, rich experience of self-worth and accomplishment. *The Performance Edge* isn't instant gratification. It is mastery."

— **Michael L. Ray,** Ph.D., coauthor of *Creativity in Business* and professor of innovation and of marketing at the Stanford University Graduate School of Business

"*The Performance Edge* is a superb contribution . . . filled with practical value. Dr. Cooper informs and instructs us on the sources of sustained top performance. Bravo!"

— **Charles A. Garfield,** Ph.D., author of *Peak Performers: The New Heroes of American Business*

"*The Performance Edge* is a treasure trove of valuable insights and immensely practical information. Dr. Cooper's work gives the reader a sense that great research has been done on his or her behalf. I have total admiration for this book's value."

— **Stephen R. Covey,** Ph.D., chairman of the Institute for Principle-Centered Leadership, adjunct professor at the Marriott School of Management, Brigham Young University, and best-selling author of *The Seven Habits of Highly Effective People*

"A *tremendous* book. *The Performance Edge* is filled with solid information and persuasive data that can help any person in achieving success. I benefited greatly from it, and I give *The Performance Edge* my total endorsement."

— **Nido R. Qubein,** international management consultant, former president of the National Speakers Association, and best-selling author of *Proven Strategies for Uncommon Achievement, How to Be a Great Communicator,* and *Get the Best from Yourself*

"Robert Cooper has written a book on human performance that is destined to become a classic — and will put him among the select few in his discipline who distinguish themselves as 'masters.' "

— **James E. Ericson,** director of the Masters of Executive Excellence Program (widely recognized as America's premier management development program)

"The real breakthrough for having America become more competitive in the 1990s will come from enhancing the human resource — making people more productive. Dr. Cooper's book *The Performance Edge* presents an exacting and comprehensive road map for achieving that critical goal."

— **F. G. "Buck" Rodgers,** former vice president of IBM, director of seven corporations, contributing editor to *Executive Excellence* magazine, and best-selling author of *The IBM Way* and *Getting the Best . . . Out of Yourself and Others*

"In today's world of mounting job demands and ceaseless challenges, *The Performance Edge* gives you advanced methods to unlock your potential for high achievement. This insightful book provides the tools you need to be on the cutting edge of personal and professional effectiveness — to get the most out of yourself *and* produce highest-quality work."

— **Brian Tracy,** president of Brian Tracy Learning Systems and best-selling author of *The Effective Manager, The Psychology of Selling,* and *The Psychology of Achievement*

"For all of us who are committed to succeeding in the world of work, yet know it can be a virtual battlefield, Dr. Cooper provides us with *The Performance Edge* — a marvelous, practical plan to mobilize our skills and to help us get control of our careers and our lives. He is a wise leader worthy of your attention."

— **Kate Ludeman,** Ph.D., president of Worth Ethic Training Company, former vice president of human resources and corporate officer at KLA Instruments, and author of *The Worth Ethic: How to Profit from the Changing Values of the New Work Force*

"Dr. Robert Cooper has written an impressive, comprehensive guide to personal effectiveness . . . covering many crucial subjects. If you want to be on 'The Performance Edge' for the twenty-first century, read this book."

— **Charles C. Manz,** Ph.D., professor of management at Arizona State University, author of *The Art of Self-Leadership,* and coauthor of *SuperLeadership: Leading Others to Lead Themselves*

"The Performance Edge is absolutely outstanding. Dr. Cooper's brilliant advice will make you a winner — at work *and* at home. In a variety of practical new ways, *The Performance Edge* teaches you how to maximize your on-the-job effectiveness and competitive advantage, while also dealing with the essential — but usually overlooked — issue of balancing the competing demands of work and family. Read — and use — this valuable book."

— **Harold H. Bloomfield,** M.D., best-selling author of *The Achilles Syndrome: Turning Your Weaknesses into Strengths* and *Life-Mates: The Program for a Lasting Relationship*

"The Performance Edge is a prescription for success. By following its suggestions, you'll achieve a clear physical, emotional, and mental advantage in business — and in life."

— **Tony Alessandra,** Ph.D., author of *The Art of Managing People, Non-Manipulative Selling,* and *People Smart*

"The Performance Edge is the most comprehensive guide to personal achievement that I've ever seen. I applaud Dr. Cooper's attention to the 'inner skills' of self-awareness explored in his Performance Turning Points, recognizing that every one of us can learn productive new responses to stress that greatly improve our potential for health and success. A powerful book!"

— **Emmett E. Miller,** M.D., stress researcher, psychophysiologist, internationally recognized developer of scientifically based audio and video programs, and author of *Software for the Mind, Self-Imagery, Optimal Performance,* and *Letting Go of Stress*

"We read in current management theory that to get the best performance in the workplace is to have an integrated approach . . . Dr. Cooper has done us all a great service by providing a book that captures this united way of living and working. *The Performance Edge* will be of great benefit to those who strive for their best."

— **Laura A. Liswood,** founder of the Liswood Marketing Group, author of *Serving Them Right: Innovative and Powerful Customer Retention Strategies,* business editor of KUOW Public Radio in Seattle, senior examiner for the Malcolm Baldridge Quality Award, and member of Bain & Company's Customer Retention/Zero Defections_{sm} Board

"The Performance Edge is thoughtful, insightful, and exceptionally practical. This is a *must* read for everyone who wants to make a difference in their organization, community, or personal life."

— **Barry Z. Posner,** Ph.D., professor of organizational behavior, associate dean, and chief service officer at the Leavey Graduate School of Business and Administration, Santa Clara University, and bestselling coauthor of *The Leadership Challenge: How to Get Extraordinary Things Done in Organizations*

"I am very impressed with *The Performance Edge.* Robert Cooper has done an outstanding job of bringing together the most responsible research in a wide diversity of topics impacting human performance. Congratulations on a superior book!"

— **James E. Loehr,** Ph.D., internationally recognized authority on performance psychology and author of *Mentally Tough*

"In today's fast-changing business world, it's more difficult than ever to capture and sustain the competitive advantage. Few of us realize that, as a complement to current management and leadership training, we need new capabilities for best health and performance. *The Performance Edge* zeroes in on these new priorities — in a clear, compelling, and practical way. This book is *must reading* for everyone who seeks the best in work and in life."

— **Marjorie Blanchard,** Ph.D., president of Blanchard Training & Development, Inc., and coauthor of *Working Well: Managing for Health and High Performance*

"Dr. Robert Cooper has done it again . . . *The Performance Edge* shows each of us how to defuse the workplace timebomb and turn stress to our advantage."

— **Peter G. Hanson,** M.D., international authority on personal and corporate stress management, publisher of "Inside Information" Newsletter, and best-selling author of *The Joy of Stress* and *Stress for Success*

"*The Performance Edge* presumes that in order to manage somebody else's business — or your own — the first step is to manage your own time and your own life. This book, more than any I have ever seen, teaches the reader just how to handle that core management skill."

— **George S. Odiorne,** Ph.D., professor of management and senior research associate at the Human Resources Institute, Eckerd College, and author of 25 business books, including *The Human Side of Management: Management by Integration and Self-Control*

"Our business evolution toward the twenty-first century requires a complete rethinking of personal and organizational performance. *The Performance Edge* is required reading."

— **Michael A. Silva,** CEO of Bennett Enterprises, global management authority, and best-selling coauthor of *Creating Excellence, The Future 500,* and *Europe 1992 and The New World Power Game*

"*The Performance Edge* will be THE business book of the 1990s."

— **Roger Dawson,** CEO of Plaza Productions and author *The Secrets of Power Negotiating* and *The Secrets of Power Performance.*

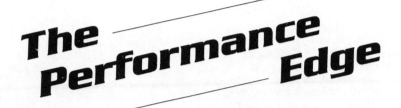

The Performance Edge

Books by Robert K. Cooper

Health & Fitness Excellence:
The Comprehensive Action Plan

The Performance Edge:
New Strategies to Maximize Your
Work Effectiveness & Competitive Advantage

Robert K.
Cooper, Ph.D.

The Performance Edge

*New Strategies to Maximize
Your Work Effectiveness &
Competitive Advantage*

HOUGHTON MIFFLIN COMPANY
BOSTON 1991

For information about permission to reproduce selections from
this book, write to Permissions, Houghton Mifflin Company,
2 Park Street, Boston, Massachusetts 02108.

Library of Congress Cataloging-in-Publication Data

Cooper, Robert K.
The performance edge : new strategies to maximize your work
effectiveness & competitive advantage / Robert K. Cooper.
p.   cm.
ISBN 0-395-53338-4
1. Success in business.   2. Performance.   3. Stress management.
4. Time management.   I. Title.
HF5386.C785 1991   90-49161
650.1 — dc20   CIP

The health information in this book is not intended as a substitute
for the medical recommendations of physicians. The author does not
directly or indirectly dispense medical advice or prescribe treatment
of any kind for illness or disease. The intent is to offer information
to help you, the reader, cooperate with your physician and other
health professionals in your mutual quest for optimum well-being.

Printed in the United States of America

DOH 10 9 8 7 6 5 4 3 2 1

Acknowledgments

Above my office desk is a small plaque that reads, "Give the world the best you have and the best will come back to you." My research for *The Performance Edge* began more than two decades ago, culminating with many months of writing, review, and editing. I would like to acknowledge that even before its publication, I *have* received the best in return, including strong support from my professional colleagues around the world.

I am deeply grateful for the insights, inspiration, or personal support from the following people who helped *The Performance Edge* become a reality:

- My wife, Leslie, for her radiant love and professional competence, and for being my best friend
- My father, Dr. Hugh Cooper, for teaching me the values of science, hard work, and common sense; and for exemplifying the courage to think creatively under pressure and the willingness to invest time and energy in rebuilding organizations and making the world a better place in which to live and work
- My mother, Margaret D. Cooper, for steadfastly inspiring me to set my sights high and trust that life always turns out best when it's lived from the inside out
- The rest of my family — my sister, Mary, my brother, David, my son, Christopher, and my daughter, Chelsea — for the love and happiness you bring to my life

- Karl H. Pribram, M.D., National Institutes of Health Professor of Neuroscience and Professor of Psychology and Psychiatry at Stanford University School of Medicine, for his friendship and for first inspiring me more than twenty years ago to view human performance potentials through an integrated scientific perspective
- Nido R. Qubein, M.B.A., my mentor and friend, for first opening my eyes to the potentials of a new kind of performance enhancement program to meet the demands of a highly competitive, fast-changing business world
- Harold H. Bloomfield, M.D., for his friendship, his leadership in the fields of health sciences and psychology, and his sage advice on media communications
- Tom Ferguson, M.D., for his friendship and award-winning medical writing that has set new standards for demystifying the language of scientific research
- Warren Bennis, Ph.D., Distinguished Professor of Business Administration at the University of Southern California, for his research on leadership at a time when our complex and rapidly changing business world needs it most
- Rosabeth Moss Kanter, Ph.D., professor of business administration at the Harvard University Business School, for her brilliant work in injecting entrepreneurial dynamism into mainstream corporate America and for her writings on creating the productive workplace of the future
- Charles A. Garfield, Ph.D., for his leadership in drawing the business world's attention to the central principles of peak performance
- Michael L. Ray, Ph.D., professor of innovation and of marketing at the Stanford University Graduate School of Business, for his friendship and pioneering work on creativity in business — and in life
- Burt Nanus, Ph.D., professor of management at the University of Southern California Graduate School of Business, for his research on leadership strategies
- Stephen R. Covey, Ph.D., chairman of the Institute for Principle-Centered Leadership, for his pioneering work on professional effectiveness and balancing the competing demands of work and family

- Emmett E. Miller, M.D., for his friendship and research on the powers of mental vision and strategic thinking
- Kate Ludeman, Ph.D., president of the Worth Ethic Training Company, for her efforts to transform corporate culture and increase productivity through trust, caring, and meaningful work
- Noel M. Tichy, Ph.D., professor and director of the Global Leadership Program at the University of Michigan's Graduate School of Business, for his advanced research on strategic change and transformational leadership
- Michael A. Silva, lecturer on global management and CEO of Bennett Enterprises, for his depth of knowledge on Europe 1992 and the sweeping, powerful changes of a borderless business world
- Mary Anne Devanna, Ph.D., associate dean at the Graduate School of Business, Columbia University, for her comprehensive insights on strategic human resource management and organizational leadership
- Craig R. Hickman, chairman and CEO of Management Perspectives Group and adjunct professor at Brigham Young University's Graduate School of Management, for his insights on the future of management and on creating tomorrow's organizations today
- Charles C. Manz, Ph.D., professor of management at Arizona State University, for his discoveries about the art of self-leadership and his concept of *superleadership* — leading others to lead themselves
- Peter M. Senge, Ph.D., director of the Systems Thinking and Organizational Learning Program at MIT's Sloan School of Management, for his enlightening research on systems thinking, personal mastery, and the "fifth discipline," the art and practice of the learning organization
- Lyle Sussman, Ph.D., professor of management at the Graduate School of Business, University of Louisville, for his practical guidelines on effective management and getting the best from yourself and your co-workers
- George S. Odiorne, Ph.D., professor of management at Eckerd College, for his revealing research on integration and self-control as key factors in the human side of management
- Barry Z. Posner, Ph.D., professor of management and director of Graduate Education and Customer Service at the Santa Clara

University Graduate School of Business, for his immensely useful ideas on leadership and accomplishment
- Robert H. Waterman, Jr., for his extensive research on corporate change and renewal
- Michael LeBoeuf, Ph.D., professor of management at the University of New Orleans, for his practical advice on results-oriented management
- F. G. "Buck" Rodgers, former vice-president for marketing at IBM Corporation, for his knowledge about individual work performance and the competitive advantage
- Tom Peters, for constantly searching out fresh perspectives and new directions for solving many of today's toughest corporate challenges
- Jan Carlzon, president and CEO of Scandinavian Airlines, for bringing the business world's attention to the critical importance of "moments of truth"
- Redford Williams, M.D., professor of psychiatry, associate professor of medicine, and director of the Behavioral Medicine Research Center at Duke University Medical Center, for his discoveries about type A behavior and cardiovascular disease
- James E. Loehr, Ph.D., for his pioneering research in performance psychology and the role of "mental toughness" in winning at work
- Laura A. Liswood, founder of Liswood Marketing Group, for her innovative, timely research on customer retention and service-directed management
- Marjorie Blanchard, Ph.D., for her insights on wellness in the workplace and on new ways to manage for both health and high performance
- Peter G. Hanson, M.D., for his perspectives on stress management and strategies for handling job pressure
- Robert S. Eliot, M.D., professor of cardiology at the University of Nebraska Medical Center and director of the Institute of Stress Medicine, for his research on the relationship between stress and heart attacks
- Esther M. Orioli, president of Essi Systems, for her research on stress management and company performance profiles
- Roger Dawson, international management consultant and CEO of Plaza Productions, for his useful advice on negotiation and performance

- Karl Albrecht, for his insights on the new service economy
- Jeanne M. Stellman, Ph.D., professor of public health at Columbia University, for her studies on environmental health and occupational medicine
- Janet Travell, M.D., emeritus clinical professor of medicine at the George Washington University School of Medicine, and David G. Simons, M.D., clinical professor in the Department of Physical Medicine and Rehabilitation at the University of California, Irvine, for their research on rapid, cost-effective treatment of myofascial pain syndromes
- Judith J. Wurtman, Ph.D., and Richard J. Wurtman, Ph.D., both of the Massachusetts Institute of Technology, for their research discoveries in neuroendocrinology and nutritional science
- Rene Cailliet, M.D., director of the Department of Physical Medicine and Rehabilitation at the Santa Monica Hospital Medical Center and professor and former director of the Department of Physical Medicine and Rehabilitation at the University of Southern California School of Medicine, for his research over the past thirty years on chronic tension and pain syndromes, exercise, and posture
- Richard A. Dienstbier, Ph.D., professor of psychology at the University of Nebraska and recent visiting scholar at Cambridge University, England, for his work on the "mental toughening" dimensions of exercise and stress
- Mauricio Padilla, D.Sc., for his friendship and scientific perspectives on nutritional biochemistry and chronobiology
- Tony Alessandra, Ph.D., for his research on nonmanipulative selling and how to deal with the differences in people
- Jim Cathcart, president of the National Speakers Association, for his ideas on developing top performers through relationship management
- Brian Tracy, for his practical perspectives on the psychology of achievement
- J. Edward Russo, Ph.D., associate professor of marketing and behavioral science at Cornell University's Johnson Graduate School of Management, and Paul J. H. Schoemaker, Ph.D., associate professor of decision sciences and policy in the Graduate School of Business at the University of Chicago, for their research and educational efforts in decision sciences
- Drs. V. P. Zinchenko, A. B. Leonova, and Y. K. Strelkov, of the

Department of Engineering Psychology and Work Psychology at Moscow State University in the Soviet Union, for their research on the psychometrics of fatigue

- Etienne Grandjean, M.D., director of the Department of Ergonomics at the Swiss Federal Institute of Technology in Switzerland, for his research on ergonomics in business
- Lisa Shoppmann, for her many hours of work as my research assistant at the University of Michigan Medical Library and Business Library
- Ruth K. Hapgood, senior editor at Houghton Mifflin, for her inspiring blend of penetrating farsightedness and down-to-earth wisdom
- John Sterling, editor-in-chief at Houghton Mifflin, for his perceptive insights in shaping *The Performance Edge*
- Others at Houghton Mifflin — Nancy Grant, Steven Lewers, Sandra Goroff-Mailly, Becky Saikia-Wilson, and Barbara Flanagan — for their straightforward advice and support
- My literary agents, Georges and Anne Borchardt

I am also especially grateful for encouragement and support from Michael Q. Patton, Ph.D., and Harold V. McAbee, Ed.D., of the Union Graduate School; and for the research insights and inspiration I have received from other leaders, including Patricia Aburdene, James L. Adams, Thomas E. Backer, Dr. Wilfred Barlow, Stephen E. Bechtold, Dr. Aaron T. Beck, John G. Belcher, Jr., Kenneth Blanchard, Robert Boguslaw, Dr. Joan Borysenko, Scott Brown, Dr. David D. Burns, Lorna Catford, Norman Cousins, William H. Davidow, Robert T. Davis, Edward de Bono, Scott DeGarmo, Dr. Marian Cleeves Diamond, Lydia Dotto, Peter F. Drucker, Charles F. Ehret, Suzette Haden Elgin, Gary Emery, Jim Ericson, Roger Fisher, Mark A. Frohman, Andrew S. Grove, John D. Hatfield, Mary Sue Henifin, Dr. William Hettler, Shozo Hibino, Thomas M. Hout, Richard C. Huseman, Masaaki Imai, Dr. David Imrie, Alice M. Isen, John M. Ivancevich, Dennis T. Jaffe, Ralph E. Janaro, Elliott Jaques, Daniel Kahneman, Donald L. Kanter, Robert A. Karasek, Tess Kirby, Suzanne C. Kobasa, Jim Kouzes, Dr. Hans Kraus, Ellen J. Langer, Dorothy Leeds, Dr. A. R. Luria, James J. Lynch, Michael Maccoby, Salvatore R. Maddi, Joseph D. Matarazzo, Dr. Vernon H. Mark, Michael T. Matteson, Michael E.

McGill, Peter Meyer, Tom Miller, Philip H. Mirvis, Dr. Hugo Morales-Ballejo, Rochelle Myers, Dr. Alf Nachemson, Gerald Nadler, John Naisbitt, Perry Pascarella, Warren J. Pelton, Michael Porter, Robert E. Quinn, Dr. Grigori Raiport, Charles Rodgers, Fran Sussner Rodgers, Robert H. Schaffer, Roger Schank, Leonard A. Schlesinger, Cynthia D. Scott, Martin E. P. Seligman, Anees A. Sheikh, Herbert Simon, David Smith, Georges Stalk, Jr., Bryant A. Stamford, Dr. Charles F. Stroebel, Rick Suarez, Richard M. Suinn, Dr. Mark Tager, Deborah Tannen, John Tropman, Amos Tversky, Peter B. Vaill, Andrew H. Van de Ven, N. Venkatraman, Hendrie D. Weisinger, Ph.D., Daniel Yankelovich, and Ron Zemke.

Finally, I want to thank the thousands of dedicated researchers throughout the world who, with little recognition, regularly bring forth vital revelations that give hope to our planet and wings to our personal and corporate dreams.

Contents

1

Introduction

At the boundary, life blossoms.

— *James Gleick,* Chaos

The only sustainable advantage that any organization is going
to have in the future is the ability of its people.

— *D. Quinn Mills, Harvard Business School*

GETTING THE JOB DONE isn't enough these days. Today's work
world demands more. More creative thinking. More communication. More customer responsiveness. More decisive action. More
risk taking. More quality control. More pull-out-the-stops performance.

The opportunities and choices are great, and they are growing.
But so is the difficulty of taking advantage of them. Markets expand and shrink overnight, driven by technologies that constantly
change. New competitors pop up from unexpected quarters.

No matter what your industry or personal position, you must
be able to work smarter and better than ever before.[1] You must be
quick and innovative enough to exploit sudden opportunities and
— at the same time — accomplish much more with dwindling resources, fewer mistakes, and shorter deadlines. Acceptable excuses
for suboptimal performance are becoming few and far between.

You're expected to achieve impressive results, not just once in a while but repeatedly, consistently, hour after hour, day after day.

This is the first book dedicated to creating — and taking full advantage of — the Performance Edge, with practical new recommendations based not on quick fixes or fads but on leading-edge scientific principles and workplace research.

Your Competitive Advantage Is Determined by Personal Performance

> What will remain true in the best organizations, whatever else changes, is that power ultimately derives from human performance.
>
> — *Charles A. Stewart*, Fortune *magazine*[2]

One reason *The Performance Edge* is crucial today is that most organizations continue to make the mistake of investing resources so heavily in *physical technology and current operations* that they overlook or neglect the need to produce *highly effective human systems*.[3] Therefore the responsibility for maximizing your work effectiveness and competitive advantage is forced squarely into your own hands.

"Most managements have largely failed to comprehend that basic performance capacity is the absolute weakest link in our struggle to be competitive," writes Robert H. Schaffer in *The Breakthrough Strategy*. "While American companies search far and wide for ever more esoteric formulas to get them back into the running, some very powerful solutions lie close at hand."[4]

"To have world-class quality and costs and the ability to assimilate new technology," says Richard E. Walton of the Harvard Business School, "we must have the world's best ability to develop human capabilities."[5]

"The key," explains Schaffer, "is that during normal times, in most organizations, unbelievably vast quantities of potentially productive capacity are untapped, undemanded, unused or frittered away."[6] In short, much of what we believe about our personal — and, in turn, corporate — performance capabilities is based not on facts, but on myths. And, worst of all, these misconceptions form iron fences in our minds. Can we break out of this trap? Yes, we can. That's the message of *The Performance Edge*.

Work Demands Are Tougher Than Ever — and Increasing

In today's relentlessly competitive, high-velocity work world, where anything is possible but nothing is guaranteed, your day-in, day-out personal advantage hinges on some formidable new priorities, including

- Continuous creative innovation
- All-out speed
- Zero-defect quality control
- On-target communication
- Mental and physical stamina to handle increased pace and workload
- Flawless teamwork
- Total customer responsiveness
- Quick-release stress control
- Balance between the competing demands of work and family

Continuous Creative Innovation

No matter what your job, finding better ways to do things has become a daily requirement. Everywhere you look, conventional wisdom and traditional procedures are being questioned — and in many cases thrown out the window.

In today's fast-changing business world, the failure to recognize — and seize — opportunities is a potentially fatal mistake. Fresh ideas are now the most precious raw materials, and your continued success depends on an inordinately high level of creative alertness and innovative problem solving — not only for management but *for every employee in your organization*.

All-Out Speed

Chances are that you're already being called on to find every possible way to work smarter and more productively every minute of the day. The way that you manage time — whether in new product development, production, sales, distribution, or service — is one of the most powerful sources of competitive advantage.[7] "Speed is becoming an increasingly important weapon in the 1990s," warns a recent *Fortune* cover story, "and managers who dawdle are likely to be swept into the dustbin of history."[8]

This high-stress management approach has become the model toward which every sector of industry seems to be striving.[9] Each of us is expected to make on-the-spot continuous improvements. According to a recent report in *Technology Review*, for example, in a growing number of state-of-the-art manufacturing companies, "no matter how well managers and workers learn their jobs, there is no such thing as establishing a comfortable pace. . . . Once the line is up to speed, each person can barely keep up with the specified job, let alone help someone else. In fact, if you can shave a few seconds off a task you *shouldn't* help fellow workers. . . . The rules mandate discipline — including firing — for 'failure to maintain satisfactory production levels.' Thus, personal stress as well as system stress drives production."[10]

Zero-Defect Quality Control

The plain truth about quality is that, for the most part, it's a human performance issue — in other words, it's up to you. And the goal at top companies has become not just fewer defects but *zero* defects. "Occasional failure is not inevitable," says Phil Kelly, vice-president of Motorola's customer response center. "*All* errors are preventable."[11]

Like many top organizations, the new aim at Motorola, recent winner of the prestigious Malcolm Baldrige National Quality Award, isn't simply to manufacture flawless products; it's to eliminate defects throughout the entire organization. Motorola's goal is to achieve plus or minus *six sigma* — an engineering term equivalent to 3.4 defects per million parts.

Put another way, the company wants to be perfect in everything 99.9999998 percent of the time. Says CEO George Fisher: "If we don't take this kind of action, we're simply not going to survive the competition around the world." Sooner or later, your own organization will probably reach the same conclusion: Even operating at the three-sigma level — an amazing 99.7 percent error-free performance — may no longer be good enough.

On-Target Communication

None of us can afford to ignore the fact that our work success depends on the ability to communicate — to listen intelligently and to get our own message across, quickly and clearly, no matter what the hour or circumstance. Any energy that's wasted arguing or miscommunicating weakens your ability to get the job done. Moreover, today's participative, partnership-oriented management requires exemplary — not just acceptable — communication. Huge chunks of time, money, and peace of mind are lost every day as a result of workplace communication mix-ups and misunderstandings that could quite easily be prevented.[12]

Mental and Physical Stamina

To handle increased speed and productivity demands, it's become imperative for every one of us to have consistently high levels of mental and physical energy and stamina. This demand raises the question How much work effort is actually enough? "In today's workplace, 'enough' is defined not by some pre-existing standard like the length of the workday but by the limits of human endurance," says Rosabeth Moss Kanter, professor at the Harvard Business School. "And this standard, in turn, changes the shape of professional and personal life."[13]

Evidence of this increased pressure is everywhere. In the past, a psychological "work contract" committed employers to providing steady employment and benefits and employees to supplying loyalty and consistent good work. But not anymore. Shaken by mergers and cutbacks, we're increasingly forced to fend for ourselves, placing our trust not in the companies we work for but in our own personal capabilities to handle pressure, adapt to change, and sustain high-level performance.[14]

Public opinion analyst Daniel Yankelovich believes that too many corporations, enamored of a lean and mean corporate policy, shortsightedly ignore the potential of what he calls *discretionary effort* — the large, usually untapped area between the minimum amount of work employees have to do to get by and the full effort they're eager to give if they receive recognition and compensation.[15]

This has driven the business world toward an individualistic work force, in which each of us must run our own career "like a privately held corporation."[16] According to Kanter, "Climbing the career ladder is being replaced by hopping from job to job. Reliance on organizations to give shape to a career is being replaced by reliance on self. Overall, the power of the position is giving way to the power of the person."[17] Here, your mental and physical stamina have a direct bearing on your achievement.

Employment security is being cast away in favor of *employability* security — the knowledge that the results you produce today will enhance your value for future work opportunities.

Flawless Teamwork

At the same time that job security is disappearing and your individual performance requires extra attention, you're faced with the conflicting demand for far greater cooperation with co-workers, no matter how hectic the pace or how competitive the situation.[18]

But, as most of us know all too well, effective teamwork is a thorny challenge. It requires decentralized management, crosstraining, greater access to information and resources, increased authority and responsibility for making decisions that affect your work, and creative new ways to provide recognition and compensation. Streamlined interpersonal cooperation depends on such Performance Edge issues as purpose-driven objectives, clear communication, effective stress management, mental and physical endurance, and innovative decision making.

Total Customer Responsiveness

Gone are the days when service just meant a smile and a money-back guarantee. Today's front-running business performers make superior customer responsiveness a priority in everything they do.

Entire organizations — from research to manufacturing, from information systems to pay incentives — are being geared toward giving customers what they want.[19] "It seems so simple," explains a recent *Business Week* cover story. "Businesses exist to serve customers and should bend over backward to satisfy their needs. But too many companies still don't get it. And in the years ahead, more customers are likely to take the opportunity to reward the ones that do."[20]

Quick-Release Stress Control

The incidence of job stress — which can be most simply defined as workplace *pressure* or *change* — is skyrocketing. Even if you survived the latest round of cutbacks, you can't breathe easy. To the contrary, the vast restructurings under way at many companies have loaded more work on those who have kept their jobs.

With managers and professionals working longer hours than ever, many are wondering whether relief is finally in sight. The answer, say bosses, is not a chance. In the latest Fortune 500 CEO poll, 77 percent of CEOs said they believe that U.S. corporations will have to push their managers and employees harder than ever to compete internationally.[21]

Job stress costs American businesses at least $200 billion a year[22]— in absenteeism, diminished productivity, direct medical expenses, employee turnover, insurance premiums, and worker's compensation awards. Put into perspective, that's already more than the profits of all the Fortune 500 companies combined.

In addition, medical researchers estimate that stress is linked to 65 to 90 percent of all illnesses and diseases.[23] Every year, for example, more than 500,000 Americans die from heart attacks — 300,000 before reaching a hospital. Many of these deaths are due to *silent heart disease*,[24] in which the victims have none of the usual cardiac danger symptoms such as high blood pressure, obesity, or elevated blood cholesterol. These people are often high achieving, physically fit, and healthy on the outside but have a time bomb tied to their hearts: Hidden stress is breaking down the heart muscle and creating a high risk of heart attack.[25]

Some leading cardiologists are even asserting that "controlling stress may be the single most important key to preventing heart attacks,"[26] and recent studies suggest that it's not only an American problem: Mismanaged stress may be killing off many of Japan's managers and corporate chiefs.[27]

Traditional, time-consuming approaches to workplace stress management have proven ineffective,[28] and researchers have found that what most of us really need are some simple, practical "quick release" methods for controlling negative stress.

Balance Between the Competing Demands of Work and Family

Although the myth about separate and nonoverlapping work and home worlds has had a long life in the corporate mind,[29] convincing new research shows that stress at home interferes with work performance and, conversely, that work stress creates or magnifies problems at home.[30] The intensity and single-mindedness that contribute to corporate achievement are often the opposite of the qualities needed to be an effective husband, wife, or parent.[31]

On top of job pressures, we're each regularly called on to deal with many home conerns, including issues involving spouse, children, aging parents, hectic family schedules, the desire for more free time, and feelings of guilt that come from too many commitments. How you handle these challenges has a direct influence on your accomplishments at work.

The preceding examples highlight the pressure-packed situation more of us are faced with every day, and, as long as these pressures exist, every conceivable strategy to help us cope becomes a matter of survival. Without the Performance Edge, fewer and fewer of us will be able to keep up with job demands.

Maximizing Your Personal Effectiveness in a Changing Work World

> Efficiency is doing things right. *Effectiveness* is doing the right things.
>
> — *Peter F. Drucker*

From both a scientific and a philosophical perspective, the "work harder, faster, and longer" idea doesn't work. In fact, it's a straight track to burnout. And that brings us to a key point. *This is not a book about living to work; it's a book about working to live.*

To begin with, quit trying harder. Research shows that doing more of the same, only harder, isn't the way to achieve more. In fact, sometimes it's a big part of the problem. You become blind to better pathways and you start producing less and less. Besides, sooner or later, you're going to reach the point where you just can't try any harder — where your current physical and mental resources are pushed to the breaking point or your spirit wanes. More effort isn't the answer. It's time to shift gears and break out of old routines.

With the Performance Edge, you can increase your personal effectiveness by taking advantage of your untapped physiological and psychological *capacities* for top performance, hour after hour, day after day.

And then — and this is critical — you can start breaking away from the job at a better hour and begin giving some of your newfound energy and time to the *other* aspects of your life — your personal fitness and well-being, your family relationships, and community concerns. Researchers are discovering that this is precisely the kind of balance it takes to strengthen your inner happiness and revitalize your mind. In turn, it further boosts your effectiveness and performance on the job.

Results Begin Right Now

> Human capacities have never been measured; nor are we to judge of what we can do by any precedents, so little has been tried.
>
> — *Henry David Thoreau*

The advice and strategies in *The Performance Edge* can be quickly learned and applied, and they cost little or no money to implement. Yet they have the power to transform your career. This book can also serve as a first step for you to join others to lift your work team or company to the next level of effective collaboration, customer responsiveness, innovation, productivity, and quality control.

I've spent more than twenty years researching human performance. In addition to earning my Ph.D. in health sciences and psychology and serving as a certified instructor for leading preventive medicine organizations, I have done graduate work in journalism, conducted computer database searches of the world's scientific and medical literature, and learned from top management authorities and researchers in the United States, Asia, and Europe. The guidelines in this book — backed by hundreds of scientific references — grew out of insights I have gained from working with leading corporations in the United States and abroad and from experts in brain science, systems thinking, performance psychology, work physiology, stress dynamics, physical and occupational medicine, nutritional biochemistry, decision sciences, ergonomics, communication, sociology, global leadership, and organizational behavior.

The Performance Edge presents you with an unprecedented opportunity to maximize your work effectiveness and competitive advantage. You'll be able to chart a more insightful, productive path into the future, and to make fundamental workplace changes that reduce unnecessary stress, maximize your personal and collaborative achievements, and improve the well-being of all members of your organization and its strategic alliances.

To do less means to fall behind. To do it haphazardly or without a plan means to burn out and ultimately fail.

As a result, you're faced with a unique challenge. Perhaps, like many of us, you've become disillusioned by the rash of business fads and quick fixes that waste your time, energy, and money. I don't blame you. But don't let this obscure the fact that researchers around the world *have* discovered some simple, practical solutions to many of today's toughest workplace performance challenges.

If you still have an unshakable commitment to being your best and are ready to learn the proven scientific principles in *The Performance Edge* — and roll up your sleeves and apply them to your work — then I have written this book for you.

2

An Overview

> Only a handful of organizations have even begun to tap into their primary resource, *their people*, much less give them the means to do what they are capable of doing.
>
> — *Warren Bennis*, On Becoming a Leader

The Performance Edge is a book of specific techniques and practical strategies that you can apply immediately. They are easy to learn. They are simple to use. And they work.

The trends that have shaken the corporate world will continue or accelerate in coming years. Global competition is certain to intensify, requiring fresh new thinking about what it takes to capture — and then hold — the advantage.

No matter how sophisticated your company's management strategies and technologies are, consistent breakthrough achievements depend on individual effectiveness and performance under pressure. The person, not the machine, will continue to be the predominant key to success in the years ahead.

Designing Your Personal Program

The way to read this book is with pen in hand. Mark it up, highlight key points, jot down ideas for your career or company in the margins, and keep a running "take-action" list. Write down your priorities and schedule them on your calendar.

You may be wondering, Do I really need to immediately learn and do *everything* in this book? My answer: Absolutely not. You can begin anywhere in this program and proceed, step by step, at your own pace, with whatever first interests you. Then, progressively, you can put together all the pieces of the Performance Edge puzzle in the most effective way for you as an individual.

Every myth you eliminate, every scientific strategy you choose, and every action step you take unlocks more of your untapped personal capabilities.

The Performance Edge is divided into two sections. Here are some highlights of what you will learn:

Part I: The Six Performance Turning Points

> Today's workforce is better educated than ever and has high expectations. There is diminished loyalty to the organization. Workers do not listen to or follow others because they are bosses. *They pay attention to the authority of competence.*
>
> — *William Sandy,* Forging the Productivity Partnership

This section focuses on maximizing your personal effectiveness under pressure — the core of the Performance Edge. Whether you realize it or not, your work performance is determined by split-second responses to minute-by-minute workplace challenges. Mismanaging these Performance Turning Points — presented in Chapters 3 through 8 — can end up driving you *away* from your goals instead of toward them.

Life and work advance through a series of decisions, and although, like the rest of us, at times you may feel frustrated or powerless, a clear-eyed look will reveal that at every turn you make a choice.

To excel, to recognize — and to capture — each successive opportunity and every perceivable competitive advantage, we each need to upgrade our level of personal effectiveness and achievement — in thoughts, emotions, words, and actions — and then sustain and expand this state. And for those times when we feel this powerful, productive level of functioning starting to slip away, we need fast, effective responses to recapture it without delay.

Again and again, in every sector of the work world, we're finding ourselves head to head with relentless new competitors whose job expertise, resources, incentives, and objectives have reached a virtual par with our own. In each of these battles, day in and day out, your success or failure hinges on the way you manage — or mismanage — the following six Performance Turning Points.

Chapter 3: Performance Turning Point #1: Stressful "Crisis Moments"

Taking Charge of Job Pressure with Quick-Release Stress Control

Scientific New Ways to Conquer Work Stress — from Daily Hassles to the Never-Ending Demand for Greater Customer Responsiveness and Fewer Mistakes, and from Unexpected Emergencies to "It's All on the Line" Performance Challenges

- Groundbreaking strategies for preventing and, when necessary, quickly rebounding from many of the conflicts and hassles that break down productivity, slow customer responsiveness, and sabotage quality control
- Ways to immediately transform "crisis moments" — including mistakes, arguments, anger, unexpected schedule changes, customer and employee complaints, confrontations, and criticism — into productive energy
- The Instant Calming Sequence (ICS), which scientifically neutralizes negative stress in less than one second and helps keep you in command of your thoughts, emotions, and actions whenever you're under pressure

Chapter 4: Performance Turning Point #2: Tension and Pain

Using NeuroMuscular Technique (NMT), the 6-Second, Medically Proven Way to Stop Tension and Pain Overcoming Persistent Barriers to Work Productivity and Quality Control

- Why stress-related headaches and backaches are the leading causes of lost work time and regularly sabotage effectiveness at work
- A remarkable new way to stop tension and pain — pounding headaches, stiff neck, tense shoulders, and back pain — in 6 to 10 seconds, using an easy, medically documented self-care skill

Chapter 5: Performance Turning Point #3: Time Pressures

Achieving "Priority Effectiveness" to Work Smarter and Faster
Why It's More Critical Than Ever to Practice Effective Self-Management: To Work Smarter and More Productively — Instead of Longer and Harder — and to Get Your Life in Better Balance so Success at Work Doesn't Have to Come at the Expense of Family Time and Personal Development

- Why time-based competition is a preeminent concern for individuals and companies worldwide — and why tough managers are insisting that "nothing short of disaster is a valid excuse for delay"
- Insights on the difference between "face time" and effective performance time
- How to develop a greater talent for getting the right things done
- New ways to stop getting sidetracked and to organize and execute around priorities
- Specific strategies to release co-workers and employees from their

dependence on you and thereby free more of your schedule for high-priority objectives
· Eight guidelines for running successful meetings in less time
· Insights on making the portable electronic office work for you

Chapter 6: Performance Turning Point #4: Communication Exchanges

Developing More Insightful, On-Target Interpersonal Skills
New Discoveries About How Eight Specific Types of Communication Interactions Sabotage — or Can Strongly Improve — Your Business Performance and Influence Your Health (and Heart Attack Risk)

· How to cut the fog out of your communication and identify and avoid "perception gaps" and other conversational pitfalls that sabotage business relationships
· Smarter questions to reduce mistakes, overcome objections, and solve problems
· New scientific discoveries about dealing with anger, arguments, criticism, and other "verbal toxins" that create tension and hostility, cut productivity, and can significantly increase your risk of heart attack
· Six steps to listen and speak with greater clarity, turning resistance into support and taking control of verbal confrontations

Chapter 7: Performance Turning Point #5: Decision-Making and Innovation Opportunities

Achieving — and Sustaining — the Mental Advantage
New Insights on Fluid Intelligence and Creativity, and the Five Most Crucial Questions for Decision Making Under Stress

· How to avoid decision-making traps and remove the most persistent barriers to innovation

• The five key mental questions that enable you to stay on top of difficult situations — remaining calm, energetic, thoughtful, and in control — whenever things at work begin to heat up, unexpectedly change directions, or start to come apart
• Specific ways to increase your ability to solve problems more quickly and effectively, dealing with competing demands and contradictory approaches
• The mindsets that block creativity and new ways to "jump the track" and free yourself from unproductive lines of thought
• The straight truth about why so much "positive" thinking is really negative — and what to do about it

Chapter 8: Performance Turning Point #6: Mental and Physical Stamina

Beating Fatigue and Increasing Your Effectiveness on the Job with 60-Second Work Breaks
    The Practical Scientific Action Plan to Relax Tight Muscles and Balance Posture, Replenish Nutrients and Fluids, Revitalize Vision, and Clear and Refocus Your Mind

• How to eliminate the four worst causes of job fatigue
• New ways to increase your mental and physical stamina during even the most hectic times at work
• Why repetitive-motion injuries — aggravated by infrequent or poorly designed work breaks — have become one of the hottest hazards of the Information Age, afflicting millions of managers and workers
• How to overcome "afternoon fatigue" and keep your energy and performance levels high throughout the day and evening
• How to take advantage of 60-second Performance Edge work break routines that quickly release tight muscles and balance posture; send a wave of relaxation through the body; replace nutrients and replenish fluids; rejuvenate vision; lift your mood; and clear and refocus your mind

Part II: The Other Pieces of the Performance Puzzle

Chapter 9: Posture: Up, Relaxed, and Energized

- Why most of us tense dozens — sometimes hundreds — of the wrong muscles when we sit, stand, and move and then suffer from fatigue, muscular pain, headaches, eyestrain, decreased blood and oxygen to the brain, and diminished productivity
- How to recognize and unlock tension patterns throughout the body — and quickly increase mental and physical vitality at any hour

Chapter 10: Exercise: How to Do It Smarter to Save Time and Increase Benefits

- Why most exercise routines are based on erroneous, obsolete, or incomplete information
- Five priorities for exercising smarter — the latest strategies to make fitness easier, save time, cut injury risks, and increase benefits
- How to ensure that your exercise program will increase your mental creativity and capacity to handle high levels of stress
- How to flatten and tone your waist using simple, scientifically advanced exercises to strengthen five abdominal muscles, including the little-known transversalis and pyramidalis
- Seven key guidelines for aerobic exercise, including why exercise can be far more effective when it's noncompetitive (self-statements like "harder," "better," and "faster" can increase hormone stress on the heart) and when to slow down the pace (when you exercise too intensively — and most of us do — it interferes with the body's ability to burn excess fat and make fitness gains)

Chapter 11: Nutrition: Healthful, High-Stamina Eating

- Which food rules to forget
- The seven newest scientific maxims for optimal nutrition

- Why eating five or six times a day (three light meals and the right kind of between-meal snacks) helps your body burn excess fat and function at its best on the job
- Why dehydration is one of the primary causes of mental and physical fatigue
- How to choose restaurant meals that promote the best health and give you a competitive edge, without counting calories or gaining weight
- Compelling up-to-the-minute evidence about the mind-mood-food connection: how certain meals and snacks may promote faster thinking, greater energy, increased attention to detail, and quicker reaction speed, while other foods may help produce a calm, focused state of mind and relaxed emotions

Chapter 12: Healthy Environments: Simple Steps to Create a More Pollution-Free, Revitalizing Work Space

- Why office work can be hazardous to your health — and what this means to your job performance
- How "techno-stress" may be steadily sapping your energy — and what to do about it
- Five simple, cost-effective ways to unpollute your personal work area and protect yourself against "sick building syndrome"

Chapter 13: Sleep and Rest: The Impact of Sleep on Alertness and Performance on the Job

- The startling extent to which the vast majority of us sleep poorly — and how this reduces alertness, cuts into job performance, and diminishes our ability to cope with stress
- The easiest ways to enhance the quality of your nightly rest, sleeping more deeply and healthfully than you do now
- How to take advantage of advice from top researchers who claim that most of us can gradually reduce our nightly sleep period by one to two hours and, at the same time, improve our health and performance

Chapter 14: Self-Renewal and Social Support: Dealing More Successfully with the Competing Demands of Work and Family

- The surprising extent to which your productivity and satisfaction on the job are determined by issues that require your attention *off* the job
- Why the company you keep has a surprising effect on your mental attitude and performance — and how to improve relationships and expand and strengthen your support network of friends and co-workers
- Practical suggestions on balancing the competing needs of work and family

Chapter 15: High-Stress Business Travel

- Why the demands of business travel are mounting and why corporate travelers are expected to get there faster, perform better, and get back sooner
- Quick-release stress control skills for business trips
- Strategies for winning the waiting game — taking maximum advantage of unavoidable travel delays
- The benefits of shifting from clock time to event time
- When and how to turn off travel-related "techno-stress"
- How to keep on track with fitness when you're on the road
- Choosing the best meals and snacks for business travel
- Practical ways to reduce air travel stress, including new advice on how to protect yourself against toxic in-flight air and high-altitude oxygen deprivation
- The latest scientific guidelines for beating jet lag and travel fatigue

Chapter 16: The Further Reaches of the Mind: More New Ways to Awaken Your Sleeping Mental Giant

- Eight little-known rules of thumb for stimulating innovative thinking

- The latest scientific insights on how to sharpen your powers of concentration and awareness — no matter what the hour or how difficult the challenge
- The most practical brain-building exercises
- Specific steps from the experts on how to form mental images that help you relax, streamline your efforts on the job, and make it easier to reach higher levels of achievement

Chapter 17: Welcome to the Future

PART I

The Six Performance Turning Points

3

Performance Turning Point #1: Stressful "Crisis Moments"

Taking Charge of Job Pressure with Quick-Release Stress Control

> The important thing is this: to be able at any moment to give up what we are for what we can become.
>
> — *Charles Du Bos*

WINNING AT WORK is determined by the choices we make — dozens every minute, thousands every day. Poor responses to stressful "crisis moments" are the primary reason for mistakes, frustration, and failure. And in today's business world, none of us can afford to be knocked off balance for long.

This brings up an interesting question. Why are some people weakened by job stress while others gain strength from it? The basic answer is simple: Those who know how to transform difficult challenges into energizing, constructive activities are able to remain alert and effective under pressure, noticing options and finding solutions that others fail to see.

Little Hassles Can Take a Big Toll

A national survey of managers found that 65 percent believed that their jobs were more stressful than the average job.[1] But the pressures that created this above-average stress level were "hassle" factors such as interruptions and interpersonal conflicts.

Nearly one-fifth of all occupational health claims are for job stress[2] — an increase of several hundred percent in only a few years. The National Council on Compensation Insurance warns that this growing number of stress-related worker compensation claims will soon strangle America's already overloaded liability system.[3] And researchers report that escalating stress is decreasing job satisfaction for the work force in general.[4]

National surveys report that effective stress management programs are the foremost concern of employees, employers, researchers, and science writers.[5] Other surveys of hundreds of corporate health programs indicate that stress management training is cited as a priority need four times more frequently than the next closest category, which is behavioral treatments for coronary heart disease.[6]

Evidence reveals that the amount of stress you feel and whether it is "good" stress or "bad" stress depends not on the *situations* you face but on how you *perceive* and *react to* them. How you respond to everyday difficult moments — involving anger, rejection, interruptions, broken appointments, the inescapable telephone, financial anxieties, bad weather, traffic jams, and deadlines — is a preeminent factor in determining your personal effectiveness.

The way you handle these "crisis moments" governs whether you stay on track to your goals and work priorities or get sidetracked into busywork and urgent but unimportant tasks. In many cases, the way you respond to hassles is a more powerful predictor of psychological and physical health than is your reaction to major life crises.[7] Recent research at Bowman-Gray School of Medicine in North Carolina confirms that mishandling these chronic, unavoidable irritations and pressures hurts health and performance.[8] More and more experts in the field of stress management are warning that "it's the little things that can make or break your relief of stress."[9]

Controlling Negative Stress Whenever It Hits

When we come face-to-face with difficult work challenges or problems, unconscious, automatic habits make us resist change and push us into negative responses of the body, the emotions, and the mind, including

Body: Tension, irregular breathing, sagging posture, fatigue
Emotions: Anxiety, anger, frustration, guilt, worry
Mind: Brain chemical changes, distraction, distorted thinking, arguments, self-doubt

Chemical and hormonal changes in the brain and body can tighten muscles and unleash negative emotions so quickly that it's much more difficult and time-consuming to reverse bad stress effects once they've occurred. But there's an alternative to these habitual, victimizing responses. According to neuroscientists, one of the most effective ways to master pressure-filled situations is to learn to *catch the first stimulus or signal of distress and then trigger an immediate control response.*

This chapter focuses on one of the simplest and most powerful stress mastery skills — the Instant Calming Sequence (ICS). The first of the six Performance Turning Points, it can be quickly learned and used to neutralize negative stress in less than one second — whenever and wherever it occurs. The *calmness* in the ICS refers to *Webster's* definition: "clearminded control in contrast with a foregoing or nearby state of agitation." This calmness factor is critical throughout the full range of human performance circumstances, from breakthrough thinking and problem solving to excelling at the most complicated, full-speed physical actions.

Identifying — and Controlling — Your Stress Hot Spots

Roller-coaster emotions and tense, anxious moments pile up, steadily breaking down your work effectiveness and magnifying feelings of distress. This situation can contribute to the elusive characteristic of many sudden heart attacks and life-threatening illnesses, says Dr. Robert S. Eliot, a noted cardiologist and stress researcher.[10] In fact, stress *can actually destroy the heart muscles,* eventually resulting in cardiovascular catastrophes.

An estimated one in every five supposedly healthy people has this faulty response to work stress, and it doesn't discriminate between the sexes: Of the 500,000 people who die each year from heart attack in the United States, nearly half are women.[11] The need for stress strategies like the ICS has become even greater with recent medical discoveries that "minor, daily mood fluctuations are associated with immune functioning"[12] and that small, persistent, unavoidable stresses of daily life may accelerate aging.[13]

All of us have stress hot spots — specific demands and situations that trigger anxiety, anger, frustration, impatience, blushing, gritting the teeth, or a physical sign such as shortness of breath, tightness in the chest or throat, yelling, clenched fists, mental distraction, or feelings of fatigue. Without a way to consistently neutralize the accumulating pressure, your health suffers. The ICS offers a practical solution.

"Moments of Truth": Problems Start in a Fraction of a Second

Every time a customer, client, or supplier comes in contact with your business, there is a *moment of truth* — an opportunity for him or her to go away with a positive impression, a neutral impression, or a negative impression. Think of the price you pay — in anger, frustration, and damage to your business — whenever these interactions are handled poorly. The same concerns are at stake whenever you interact with your boss, co-workers, staff members, and employees.

The moments of truth concept was recently brought to light by Jan Carlzon, CEO of Scandinavian Airlines (SAS).[14] Carlzon observed that every day in his company employees came into contact with SAS customers some 50,000 times, and the way these moments of truth were handled was a pivotal factor in determining SAS's success or failure as a company.

By drawing attention to these brief, crucial human interactions,

Carlzon inspired SAS managers and employees to take a different view of their performance and service to customers. This action caught SAS's competitors napping, and business-class travelers — Carlzon's marketing target — recognized the improvement. By combining the moments of truth focus with other strategic changes, Carlzon turned SAS around.

Over the past few years, the moments of truth idea has been applied by hundreds of companies in various service and manufacturing industries. But results have generally been modest at best. Inspiring people to pay attention to moments of truth is a smart step to take, but it's not enough, because your toughest competitors are increasing their awareness, too.

What's missing is the *execution,* the Performance Edge — the physiological and psychological capabilities required to calmly and effectively deal with moments of truth in every kind of human interaction and work procedure.

Too Rushed to Relax: Why Traditional Approaches Usually Don't Work

Studies show that one of the main problems with most popular stress management techniques — including biofeedback, relaxation training, and passive meditation — is "lack of transference."[15] That is, techniques that may work well when you're on vacation or alone in a quiet meditation room or doctor's office are extremely difficult to apply to situations in the real work world.

It seems all but impossible to calm down when you're hit with problem after problem all day. And there's also the issue of *time* — when can you afford to take twenty or thirty minutes twice a day to relax or meditate? The ICS helps solve this problem and is one of the simplest ways to make stress management an automatic part of your work life. "Poorly handled stress is one of the greatest impediments to creative productivity," says Dr. Thomas E. Backer, stress researcher and associate professor at the UCLA School of Medicine.[16] He warns that formal relaxation or meditation methods can actually be anxiety producing for some high-energy, achievement-oriented people.[17]

"Keeping your cool under fire" is a top priority for effective corporate leadership, according to a recent international business survey. "While crisis isn't the only test of leadership, it's the acid test. By demonstrating grace under pressure, the best leaders inspire those around them to stay calm and act intelligently."[18] In short, skills like the ICS enable you to perform at your best in difficult situations, confirming that you are willing and able to assume responsibility and leadership at critical moments.

Scientific Approach to Mastering Pressure

Because an ICS is performed while you are fully alert, with eyes open, the technique may be used unobtrusively in a wide range of circumstances — from all-out physical challenges requiring quick reflexes and sudden bursts of speed or power to the cognitive demands of corporate strategy sessions. The ICS can be used successfully whether you're standing, sitting, or moving. The process begins with learning to recognize your own stress cues at work and then knowing how to take immediate action to remain calm and in control. Your own reactions — or overreactions — are the key.

Recent research confirms the benefits of each of the five ICS steps. The "instant" and "automatic" stress management concept is verified through successful results with thousands of behavioral medicine patients and seminar and workshop participants and is endorsed by experts in the United States and Europe.[19]

The best moments — in work and in all of life — usually occur when your body or mind is stretched to its limits in a voluntary effort to accomplish something difficult and worthwhile. No matter what pressures you face — major performance challenges and on-the-spot responses to work problems or quiet, haunting self-doubts that flare up every time something or someone reminds you of past job mistakes or present weaknesses — the ICS is a powerful skill you can begin using right away. Its applications can be grouped in two basic categories:

1. *Dealing with sudden unexpected problems or challenges,* such as when you are

- forced to make a sudden decision and "it's all on the line";
- being criticized;
- on the verge of plunging into an unnecessary argument or negative self-statements (put-downs);
- receiving unexpected bad news or a customer complaint;
- asked to undertake a major assignment or task;
- feeling pressed for time and are reminded about a deadline;
- making an obvious mistake;
- feeling busy or rushed and then are suddenly forced to wait for someone else;
- caught in a traffic jam or at a red light when you're late for an appointment;
- feeling overloaded or pushed to the limit with job tasks or responsibilities;
- first hearing that your airline flight has been delayed or canceled;
- being asked to reprimand or fire an employee;
- starting to feel guilty about something in the past or anxious about the future;
- feeling frustrated about having "bad luck" or getting a "bad break";
- feeling that you don't get enough appreciation or recognition for work you've done well.

2. *Handling scheduled peak pressure situations,* such as

- making a key phone call;
- entering a job interview;
- making a crucial point in selling your idea or product;
- presenting your work for evaluation;
- answering a difficult personal question;
- beginning a complicated problem-solving process;
- negotiating a sensitive issue;
- standing up to give an important speech;
- communicating what's on your mind — with your boss, co-workers, customers, clients, or employees.

In short, the ICS is effective whenever you don't want work pressures twisting your thinking, lowering your mood, or obstructing your actions.

Using Fluid Intelligence

With practice, your brain and nervous system can enact the five-step ICS in a fraction of a second, using *fluid intelligence* pathways in the nervous system, where messages travel at speeds measured in thousandths and ten-thousandths of a second and produce complex interactions in perception, attention, neuromuscular activation, and responsiveness.[20] The power of this phenomenon is exemplified by the fact that the brain can recognize the meaning of more than 100,000 words or images in less than one second.[21] It takes only one-hundredth of a second for the eye to blink completely, and at least six hundred individual muscular actions can occur in a single second, "and the number may be much higher," say researchers.[22]

Some scientists believe that skilled actions — such as the ICS — may be stored in the nervous system as "chunks of instructions . . . that can be called up and executed by a single command."[23] This may in part account for the deep relaxation and control — the "flow state" — felt by top musicians, jet fighter pilots, and athletes.[24]

Further confirmation of our untapped ability to master stressful moments comes from Dr. Karl H. Pribram, a National Institutes of Health professor of neuroscience, professor of psychology and psychiatry at the Stanford University School of Medicine, and director of Stanford's Neuropsychology Laboratory. Dr. Pribram is an expert on perception and reactions. His research indicates that the human brain and nervous system can use what he calls "holonomic parallel processing" to function outside many time-space limitations — and instantaneous *performance reflexes* such as the ICS can indeed be created with practice.[25]

Best of all, the ICS can be quickly learned and used at the first sign of irritation, anger, tension, or anxiety. At first, the five steps have to be practiced consciously, but they soon become automatic.

The Instant Calming Sequence (ICS)

1. **Uninterrupted breathing**
2. **Positive face**

3. Balanced posture
4. Release muscle tension
5. Mental control

ICS Step 1: Uninterrupted Breathing

Surprisingly, most of us halt our breathing for several seconds or more at the start of a stressful situation. This reduces oxygen to the brain and pushes you toward feelings of anxiety, anger, frustration, panic, faulty reactions, and a general loss of control.[26] The ICS command is simple: continue breathing — smoothly, deeply, and evenly, no matter where in the inhalation or exhalation cycle you happen to be when the pressure cue first captures your attention.

ICS Step 2: Positive Face

In addition to breathing control, a "positive face" can make a difference during stressful, turning point situations. New evidence suggests that the slightest smile — an upturn at the corners of your eyes — *even when you don't feel like smiling* may increase blood flow to the brain and help "reset" the nervous system so that it's less reactive to negative stress.[27] Learn to flash a slight smile — or at least don't scowl or frown — whenever you enter a difficult moment.

ICS Step 3: Balanced Posture

Your posture mirrors and affects your reaction to work pressure. "You will notice that even thinking of a stressful issue causes you almost automatically to tense up," warns a recent commentary in *Management Solutions*. "Your neck or back muscles become knotted."[28]

A common self-victimizing response to stressful moments is known as *somatic retraction,* a slight slouching posture characterized by tightening or collapsing the chest, rolling the shoulders forward and down, and tensing the abdomen, back, or neck.

Somatic retraction not only restricts breathing and can reduce blood flow and oxygen to the brain and senses but also adds needless muscle tension, slows reaction time, and magnifies feelings of panic and helplessness.[29]

The solution to this problem is easier than most of us think. With balanced posture, you have an exhilarating sense of no effort in action, of moving buoyantly, comfortably in space. Your head is up, with neck long and chin slightly in; jaw and tongue are relaxed; shoulders are broad and loose; pelvis and hips are level; back is comfortably straight; abdomen is free of tension. An imaginary sky hook is gently lifting your whole spinal column upward from a central point on top of your head.

During an ICS, the key is to keep your posture buoyant and "up"; don't let it become tense or collapse even slightly. (For more on posture, see Chapter 9.)

ICS Step 4: Release Muscle Tension

One common habitual response to stressful situations is to resist the pressure by unconsciously tightening muscles in the jaw, neck, back, shoulders, or abdomen. But this needless tension immediately drains energy, slows reaction speed, and clouds the mind.

In this step of the ICS, you perform a tension check by scanning all of your muscles in one fast sweep of your mind — from your scalp, jaw, tongue, and face to your fingertips and toes — to locate unnecessary tension. At the same time, you flash a mental "wave of relaxation" through your body, as if you're standing under a waterfall that clears away all excess tension. Your mind remains fully alert, your body calm.

ICS Step 5: Mental Control

The most critical step in directing your mind for the first response to a sudden business challenge is to *acknowledge reality*.[30] It's essential to what psychologists call the "flow state," in which elite athletes, artists, and creative thinkers perform at their absolute best by avoiding the paralysis of analysis.[31]

Of course, to acknowledge reality we must first *perceive* it — quickly, objectively, and accurately. As discussed in Chapter 7, surveys show that under stressful job conditions many managers and workers have difficulty doing this, and they wind up misreading data, making false assumptions, leaping to conclusions, and solving the wrong problems. It's an enormous waste of time and energy to keep digging ourselves out of these traps when we repeatedly fall into them.

Changing counterproductive responses to job pressure takes practice. To be successful, first you must create an unshakable open-mindedness combined with well-developed powers of alertness and concentration (see Chapter 16).

Second, you must develop a keen understanding of your own organization — including its culture, mission, management style, performance appraisal system, and whatever power structure and psychopolitical pressures you're up against in your department or office.

Third, you must sharpen your ability to perceive — and then effectively deal with — differing perspectives, competing objectives, and difficult personality traits in the people you must interact with. You must also get past another stumbling block — the tendency to *deny the stressful circumstance that's suddenly staring you in the face.*

By failing to acknowledge the reality of a peak-pressure situation — that is, by wishing it weren't happening, regretting you didn't have more time to prepare, wanting to be somewhere else, or anguishing over your job's unfairness — you set off a biochemical avalanche of victimizing thoughts and feelings. Without realizing it, you actually *help* yourself lose control and get loaded up with anxiety or anger, and this weakens your performance. A single difficult moment can disrupt an entire day.

Studies confirm that individuals who deal most effectively with peak-stress situations have what is called *unself-conscious self-assurance*.[32] This means that they are confident but not self-centered; are aware of ethical, professional behavior but not consumed by worries about their own personal gain; and are not directing their energy toward dominating their stressful circumstance as much as on acknowledging challenges and finding ways to function within them harmoniously and productively.

One helpful strategy is to sharpen your awareness that *each and every problem is unique*. Practice immediately identifying the distinctive aspects of whatever challenge is at hand, rather than getting caught up looking for similarities with previous experiences you may have had. Researchers claim that this helps you remain mentally alert and flexible and can head off negative habitual patterns of response.[33] When you take charge of Performance Turning Points, your key thought is *What's happening is real — and unique — and I'm searching for the best possible solution right now.*

In case you're thinking that this momentary pause might sacrifice some flash of competitive advantage, there's no need to worry. Scientific research on reflex-reaction speed shows that when dealing with high-pressure situations at full speed, in the critical first instant of a challenge you're better off *pausing for a moment* to acknowledge reality and clear your mind and *then* making a quick, appropriate response, rather than reacting too quickly with a hurried, less focused response.[34]

The second mental response priority of the ICS is to *focus your mind*. In large part, what you do with your mind in the initial moments of a turning point situation determines the outcome. If you look back at times on the job when you reacted poorly to pressure, it's probably apparent that, in many instances, had you remained calmer and more flexible and had you been able to think more clearly during the first moments of the situation, you could have chosen a better response. That's the key to this ICS step — *learning to insert that calm, clear-mindedness in precisely the right place at the very beginning of each stress scene.*

"People who know how to transform stress into an enjoyable

challenge spend very little time thinking about themselves," says Mihaly Csikszentmihalyi, professor and former chairman of the Department of Psychology at the University of Chicago. "They are not expending all their energy trying to satisfy what they believe to be their needs, or worrying about socially conditioned desires. Instead, their attention is alert, constantly processing information from their surroundings."[35]

With practice, you can train your mind to seek solutions quickly instead of getting locked on resisting problems and to focus on what you can control rather than what you can't. This is the place to choose an *intent to learn* instead of your old reactionary habits; to pause for a moment, to listen with an open mind instead of blindly talking back; to resolve, rather than ignite, conflict; to apply your personal golden rule or spiritual philosophy in place of a rush of anger, impatience, or anxiety; to be skilled enough to protect yourself without harming other people; and to think clear, honest thoughts instead of distorted ones.

The central principle in this step is to quickly scan each new situation, noticing whatever is unique, drawing out your options for dealing with it most effectively. The remaining chapters of this book provide a variety of useful suggestions and recommendations. Chapter 7, for example, presents key questions for improved problem solving and decision making, such as What is the *heart* of this issue or problem? Is what I'm seeing/hearing/feeling/thinking accurate? How important is this going to be in the long run? What can I *do* about it right now? (that's the reason it's so critical to ask What next? rather than Why?) and What's the best way to express my thoughts or feelings?

ICS Examples

Take a quick inventory of your own crunch times — the most stressful hot spots at work. Select one particular kind of problem or challenge where you'd especially like to see improvements right away.

Then begin gaining control of it by using mental imagery.[36] Sit down, relax, and vividly imagine the circumstance. Roll the slow-motion mental videotape backward in your mind's eye until you catch *the very first signal* that you're entering the stressful situation. *This* is the key moment — the first clue that a stress onslaught feels imminent. This is exactly the place where you need to begin inserting an ICS.

Imagine — in extra-slow motion — that this particular stressful situation is just beginning to happen. Stall the stress signal right there. Now picture yourself effortlessly, successfully going through the ICS: (1) uninterrupted breathing, (2) positive face, (3) balanced posture, (4) release muscle tension, (5) mental control.

Now repeat the process, a little faster. Remember, this is a natural, flowing sequence. You unleash it; you don't force it. Practice several times a day, using different stress cues, increasing the vividness of the mental images and the speed of the ICS.

If at first you have difficulty with any of the steps, practice them one at a time until they become comfortable. If you get partway into the ICS and feel yourself starting to lose control, back the sequence up and slow things down. Be absolutely certain that you freeze the image of the pressure signal at the first instant — don't let the stressful image keep rolling to the point at which you become anxious.

You are learning to automatically slip the ICS into the situation right behind the first sign of stress, and this makes all the difference in the outcome. When rehearsing for especially intense situations, you might try lightening the image of the stress signal (by seeing yourself move farther away from it in your mind or by dulling the vividness of the scene) until you're at ease with using the ICS to handle it.

Here's an example: Let's say someone is starting to criticize you for something you've done. Imagine the scene in slow motion: You catch the first critical remarks coming and trigger the ICS — uninterrupted breathing, positive face, balanced posture, release muscle tension, acknowledge reality. Then, as you reach the mental control part of this final step, pause.

Your past habits are probably primed to push you into old responses — getting down on yourself, blurting out an excuse, bracing yourself to angrily lash back at the critic, and so on. But if you don't learn to substitute a new mental focus right here, at the turning point, you may be stuck repeating these old victimizing responses for the rest of your life.

The alternative — if we keep our example in slow motion and you choose the outcome you really want — paints an entirely different picture: Your mind zeroes in on the specifics of the challenge, putting the importance (or unimportance) of the criticism in immediate perspective, and you scan for every possible way you can benefit — or at least learn — from the situation. In short, you're neurologically derailing negative habits and turning a potential blowout into a moment for self-improvement or leadership. It takes practice, but it works. Almost every situation we encounter at work and in the rest of life presents possibilities for growth and advancement.

If this all sounds a bit overoptimistic, note that it doesn't mean that you have to *pay attention* to criticisms that are irrelevant or that ridicule, accuse, or threaten. If you do opt to stand there while your boss, co-worker, or customer is berating you, you might elect to send your mind on a short, pleasant mental vacation and leave your body relaxed and emotions calm. However, you give up this option whenever you've already launched into a self-victimizing reaction.

Present-Moment Awareness

We grow up believing that what counts most in our lives and work is what will transpire in the future. In contrast, as a reality of business, we also know that even a momentary lapse of concentration on the job can spell defeat.

Yet by and large we fail to take advantage of the fact that whenever we allow ourselves to become distracted by the past or future we severely limit our effectiveness in the present. And there are growing indications that our increasingly chaotic business environment is pulling us farther and farther away from what researchers call *present-moment awareness* or *mindfulness on the job*.[37] A recent Stanford University study, for example, estimated that people in some workplaces may spend an average of nearly 58 minutes of every hour forgetting the past or anticipating the future and *only about 2 minutes* dealing with the present.[38] The ICS is a simple, effective tool to help you gain more complete, mindful control of your work.

Present-moment awareness is also a prerequisite to achieving what Csikszentmihalyi calls *flow* — the optimal experience state with a sense of mastery and seemingly effortless movement exhibited by peak performers in a wide range of occupations and avocations.[39] After more than two decades of research on this phenomenon, Csikszentmihalyi has found that regardless of the task or circumstance, every one of us can increase the ability to experience flow in our work.

For this to occur, however, we must first overcome a common obstacle: excessive self-consciousness. People who are worried about how others will perceive them, who are afraid of creating the wrong impression or of doing anything that may be viewed as inappropriate, are blocked from flow experiences, says Csikszentmihalyi.

"Contrary to what we tend to assume," he explains, "the normal state of the mind is chaos. Without training, and without an object in the external world that demands attention, people are unable to focus their thoughts for more than a few minutes at a time. . . . It is amazing how little effort most people make to improve control of their attention."[40]

It takes sharp concentration skills to use the ICS most effectively during stressful work situations. Chapter 16 presents a variety of simple ways to increase these mental attention powers.

Developing the ICS as an Automatic Response

Begin applying the ICS to everyday situations. Be patient with yourself, especially during the first weeks. Some types of challenges will require quite a bit of rehearsing before you can handle them with ease every time. Remember, most of us have had years of practice strengthening the unproductive reactions that the ICS will replace.

If you try to deal with a particularly difficult challenge and happen to get impatient and revert to an old, ineffective response, don't worry about it. Simply take some time later that day to sit down for several minutes in a quiet place, relax deeply, and replay the beginning of the scene in slow motion in your mind. But this time, bring in the ICS early and see it succeeding in your mind's eye. Each time you use it, the sequence will flow more easily and become more automatic.

As Albert Einstein often said, "In the middle of every difficulty lies opportunity." With your senses alert, your breathing steady, your posture erect, your emotions controlled, and your mind clear and looking for solutions, you're far better prepared to maintain a steady course to your dreams and to win the moment-by-moment skirmishes that greet you every hour of the workday.

4

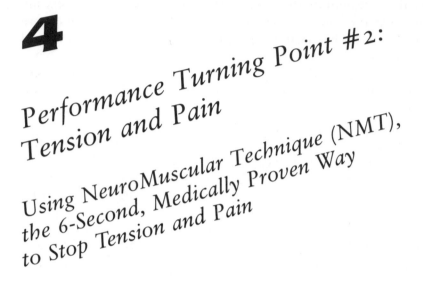

Performance Turning Point #2: Tension and Pain

Using NeuroMuscular Technique (NMT), the 6-Second, Medically Proven Way to Stop Tension and Pain

POUNDING HEADACHES, stiff necks, tense shoulders, and back pain. For millions of us, these afflictions regularly sabotage our effectiveness at work and leave us frustrated and fatigued. Yet preventing and correcting these conditions usually receive scant attention by management — and we're paying a high price for this oversight.

Stress-related headaches are the leading cause of lost work time in American industry,[1] followed by back pain.[2] On any given day nearly 7 million Americans are under some form of treatment for lower back pain.[3] It is estimated that 3 percent of American workers are absent every business day of the year, and in wages paid the annual cost of this absenteeism is estimated to be $30 billion.[4] The total annual loss, including the cost of diminished productivity, may be $150 billion or higher.[5]

Three work stress–related disorders — chronic pain, hypertension, and headache — are estimated to account for 54 percent of these absences, or $15.7 billion of the $30 billion lost in wages every year.[6] Upper and lower back pain, neck pain, and shoulder pain account for an estimated 33 percent of absenteeism.[7] And none of these figures take into account the reduced productivity cost of those workers who suffer from these conditions but don't take time off. Nor do they include the cost of absenteeism resulting from related disorders, such as fatigue and depression, that can be brought on by headache, hypertension, and chronic tension and pain syndromes.[8]

Poorly designed, ill-fitting office equipment, manufacturing tools, work stations, and furniture force the body to assume stressful postures throughout the day. These cramped, inefficient body positions cause or aggravate tension and pain problems.

In addition, nearly half of the work force in North America, Europe, and Japan is now susceptible to what experts call *repetitive-motion injuries* or *cumulative trauma disorders* (CTDs), caused by jobs such as typing at a computer work station or performing high-technology assembly operations that strain muscles and tendons and lead to painful, debilitating conditions in the hand, wrist, shoulders, back, and neck. These tension-related ailments already affect 5 million Americans, and the National Institute of Occupational Safety and Health projects that by the year 2000, half the work force will be vulnerable.[9]

Think about it. Even if work conditions are ideal and your motivation is high, tension and pain conditions wear you down, weakening your concentration and sapping your stamina. They also make it more difficult for you to handle even minor stress situations. Job errors increase, and so do interpersonal conflicts.

Unfortunately, thus far few companies have taken action, either in terms of workplace *ergonomics* (which, as discussed in Chapters 9 and 12, means an environment "engineered to meet human needs") or education for employees on medically sound self-care treatments to reduce or eliminate job-related pain and tension syndromes. No matter how you look at it — in terms of medical expenses, productivity measurements, teamwork, customer responsiveness, or quality control — this is a costly management oversight.

Moreover, chronic pain and tension are lonely experiences, locking us away from many of the rewards of work and life. And if the pain or tension continues for days or weeks on end, fatigue and anxiety can turn into depression.

Your options? First, you can try to ignore or resist the tension and pain, which tends to make it worse. This struggle transforms many of us into grumps and grouches, a fact readily acknowledged by those who have to live or work with us.

Second, you might gain temporary relief by taking a painkilling medication, but this leaves the cause of the pain or stiffness untreated. When all else fails, you may be advised to take more drastic measures — time off from work, a change in jobs, doctor appointments, even surgery. But in many cases, there's another, better alternative that few of us have learned about, and that's the subject of this chapter.

One of the fastest, most effective, drug-free ways to stop tension and pain is a simple method of pressure-point therapy that you can do right where you are now. It is called NeuroMuscular Technique (NMT), a method that, in just 6 to 10 seconds, treats a predominant cause of tension, aches, and pain. NMT is gentle, easy to learn and apply, and based on solid scientific and medical research.[10]

Trigger Points

NeuroMuscular Technique is focused on tiny distress spots in the body called *myofascial trigger points*. (*Myo* means muscle and *fascial* refers to a protective tissue that wraps the muscles.) Any one of the body's nearly 700 muscles can develop trigger points.

Active trigger points can cause debilitating, sometimes incapacitating, pain. *Latent trigger points* cause stiffness and restricted movement but are not painful except when pressure is applied to them. Usually, the discomfort occurs at or near the trigger point itself. But in some cases, the pain shows up at a site in the body far distant from where the trigger point actually originates. For example, a hidden trigger point in the shoulder muscles might cause neck pain or headaches. This is called *referred pain*.

How many of us have trigger points? "Trigger points are extremely common and become a distressing part of nearly everyone's life at one time or another," say two national experts, Dr. Janet G. Travell, emeritus clinical professor of medicine at George Washington University School of Medicine, and Dr. David G. Simons, clinical professor in the Department of Physical Medicine and Rehabilitation at the University of California, Irvine.[11] One study of young adults found latent trigger points in the shoulder muscles in 54 percent of females and 45 percent of males.[12] Another research team discovered that the greatest number of trigger points are found in people between the ages of thirty-one and fifty.[13]

"Individuals of either sex and of any age can develop trigger points," observe Drs. Travell and Simons. "It is our impression that the likelihood of developing pain-producing *active* trigger points increases with age to the most active, middle years. As activity becomes less strenuous in later years, individuals tend to exhibit chiefly the stiffness and restricted motion of *latent* trigger points."[14]

You may be wondering, "Why haven't I heard about trigger points before?" It's because until very recently, they have been one of the most overlooked causes of muscular tension and pain. But leading medical experts are determined to change that.

Most trigger point problems can be relieved by simple detection and treatment, researchers say. But there's a problem — few health professionals have been trained to recognize trigger points. The total cost of this oversight is "enormous," say Drs. Travell and Simons, and other authorities agree. "When patients mistakenly believe that they must 'live with' trigger point pain because they think it is due to arthritis or a pinched nerve that is inoperable, they restrict activity in order to avoid pain. Such patients must learn that the pain comes from muscles, not from nerve damage, and not from permanent arthritic changes in the bones. Most important, they must know it is responsive to treatment."[15]

What causes trigger points? Injuries, including life's bumps, bruises, twists, and strains; imbalanced posture; chronically tensed muscles; overwork fatigue; emotional distress; poor sitting or sleeping positions; lack of sleep; or chilling, exposing the body to cold temperatures when fatigued or following an intensive exercise session.

Trigger points vary in irritability from hour to hour and day to day. But once formed, they tend to remain in your muscles unless treated and released. The reason is that, when injured, most body tissues heal, but muscles "learn" to avoid pain. Trigger points cause you to hold tension and "guard" muscles by limiting their motion.

In addition to producing pain, stiffness, fatigue, and restricted range of motion, trigger points also reduce circulation and can cause weakness in the affected muscles, loss of coordination, dizziness, and other symptoms.

Easy 6-Second Therapy Skill

One of the most effective ways to relieve trigger points is a pressure-type therapy. You can quickly learn to use this simple technique on your own muscles or by spending a few minutes exchanging "therapies" with a co-worker or loved one. Health professionals trained in NeuroMuscular Technique frequently recommend that their clients learn this method for self-treatment.[16]

To locate trigger points, first be certain your muscles are warm and relaxed. Otherwise, it's difficult to distinguish tense bands of muscle — where trigger points are usually located — from adjoining slack muscles. Once you've located a taut band or cord of tense muscle fibers, press or squeeze it with light to moderate pressure until you locate the spot of maximum tenderness with minimum pressure — the trigger point.

In most areas of the body, you can press the muscle against underlying bone using your fingertip or thumb. Even a tennis ball placed behind you in a chair may be used to reach some points on the back.

There are a variety of ways to use pressure to treat trigger points. The most common treatments use the pad of the thumb or knuckle of the index or middle finger. In the temple areas of the forehead and the hinge joint of the jaw, the pad of the index finger (which may be covered or reinforced by the adjoining middle finger) is used to apply pressure. The eraser on a pencil is also recommended by some therapists as an on-the-job treatment tool.

In addition to straight-on pressure, certain muscle areas can be checked for trigger points using a spiral pattern of pressure: First press down in the center and then press down successively on different points in a circular pattern until you have checked the whole area. Each time you locate a trigger point, treat it by holding steady pressure for 6 seconds and then releasing.

There are dozens of everyday applications for NeuroMuscular

Technique on the job and during corporate travel. You can locate and treat trigger points in any of the major muscle areas of the body — the back of the head, the neck, jaw, shoulders, arms, forearms, hands, upper back, lower back, hips, buttocks, upper and lower legs, ankles, and feet.

Here's the essence: If you feel tense, tight, or uncomfortable in one of these areas, take a few moments to use finger, thumb, or knuckle pressure to search the area. Once you have located a trigger point, apply pressure that is gentle enough so that it creates only mild discomfort. Hold the trigger point for 6 seconds and then release. Go on to another trigger point, treat for 6 seconds, and then release. And so on. You can repeat the therapy at each trigger point twice in one day if desired.

With practice, you can learn to quickly notice when trigger points are aggravated — sensing your muscles becoming tense from poor posture or an uncomfortable seating position, for example — and then take immediate action to relax the affected area by balancing your posture, changing the way you're sitting, and releasing tight muscles. If necessary, you can go ahead and treat any other irritated trigger point areas.

In many cases, trigger point therapy gives immediate benefits, including reduced tenderness or stiffness in the muscles. Relief is likely to be more lasting if the area is kept warm after treatment and if you balance your posture (see Chapter 9) and go through several gentle range of motion exercises for the affected area.[17]

Of course, all persistent or severe pain requires medical attention.

Several Examples to Try Right Now

Here are two examples of common trigger point locations and treatments.

First, place your right forearm, palm down, on the desk or table in front of you. With the pad of your left thumb or the knuckle of your left index or middle finger, press straight down on the top of your forearm about one-half inch toward the wrist from the fold of skin at the elbow. Press in slowly and firmly.

In most cases, you will find a sensitive spot that will become more sensitive the harder you press on it. Hold moderate pressure here for 6 seconds, and then release. You have just located and treated a trigger point.

Now move your left thumb or knuckle several inches toward your right wrist and press again on this new spot on your right forearm. Unless you have chronic pain or tension in your forearm, wrist, or hand, you will feel pressure, but no pain. When an area of your body is free from trigger points, all you will feel when you press down on the muscles is pressure, not sensitivity or pain.

Second, explore the area at the base of the skull for trigger points— the site of trigger points in my headaches. Gently place the pad of your right thumb — or, if you have weak thumbs, use your index finger reinforced or covered by your adjoining middle finger — on the back of your neck just to the right of your spine. Glide up to find the natural "notch" at your hairline at the base of the skull. Apply moderate pressure upward against the bone to locate any trigger points.

Search the area from right next to the spine outward along the base of the skull to just behind your ear. Treat any trigger points for 6 seconds and then release. Repeat the process for the matching area on the left side of your neck where it meets the skull.

A third area where trigger points are commonly found is the trapezius muscle that attaches from your shoulders to your neck. Reach up with your hands and squeeze the uppermost muscle midway between the crest of your shoulders and the sides of your neck. Squeeze with a thumb on the front side and your index and middle fingers on the back side of this muscle. Squeeze slowly and firmly. If you find a sensitive area, hold the pressure on that spot for 6 seconds and then release. Move a finger width at a time toward the sides of your neck and then out toward your shoulder crests, locating and treating any trigger points along the way.

Key Supportive Factors for Best Results

To prevent the formation and recurrence of trigger points, it's important to follow a balanced plan for improving your overall health

and fitness. One such program is presented in my book *Health &*
Fitness Excellence: The Comprehensive Action Plan (Houghton
Mifflin, 1990).

Researchers note that the following factors are of special importance in preventing trigger points.

Correct posture. For standing, sitting, bending, turning, and all
work-related movements. As discussed in Chapter 9, by paying
attention to muscle strain you can develop a high degree of sensitivity to body balance. You can learn to have maximum freedom
of movement with minimum tension, the hallmark of good posture. This helps prevent the formation of new trigger points.

The following postural imbalances have been linked to trigger
points: slouched reading positions; tension held in the abdomen,
back, neck, shoulder, arms, or legs; prolonged sitting at a poorly
designed work station or in ill-fitting office furniture; neck held
forward during driving or television viewing; sleeping with the
shoulders creeping up toward your ears or with too few or too
many pillows; and excessively abrupt, jerky movements of any kind
(which can overstress the muscles and joints).

Regular exercise. Individuals who exercise regularly are less likely
to develop trigger points than sedentary people or those who exercise vigorously only on occasion.[18] A recent medical study directed by Dr. Alf Nachemson, chairman of orthopedics at Goth-
enburg University in Sweden and a leading researcher on back pain,
concluded that individuals who were out of work because of back
pain and who participated in a moderate program of regular exercise, gradually building up their endurance, returned to work far
sooner than, and outperformed, those who were inactive.[19]

Some authorities contend that trigger points are irritated and
perpetuated by sedentary living. As noted in Chapter 10, a safe,
progressive exercise program can pay great dividends in this respect.

Ability to relax deeply. Trigger points are aggravated by chronic
holding of muscle tension. Heavy purses, briefcases, and luggage;
tight shirt collars, neckties, bra straps, and belts; and ill-fitting furniture — in which you must strain to sit upright — all contribute
to forming and irritating trigger points. The solution is, first, to
take action to prevent these postural problems and, second, to spend
a minute or two each day releasing tension by progressively relaxing all the muscles of the body.

Good nutrition. Medical researchers report that vitamins, minerals, and other nutrients may be important in the correction and prevention of trigger point pain syndromes.[20] As noted in Chapter 11, the priority is a widely varied diet of wholesome, fresh foods consumed in five or six small meals and snacks per day. In some cases, it may also be wise to take a basic multivitamin-mineral supplement that does not exceed 150 percent of the U.S. Recommended Daily Allowances (RDAs). Other nutritional supplements may be recommended by your physician or registered dietitian based on your personal needs.

Frequent work breaks. One of the smartest ways to increase your mental and physical stamina, relieve routine job-related tension, and help prevent repetitive-motion injuries is to take frequent short work breaks throughout the day, as discussed in Chapter 8.

Psychological well-being. Anxiety, mismanaged anger, chronic muscle tension, and other poor responses to stress cause fatigue and contribute to trigger point symptoms. In addition, a primary factor in the psychological treatment of these pain syndromes is clearing up misunderstandings about the cause of the symptoms.

"Patients who have been erroneously convinced that their pain is due to untreatable physical factors," warn Drs. Travell and Simons, "such as degenerative joint disease, a 'pinched nerve' that is inoperable, or 'rheumatism' that they must learn to live with, often live in dread of aggravating their condition by any movement or activity that elicits the pain."[21] When the pain and other symptoms are due to trigger points, curtailed movements and inactivity actually aggravate the trigger points and make the problem worse.

With the simple, scientific technique presented in this chapter, you can quickly and safely identify and relieve most trigger points. In busy workplaces where stress, tension, and pain block many of us from being our best, this is one of the most important Performance Edge skills you can learn.

5

Performance Turning Point #3: Time Pressures

Achieving "Priority Effectiveness" to Work Smarter and Faster

> Things which matter most should never be at the mercy of things which matter least.
>
> — *Goethe*

IT'S ONE OF THE AXIOMS of modern business life: There's never enough time. However fast the work world was spinning just a few short decades ago, it seems to be spinning twenty times faster today. Markets have gone global, competition has turned fierce, and resources — including time — have grown scarce.

Fax machines, cellular phones, international overnight mail, satellite pagers, supersonic jets, ground-to-air telephones, laptop computers, modems, pocket-size organizers, voice mail, and electronic mail can reach nearly all of us at all hours of the day and night.

This sense of tremendous acceleration and urgency is not just some vague impression. According to a recent Lou Harris survey, the amount of leisure time enjoyed by the average American has shrunk nearly 40 percent in the past twenty years. Over the same period, the average work week has expanded from 40 to 48 hours, and in some professions 80-hour work weeks are becoming common.

"These are the days of the time famine," warns a recent cover story in *Time* magazine. "Time that once seemed free and elastic has grown tight and elusive, and so our measure of its worth is dramatically changed."[1]

Competing Against Time

The number of minutes and hours available each day is the one resource we all have in common. How individuals and companies manage time — in innovation and new product development and in production, sales, distribution, and service — represents one of the most powerful new sources of competitive advantage.

"Senior management must shift its focus from cost to time, and its objectives from control and functional optimization to providing resources to compress time throughout the organization," says George Stalk, Jr., author of an award-winning article for *Harvard Business Review*. "Time is now the organization's number one competitor. In fact, as a strategic weapon, time is the equivalent of money, productivity, quality, and even innovation."[2]

"Speed is catching on fast," adds a report in *Fortune* magazine. "A recent survey of 50 major U.S. companies found that practically all put time-based strategy, as the new approach is called, at the top of their priority lists. Why? Because speed kills the competition. . . . No wonder — it influences virtually every operation in every company. Managers must make clear that *nothing short of disaster is a valid excuse for delay*."[3]

"Face Time" Versus Effective Performance Time

Managers and professionals seem to agree universally that to get ahead, to make it to the top of a company, there's no substitute for working beyond-normal hours. But regardless of the career track, there's a point of diminishing returns for the extra hours spent. Despite the fact that the "80-hour manager" still *sounds* like a peak performance descriptor, the truth is that a growing number of "50-hour top achievers" can outsmart, outinnovate, and outproduce them.

Cary Cooper, a professor of organizational psychology at the University of Manchester in England, recently interviewed more than a thousand executives and managers in the United States and Britain about their work habits. His conclusion: "Any manager who works over 50 hours a week in my view is turning in less than his best performance."[4]

Another problem with bosses and managers who get caught up on the get-here-early-stay-later-than-everyone-else treadmill is that they inadvertently trap others into equating hours worked with services rendered. Staff members and employees who feel obligated to emulate such an example may end up logging extra hours that amount to nothing more than "face time" — an ethic that still applies in far too many corporate environments. Face time is the low-productivity time people spend hanging around the office — early in the morning, late at night, and on weekends — just to make sure they're seen by those with the power to promote them.

Unfortunately, most people still equate time spent on the job with performance, but the correlation between the two is often negative. More and more companies are starting to evaluate and compensate their managers and employees on the basis of the question How *effectively* did you work? instead of How *long* did you work?

There's a gradual shift in the basis of pay, from *position* to *performance,* and from *status* to *contribution.*[5] With stakes so high, it's a long overdue recognition of an age-old fact of honest, ethical business: *It's not what you do, it's what gets done.*

The Ultimate Time Savers

To begin with, don't let time management be a waste of time. It's not something you can learn easily from most books on the subject. Elaborate list making, minute-by-minute scheduling, and neurotic watch watching can use up more time than they save — and result in a rigid set of expectations that can rarely be met in the modern work environment. Time effectiveness is the goal, not time warfare.

"A manager can schedule as much as he wants," says William Oncken, Jr., author of *Managing Management Time.* "But schedules often get blown to hell within 10 minutes of showing up for work."[6]

Peter F. Drucker has said that while successful managers vary widely in their interests, temperaments, and abilities, they have one trait in common: *a talent for getting the right things done.* Effective self-management requires knowing how to juggle your time without becoming a slave to the clock — having the guts and farsightedness to concentrate on the most important tasks rather than attempting to do everything. The following are several key concerns.

1. Set — and Schedule — Priorities

"If the pressures, rather than the person, are allowed to make decisions," writes Drucker in *The Effective Executive,* "the important tasks will predictably be sacrificed."

Being *busy* often creates the illusion of being *productive,* but they're not at all the same. You can be maximally efficient — in motion every moment of the day, accomplishing long lists of tasks — and get nowhere in terms of your highest priorities and most important goals.

• *Clarify your mission and set specific purpose-driven objectives.* One of the most powerful ways to unlock personal work energy is to create a detail-rich, crystal-clear picture of what you want to accomplish. Despite all the corporate chatter about visions and values, few of us operate with a sharply defined mental image of the outcomes we seek.

"The essence of the best thinking in the area of time management," says Stephen R. Covey, chairman of the Covey Leadership Center, "can be captured in a single phrase: *Organize and execute around priorities.*"[7]

Take a fresh, hard look at your work and your life, and then write out a personal purpose statement or mission statement.* First, define what you want to *be* — what character strengths you want to have and what qualities and skills you want to develop. Then describe what you want to *do* — specify in detail what you want to accomplish and what specific contributions you want to make.

Next, reflect on what you've written and make any revisions that come to mind. Ask yourself, Is my mission based on timeless, important principles? Does it represent the best within me? Do I feel motivated when I read it or think about it? Am I aware of the strategies and skills I'll need to accomplish my objectives?

Then, most important of all, ask, What, specifically, do I need to do today to reach where I want to be tomorrow? What are the most important activities for me to do now to reach my longer-term goals? As a manager/professional? As a husband/father or wife/mother? As my other roles in life? Write down these priorities.

Taking this process to a company-wide level depends on creating an effective corporate or division mission statement † spelling out specific purpose-driven objectives. One of the most pressing challenges is defining your company's strategic priorities — drawing together participation and insights from all corporate levels and then integrating these into day-to-day management decisions and operations.

Key questions include What is our corporate reason for being? What is the focus for our future business development? What is the range of products, services, and specific markets to be considered? What priority *capabilities* are required to be successful in achieving these objectives? What specific actions should be planned and scheduled now?

• *Schedule your priorities instead of prioritizing your schedule.* Contrary to the advice doled out by most time management gu-

---

* For exploring this process in detail, two of the best books are *Peak Performers* by Charles A. Garfield (Morrow, 1987) and *The Seven Habits of Highly Effective People* by Stephen R. Covey (Simon and Schuster, 1989).
† See *Vision in Action: Putting a Winning Attitude to Work* by Benjamin B. Tregoe et al. (Simon and Schuster, 1989) and *The Purpose-Driven Organization* by Perry Pascarella and Mark A. Frohman (Josey-Bass, 1989).

rus, don't spend too much time drawing up a detailed schedule, advises Stephanie Winston, author of *The Organized Executive*. "That isn't realistic or desirable for most managers." Instead, Winston advises scheduling at least an hour every day to isolate yourself from other demands and concentrate on one or two of your top priorities. This guarantees that they'll receive your up-front attention and not get lost in the shuffle of urgent but less important tasks.

Alec Mackenzie, author of *The Time Trap*, suggests making goals as specific as possible and, above all, setting a deadline. "People don't take anything seriously until there's a deadline."[8] That's when we put away our excuses, says Mackenzie, and get down to the business of making things happen and getting things done.

• *Stop getting sidetracked*. Time competency combines calm, attentive awareness to whatever task is at hand and periodic time checks — keeping track of planning, scheduling, and completing your priorities. Obviously, you'll get sidetracked sometimes. But many of us seem to spend most of our work hours on urgent, but non-priority, tangents. Nearly all of us can free up at least three or four hours a week of productive time by learning some simple new skills (see Chapters 3, 6, and 7) to prevent the inevitable onslaught of daily hassles and "crisis moments" from turning into major distractors and time killers.

Throughout the day — and especially on each work break — ask yourself, What's the best use of my time right now and in the hour ahead? By frequent mental check-ins, you can lose less time to nonproductive, nonfulfilling activities.

• *Expand your "time horizon": Schedule some strategic thinking time every day*. If you're in a leadership position, you probably wish you had more time in your daily schedule for deep thinking — the kind of strategic contemplation that helps you define priorities and plan fresh new initiatives — instead of getting bogged down with busywork. In fact, the toughest habit for many executives and managers to break is always being in motion.

Abraham Zaleznik, Matsushita Professor of Leadership at the Harvard Business School, argues that U.S. managers are "too interactive, too structured, too organized. They suffer in their lack of ability to be imaginative."[9]

Zaleznik believes that managers and professionals should periodically close the office door, unplug the phone, sit back, and think deeply. Where is the company going? Where should it be headed? What business do we want to be in five years from now? And how do we plan to get there? What am I doing well? What could I be doing better — and how, specifically, can I make improvements? Are my priorities still the same? Am I staying on track to accomplish them? "Life is a combination of action and reflection," Zaleznik observes, "and if managers are only going to act, they cheat themselves" — and, by implication, their companies.

Evidence is growing that the further into the future your brain can see itself functioning, the more competent you'll become right now in handling complexity, ambiguity, change, and paradox. Your *time horizon* is the maximum cognitive period in which you can plan and execute specific, ongoing, goal-directed activities. (This is different from "strategic thinking" or "strategic planning.") Time horizons of five to ten years (discussed in Chapter 7) can be readily developed, and this is one of the missing scientific pieces to effective time management.

• *Make personal and family time top priorities — it pays work dividends.* The myth about separate and nonoverlapping work and home worlds has a long history in corporate thinking.[10] But convincing new research shows that stress at home — often caused by a lack of family time owing to unnecessarily long work hours — interferes with work performance. Conversely, work stress and the inability to release job-related pressures on nonwork hours when you are together with your family create or magnify problems at home.[11]

Begin by elevating your family and personal time to a level of equal importance to your highest work priorities. Block out these nonwork times and commit to them in indelible ink — a full year in advance whenever possible. If you and your family don't plan for this time together, you'll rarely get around to it and you'll soon be plagued by feelings of guilt over neglecting your personal development and important relationships.

As your effectiveness and stamina increase with the Performance Edge, resist the temptation to work longer hours and run a few extra circles around your beleaguered colleagues. Instead, do whatever you can to encourage or initiate actions to move your organization or department toward compensation that is based at least in part on performance, and then strategically work *fewer* hours whenever possible. Devote this newfound time to balancing out the *off*-work areas of your life. This, in turn, will further improve your effectiveness on the job.[12] For more details about balancing the competing demands of work, self, and family, see Chapter 14.

• *Planning notebooks and software: Look before you leap.* If you feel you may benefit from something more elaborate than a yellow legal pad and some file folders to organize your life, take a hard-nosed look at the full range of options. Feature-loaded, pocket-size electronic organizers, discussed in the final section of this chapter, are rapidly gaining popularity. More traditional pocket-size organizers and desk planners that use paper and pencil are available in a variety of formats.*

Organizational software for your personal, laptop, or notebook-size computer is a powerful way to help you keep track of objectives and appointments. Some sophisticated versions mix quick, random-access data management with first-class schedule tracking. Another breakthrough, known as groupware,† can coordinate individual and team schedules and put everyone in a system that categorizes electronic messages — requests, proposals, offers, responses — and notes what action needs to be initiated. At any point, each individual can see what commitments he or she has made in communications to others and what commitments are due.

2. Say No

Once you've set out your highest priorities, have the courage — pleasantly and nonapologetically — to say no to other things. Don't

---

* Pocket-size organizers and desk planners are available from (alphabetically): Stephen R. Covey and Associates (3507 North University, Suite 100, Provo, UT 84604; 800-331-7716); Day-Timers, Inc. (Allentown, PA 18001; 215-398-1223/395-5884); Personal Planning System (R. Webster Systems International, Inc., Suite 260, 500 W. Wilson Bridge Rd., Columbus, OH 43085; 614-436-5300); and Time/Design (11835 W. Olympic Blvd., Suite 450, Los Angeles, CA 90064; 800-637-9942).
†To learn more, see *Groupware: Computer Software for Business Teams* by Robert Johansen (Free Press, 1990).

be defensive. Where appropriate, give an explanation — but not an excuse. Saying no means displeasing people regularly, yet by doing it honestly and diplomatically you can minimize friction and accomplish the things you value most in life.

- *Overplan if you must, but don't overcommit.* There's a dramatic difference between overplanning and overcommitting. Overplanning — planning to do more than you can realistically accomplish — is something many of us do to make sure we have a backlog of projects we feel are important. It may waste some immediate time, but in general it's a benign habit. Overcommitting, in contrast, is deadly. You say yes to too many people and too many projects and begin to flounder — and then drown — in to-do memos and meetings. Your moods start going up, down, and sideways. Family time suffers and your loved ones let you know it. And then burnout rears its ugly head.

  To break out of this trap, do some task pruning and begin to commit yourself to *less* than you can accomplish and do *only* those major projects that are most important to you. Next, make saying no a strategic part of your new approach to work. Many top achievers credit their career success to learning to say no — with sagacity, warmth, and finality.

- *Delegate, delegate.* The ability to delegate is one of the most important tools for strategic time management. Instead of asking yourself, Who can best tackle this project or assume this responsibility? — to which you'll usually answer, "I can" — begin asking, Who *should* handle this? Usually, it *isn't* you.

  Do your best to get rid of many of the busywork tasks you don't enjoy. Rate your planned daily activities with a priority code. Make it a habit to evaluate every urgent-looking activity you're faced with. Is it really important or urgent? In what ways will it help you achieve your objectives? Can it wait until later? Does it require *your* attention or can you delegate it?

  Combat the tendency to assume the workload of co-workers and subordinates. Begin with awareness. When people come to you with a question, whenever possible stop offering answers. And resist the natural inclination to be helpful and say, "I'll get back to you." Instead, as noted in Chapter 6, respond with smarter answers, such as "What do *you* recommend?" or "See what you can do about it" or "Look into it and get back to me with your personal advice."

Before long, the parade up to your work station or into your office will thin out. Your colleagues and staff members will start to think through more of their own questions and possible solutions before tying up your time. And, more often than ever, they'll come up with their own answers. This promotes a healthy reliance on self-management and strategic thinking.

When delegating a task, first "create a clear, mutual understanding of what needs to be accomplished," advises Stephen Covey, "focusing on *what*, not *how; results*, not *methods*. Visualize the desired result. Have the person see it, describe it, make out a quality statement of what the results will look like, and by when they will be accomplished."[13]

• *Deal decisively with interruptions.* Once you start a project, you develop a flow, or momentum, toward results. For each interruption, it usually takes a few minutes to recapture that momentum, and you have to cover some of the same ground twice.

"Interruptions are *people* — people who want to shift your attention from what you're doing to something else," say Merrill Douglass and Larry Baker in *The New Time Management*. "While people are important, many of the issues they call or walk through your door with are *not* important. Learning to separate people from issues and then dealing with the issues makes it easier to cope with interruptions. Be gracious with people, but be serious about time."[14] When faced with frequent interruptions, act decisively to prevent, intercept, consolidate, or delegate them.

A good place to begin is screening out extraneous phone calls. The telephone is a blessing, but most managers and professionals curse it at least once a day. The most effective people make it into a tool instead of a burden.

The average middle manager is interrupted by the phone every five minutes or so all day. To curb this interference with your concentration, have your calls held for an hour or more at a time whenever you're working with momentum on top-priority projects. During this time, have your assistant, secretary, or receptionist tell callers, "I'm sorry, he or she is in a meeting." Then schedule out a block of time for returning the important phone calls yourself and asking your assistants to return the rest. If you don't have a staff to help you, your best final lines of defense are turning on your answering machine (or unplugging your phone) and closing your door.

Studies show that it also pays to take a few key seconds to plan every single phone call you make — jotting down some notes on what you want to say before dialing. Unplanned calls tend to take at least five minutes longer than planned calls, so if you make a dozen calls a day you could presently be wasting a full hour or more of your work time.

• *Spend some strategic interpersonal time now to save a bundle later.* Instead of getting stuck with a strict scheduling approach to increase your productivity, William Oncken suggests trying a "relationships" gambit,[15] a kind of lateral switch of your attention for about 5 percent or more of your schedule time. For example, use some of these minutes during the workday to improve rapport with your boss and co-workers so that their intrusions become less frequent and don't throw you too far off balance. Establish more stable working relationships with your staff and subordinates. And stop doing anything that they are responsible for, says Oncken. Make delegation work.

3. *Rest Better, Sleep Less: The Newest Time-Saving Frontier*

How often have you said to yourself, "I just wish I had more time." One of the most overlooked ways to gain more free, discretionary hours each week is sleep.

Few of us realize the extent to which our personal effectiveness depends on the *quality,* not quantity, of our nightly rest. Researchers have discovered that the majority of us are suffering from various kinds of *chronic partial sleep deprivation*[16] — we don't get enough sleep or, more often, we sleep poorly night after night.

You may be able to find a treasure chest of extra waking minutes by learning to sleep more deeply and in fewer hours a night. In fact, most of us can gradually reduce nightly sleep by about an hour and a half to two hours, says James A. Horne, a sleep researcher and psychophysiologist at Great Britain's Loughborough University.[17] (To learn more, see Chapter 13.)

4. *Expand Your Capability for Consistent, Top-Level Achievement*

The more effective you are, the greater your output and the less time you have to spend after hours when your productivity starts to wane and you're cutting into family time. Survey your current daily work level to locate a particular time slot when you traditionally do your best work. To maximize your return on energy — and stop spending additional after-5:00 hours on the job — start accomplishing more in less time by scheduling your toughest high-priority tasks during this peak period. When possible, block out enough time to accomplish at least one specific objective in one sitting, thereby reducing the setup time that most of us need when refocusing on a project after each interruption.

Organize your work space; take regular, effective work breaks (see Chapter 8); use decision sciences guidelines (see Chapter 7) to reduce the number of errors you make, both charging off in nonproductive directions and becoming involved in interpersonal mix-ups that force you to spend extra time fixing or redoing botched projects; and incorporate other Performance Edge tactics to increase your work effectiveness. Then start heading home earlier to spend more time with your family and on personal priorities.

5. *Deal with Other Major Time Wasters*

• *Streamline your paperwork shuffle.* Some time management specialists insist that clients sweep their desks clean of everything except what they're working on. But no studies to date show a correlation between how your desk looks and how much you actually accomplish.

The most important thing seems to be developing the discipline to quickly, decisively deal with incoming paper. Identify the correspondence you need to take action on, and then schedule that action. Sort materials you want to read, send to others, or file. *All* other paperwork and mail should be thrown out immediately and with finality — otherwise the ocean-of-paperwork syndrome can lead to lost time when you're forced to shuffle around searching for what you do need for your work at hand.

• *Read faster, listen and learn, and remember more.* If you're inundated with important or potentially important reading materials that you may never catch up on, there's a good chance that you're suffering from *information anxiety* — the black hole between data and knowledge that one expert describes as being "produced by the ever-widening gap between what we understand and what we think we should understand." [18]

One wise way to accomplish more in each "information update" slot on your schedule is by increasing your reading speed and expanding your memory power.

I know. I made a decision twenty years ago to take a variety of speed learning programs. From these, I developed a personalized system for accelerative reading — and greater retention — of important information.

While most of my colleagues felt good if they could manage to glance over the daily paper and scan half a dozen periodicals each week, I was able to spend the same amount of time in a far more effective way, previewing computer databases in a dozen different scientific fields and then reading at least fifty professional articles and four or five new books every week of the year. I felt solidly in control of my time, with considerably less frustration. And this new learning capability opened my eyes, changed my perspectives, and redirected my career.

Studies suggest that most of us can at least double our reading speed and increase our memory capabilities in six to eight weeks by following some simple recommendations. The most popular speed-reading program is Evelyn Wood Reading Dynamics (now available in book and audiocassettes from Nightingale-Conant, 7300 North Lehigh Ave., Chicago, IL 60648; 800-525-9000).

One popular way to turn commuting "downtime" into learning time is to listen to audiocassette tapes. Thousands of audio programs are now available on a wide range of subjects. This learning method can be an efficient and enjoyable way to stay in touch with some of the latest information on leadership, quality control, customer service, marketing, and sales techniques; to learn about personal development issues such as health, family relationship skills, and new hobbies; to listen to popular books on tape, including novels and nonfiction; to catch an extra lift of enthusiasm from a motivational speaker; to explore new strategies in financial investment; to practice speeches; and even to learn foreign languages.

- *Organize and run meetings that make sense.* Every day, an estimated 20 million business meetings are held in America. The average upper manager or executive spends four hours a day (which translates into twenty-one weeks a year) running or attending meetings, with up to half of that time totally wasted.

  The factors that make meetings fail — unclear objectives; lack of proper preparation; problems in communication; absence of leadership and control; confusion and inefficiency; time wasted on *why* instead of *how;* poor handling of conflict, critique, and feedback; weak decision making; and no follow-through — are the same ones that can undermine a company's entire operation.

  Researchers suggest a number of ways to make meetings take less time and produce better results:[19]

1. *Determine if a meeting is really necessary.* There's no need to call a meeting if you can accomplish or delegate the task yourself through an informal talk with another person or if a telephone call, fax, or memo would be more effective. Routine meetings are warranted only as long as each one continues to fulfill your objectives.

    Lynn Oppenheim, vice-president of the Wharton Center for Applied Research, suggests, "Instead of having a weekly staff meeting, which is often the most disliked of all meetings, propose a more flexible meeting schedule, depending on what needs to be done next."[20]

2. *Establish the meeting's purpose and stick to it.* "A meeting without a clear-cut objective is a trip to nowhere," says Milo O. Frank.[21] Set clear, specific priorities for every meeting and make sure the minutes you spend together are focused and productive. Force the leaders of all meetings to determine what three or four points they want to make.

3. *Get the right people to attend — those who are essential to the meeting's success — and no one else.* Make sure that all the principal people who can influence the fulfillment of the meeting objectives are invited to attend. Then consider bringing in

a few key experts who can provide answers and lend an outside perspective to the discussion. This can help save time. But remember, the number of people who attend is directly proportional to the length of most meetings.

4. *Prepare for the meeting by sending the participants a formal agenda with backup materials.* Use a written agenda as a blueprint for action for every meeting. It should state the objectives and specific issues, the time the meeting will begin and end, the place, the participants involved, and what is expected of each of them in the way of preparation. Make sure everyone does some homework before the meeting.

5. *If you are the leader, beware of expressing your opinion too early.* Even when you're well versed on a meeting's agenda, if you're genuinely interested in what others have to say, don't participate too early. Get everyone else involved, beginning with those lower on the corporate ladder. Ask questions, probe, and invite dissenting views, encouraging what diplomats call a free and frank discussion. Have the opposing sides blast away — at issues and methods, not people — secure in the knowledge that they need not take their differences personally. Discuss only one issue at a time. For formal presentations, each participant should be expected to present his or her viewpoint in a concise manner within the designated time limits.

6. *Stick to the schedule and structure the meeting so participants can leave when no longer needed.* Start exactly on time and end on time. Rod Canion, CEO of Compaq Computer, speaks for many managers and executives when he says that his biggest time waster is "waiting for meetings to begin."

7. *Review the results — and never end a meeting without deciding on the next action.* People too often leave meetings unclear about how it connects to what comes next. Set specific action guidelines and deadlines for accomplishing them.

8. *Consider using teleconferencing, video conferencing, and computer-aided meetings on certain subjects.* Teleconferencing has been on the business scene for years, and when wisely used it can drastically reduce travel time to meetings. Video conferencing adds the visual element to a telephone conference and has become popular in some major corporations.

A new twist on this theme is known as computer-aided or

electronic meetings. These high-tech get-togethers are winning support for specialized purposes at leading companies worldwide. The participants sit in silence side by side — or on opposite sides of the globe — in front of personal computers, typing anonymous messages that flash on a projection screen. A complex, local-area network tracks and sorts by topic and order of response every sentence typed in by attendees. When participants want to vote on an issue, the computers tally the results and display them immediately. At the end of the meeting, everyone gets a printed synopsis.

A recent study by IBM and the University of Arizona[22] confirms that electronic meetings are fast — up to 55 percent faster than traditional ones. A lot of people can "talk" at once without stepping on toes, chitchat is eliminated, and discussions don't digress. Perhaps most powerful of all, participants can be brutally honest. This can produce a gold mine of valuable, unfiltered information. But there are shortcomings. The anonymity makes it impossible for people to get credit for good ideas, and computer-shy attendees often have trouble keeping up with others. Yet when used appropriately, computer-aided meetings can serve a valuable purpose in group work achievement.

- *Implement at-home strategies for saving time.* Professional organizers report that some extra hours of discretionary time can usually be freed up every week by experimenting with typical personal time wasters at home. Examples include watching less TV; shopping by phone; cooking in larger quantities and freezing separate meals; buying low-maintenance clothes and appliances; screening calls with an answering machine; consolidating errands and household tasks instead of making small, frequent, one-item trips to the store; combining activities to satisfy varied needs (example: take an exercise walk with a loved one or friend, strengthening both the relationship and your fitness at the same time); making it a point to connect with loved ones during routine family tasks (when cooking, riding in the car, and so on); and taking a bit more lax attitude toward lawn care and housekeeping.
- *Take full advantage of travel wait time.* Part of strategic time planning is finding ways to reduce time urgency. Unexpected de-

lays and traffic jams are a poor excuse for tying yourself up in stress knots. During business travel, in particular, waiting occurs frequently and it's a learned aggravation. As noted in Chapter 15, it pays to develop a personal collection of valuable things you can be prepared to do in order to turn down — wait — time into highly productive breaks.

The Portable Electronic Office — Making It Work for You

As time pressure builds, so does your need to organize time better. Fortunately, the technology that helped create the problem can also help solve it. The shift to an electronically assisted lifestyle is gathering momentum. We are departing from many of the attitudes and structures of the industrial age and are flattening organizations, eliminating much of the hierarchy that permitted only those at the top a view of the entire corporation. As mentioned earlier in this chapter, computer networks and organizational software are bringing sweeping changes to many companies. Other developments are also making it possible to work and stay in touch 24 hours a day from anywhere in the world.

Cellular phones, voice mail, and electronic mail. For some managers and professionals, cellular phones have added as many as a dozen productive hours a week to their work schedule — transforming commuting time into a chance to take phone calls they would normally miss, return calls, make immediate follow-up calls after appointments, check in for messages, cross time zones to connect with distant contacts as they drive to or from work, make appointments, keep in touch with their families, and brainstorm with colleagues and customers.

Electronic mail (E-mail), or computer-to-computer exchange of messages, is already a favorite of big corporations with extensive computer networks. And it's catching on fast with smaller firms. Because, on average, E-mail costs 90 percent less than overseas calls and letters and 75 percent less than telex, the savings add up in a hurry.

Voice mail systems allow you to join a toll-free network in which you can communicate with others without actually talking directly. The voice mail system digitizes voice messages and stores them in a computer. You can retrieve your messages from any touch-tone phone — anywhere in the world — and replay them one by one. After hearing each message, you can either store it, replay it, forward it to someone else on the system, or delete it. If the caller is on the same voice mail system that you are, you can immediately record an answer to the message and forward it to his or her voice mailbox. Voice mail can also be used to relay the same message to a large number of representatives in the field.

By some estimates, two out of three traditional business telephone calls don't go through on the first try. So in many cases, E-mail and voice mail systems can help you end the annoyance of telephone tag — at least with your suppliers, closest colleagues, and most important customers.

Laptop and notebook computers and fax machines. In the past several years, advances in facsimile machines, laptop computers, and unbelievably powerful miniaturized, notebook-size computers have helped make working anywhere a reality for millions of us. One of the hottest technology markets is for after-hours home workers — often parents of young children who leave the workplace at five and finish work projects at home on a PC or laptop PC after they put the kids to bed and spend some quiet time together. These flextime workers can also use their computers to read and answer E-mail from anywhere at any hour.

Pocket file cabinets. Pocket-size electronic organizers continue to grow in popularity. More than a glorifed address book, these audiovisual memo pads and calendars have a powerful memory and can now perform hundreds of sophisticated scheduling and organizational functions and may include a calculator, telephone number and address directory, monthly appointment calendar and daily schedule (programmed for decades into the future), time/expense budget ledger, dictionary, spelling corrector, thesaurus, abbreviation expanders, digital world time clock, electronic memo/notepads, city guides, language translators, schedule alarms, programmable financial calculator with spreadsheet functions, and more. In fact, some versions can store up to an entire file cabinet's worth of material and can interface or link with organizational software on your office PC.

The number one priority in designing a portable electronic office is to get to the heart of your personal needs. Read critical reviews of products in a variety of periodicals. Talk to other users. Some electronic breakthroughs can be more of a burden than a help, depending on your unique business objectives and corporate structure. Arrange to have a trial period to test any product that looks as if it might fit your needs. And make certain that you have fast, reliable service available since unforeseen repair headaches can quickly turn electronic marvels from time savers into time wasters.

In more and more front-running companies, work-hour *effectiveness* — in innovation, customer responsiveness, quality control, and productive outputs — is becoming the criterion for promotion and compensation. Ultimately, your ability to get things done is determined more by *self*-management than by *time* management. Remember, there's no point trying to manage your time unless you're willing to change the way you spend it.

6

Performance Turning Point #4: Communication Exchanges

Developing More Insightful, On-Target Interpersonal Skills

Language is the picture and counterpart of thought.
— *Mark Hopkins*

Communication is the most important source of personal power.
— Fortune *magazine*

EFFECTIVE COMMUNICATION is a cornerstone of the Performance Edge. The way we perceive and talk to each other at work — about goal setting, job performance, quality control, service improvement, interpersonal relations, career development, and other important issues — is a major determinant of the profitability of our organizations. Communication also sets the tone for individual and work team motivation and for job satisfaction in general.

Communication mistakes and misunderstandings not only create stress[1] and cause or aggravate interpersonal conflicts; they also reduce productivity, weaken quality control, and lead to anger, resentment, mistrust, and cynicism.[2] Even worse, communication-related stresses are linked to "silent heart disease" and increased risk of sudden death from heart attack.[3]

In today's fast-paced work environment, projects rush forward, requiring tremendous amounts of mental and physical energy. Think of the time, money, and peace of mind lost as a result of communication misunderstandings, inaccurate or incomplete messages, and related problems. When interpersonal communication is on target and constructive, work is more enjoyable, information flows more freely, disagreements are more readily resolved, and greater trust is generated. Research confirms that, in general, the better the business communication, the greater the work productivity.[4]

"Whenever a group works together on a developmental (or other) task," observes Rosabeth Moss Kanter, professor at Harvard Business School, "their ability to share this rapidly accumulating knowledge makes a difference in how effectively they can work toward the common goal."[5] Today's participative, partnership-oriented management and supervisory positions carry with them the requirement for greater communication and interaction. People at every corporate level "need to spend more time explaining goals, keeping staff or allies up to date with timely information, and making sure they understand where their responsibilities fit into the whole task."[6]

In the latest *Fortune* magazine/CNN/Moneyline poll of the chief executives of Fortune 500 and Service 500 companies, fully three-fourths of the CEOs claim that, compared with the past, they are more participatory and more consensus-oriented and rely more on communication than command.[7] Research also indicates that the greatest proportion of work time for every executive and manager is now spent communicating, usually in short interactions with a large number of people and on a great variety of business topics.[8]

But many of us need to do more: A. Foster Higgins & Co., an employee benefits consulting firm, recently found that while 97 percent of CEOs it surveyed believe communicating with employees has a positive impact on job performance and satisfaction and 79 percent think it benefits the bottom line, only 22 percent actually do it weekly or more often.[9]

The Competitive Advantage Comes
Through People

To achieve outstanding communication in the workplace, we must overcome all kinds of obstacles in dealing with our co-workers, bosses, employees, suppliers, and customers — all of them individuals with their own concerns, sensitivities, and desires. Any energy that you or your work team members expend arguing or miscommunicating weakens your ability to get the job done. In fact, stress researchers report that carrying an extra load of work pressure, even for weeks at a time, isn't nearly as stressful as interpersonal conflict with a colleague or loved one.[10] And the most frequently cited source of person-to-person conflict is poor communication.[11]

A major study conducted at the Center for Creative Leadership discovered that "specific performance problems" were only one of the ten most commonly cited reasons for managerial failure. The other nine reasons all had to do with interpersonal communication and the way work was done.[12] A recent survey of nearly 1,200 CEOs, presidents, and executive vice-presidents of major American corporations reported that communication problems are the primary reason that many of the most capable businesspeople flounder.[13]

In decentralized, customer-driven companies, effective leaders — at all levels — must regularly communicate with two main groups of people:

- *Co-workers and employees:* To keep everyone aligned with organizational purpose and direction, in touch with management, and focused on specific work goals and to gain their input and involvement in decisions
- *Clients and customers:* To keep them up to date with the company's newest activities, products, services, and support

Rather than merely issuing reports and delivering messages, effective communicators use clear, straightforward language to establish targets that everyone can envision and work toward, and they choose words and body language that let people know that their input is welcome and valued.

Yet "to the extent that managers currently communicate expectations at all," observes Michael E. McGill, professor of organization behavior at the Cox School of Business at Southern Methodist University, "they focus on the bottom line — the results to be achieved. In fact, the process, the *how* of getting there, is just as important in most companies, although it is rarely acknowledged in performance pronouncements."[14] McGill further says that "to be responsive, managers must open themselves to experiencing the organization as employees experience it — managers need to listen."[15]

Communication Also Affects Health

Few of us realize that the way we communicate is a significant health factor and that poor communication is linked to high blood pressure (hypertension) and heart disease. Chronic misunderstandings and mismanaged anger not only create resentment and cynicism but can break down the heart muscle and lead to heart attack.[16] Communication may also be the most profound way to change brain chemistry, says Steven Paul, chief of clinical neuroscience at the National Institute of Mental Health.[17]

Simple human dialogue — the process of talking and listening — dramatically affects the heart and blood vessels, say researchers, and, in turn, every aspect of our health and well-being.[18]

As people begin to speak, their blood pressure goes up, and microscopic blood vessel changes are detectable at far distant points in the body. Conversely, when people listen attentively or tune in to the external environment in a relaxed manner, their blood pressure falls and heart rate slows, often slightly below normal resting levels.

One recent research project[19] reviewed forty-eight studies from the previous decade and pinpointed three primary characteristics associated with hypertension:

1. Anger and hostility
2. Difficulty with interpersonal communication
3. Frequent use of denial when responding to criticism

"Study after study reveals that human dialogue not only affects our hearts significantly but can even alter the biochemistry of individual tissues at the furthest extremities of the body," reports James J. Lynch, codirector of the Psychophysiological Clinic and Laboratories at the University of Maryland School of Medicine. "Since blood flows through every human tissue, the entire body is influenced by human dialogue. Thus, it is true that when we speak we do so with every fiber of our being. The 'language of the heart' is integral to the health and emotional life of every one of us."[20]

For good health, the *rise* in blood pressure experienced when you speak must be balanced by the *lowering* of pressure that occurs when you listen in a relaxed manner. (This means *real* listening. If you're on the edge of your seat waiting to grab your turn to speak or are rehearsing in your mind what you're going to say, you won't receive the benefits of lower blood pressure, slower pulse, and other biochemical balancing processes.) This talk-listen combination helps keep blood pressure evenly regulated. Unfortunately, most of us have learned to listen defensively and talk too much.

Key to Participative Management

The Latin root of the word *communicate* means "coming together," and today's management style calls for pushing authority down, speeding up decisions, getting closer to employees and to customers, and learning new ways to deal with difficult people. None of us can afford to let hidden dialogue conflicts and misunderstandings leave us feeling frustrated, fuming, or tongue-tied.

This chapter of *The Performance Edge* introduces a new way of thinking about work-related communication. The latest research on the subject can be divided into eight priority areas:

1. **Listening**
2. **Language and time management**
3. **Smart questions**

4. Clear perceptions
5. Precise language
6. Dealing with difficult people
7. Compliments, anger, and criticism
8. Verbal self-defense

---

1. Listening

> The key to effective interpersonal communication is this:
> Seek first to understand, then to be understood.
>
> — *Stephen R. Covey, Ph.D., chairman of the Institute for Principle-Centered Leadership*

"It can be stated with practically no qualification that people in general do not know how to listen," says Dr. Ralph G. Nichols, who developed innovative programs on listening at the University of Minnesota. "They have ears that hear very well, but seldom have they acquired the necessary . . . skills which would allow those ears to be used effectively for what is called listening."[21]

Leaders at every work level know how to listen. They know that listening to people builds their self-esteem and can result in an honest pride that promotes innovative, dedicated work. These leaders — in management, sales, service, and production roles — take the time to sit down with their work team members and customers, use questions to stimulate thought and solicit information, and then pay full attention to the answers. And, just as important, they encourage silent employees to speak up and keep talkers from monopolizing meetings and discussions.

However, most corporate corridors are still gridlocked by people unable or unwilling to change the way they respond to questions and feedback. "Token tours (management by walking around) may put managers within physical reach of employees," warns Michael McGill, "but just *being* where employees can be heard is not enough; managers must *behave* in ways that allow employees to be heard.

"Managers often fall into behaviors that actually discourage hearing from employees. Many managers personify the organization to the point that any criticism is viewed as a personal attack. Debating, denying, or discounting employee input are frequently used defensive tactics and certain signs of a closed managerial 'ear.' Some managers simply give the clear impression that they are 'too busy' to concern themselves with what employees have to say. One of the strongest deterrents to encouraging employees to share their experience is the failure of managers to act on undesirable conditions or practices that employees have previously brought to their attention. Once denied a 'hearing,' employees are reluctant to press the point. Fear of retribution (shoot the messenger) runs deep in subordinate/superior relationships."[22]

Be exquisitely careful about how you receive less than good news. Even if the message is incendiary or sinks your hopes, it's best not to show it — no tirades, no sarcasm, no rigid body language, no eyes rolling upward. Elicit recommendations, asking a calm question such as "What do you think we ought to do?" And then, with a sincere heart, tell the messenger, "Thank you for bringing this to my attention." It will also help substantially if, long before waves of discontent or bad news arrive, you have established an atmosphere in which co-workers and subordinates feel comfortable speaking up.

Here are the key components of effective listening:

Choose a nondistracting environment. Go somewhere free of ringing telephones, background noise, or desktops full of distracting, unfinished work. Pick a place where the speaker can relax, since this helps people let go of tension and open up honest communication.

Select a listening posture. Good listeners communicate attentiveness through the relaxed alertness of their bodies. They face the other person squarely and incline slightly, with arms and legs uncrossed, leaning toward the speaker with a warm — or at least nonthreatening — facial expression.

Use attending skills. Attending consists of giving your physical attention to another person, demonstrating that you are truly interested in what is being said. Nonattending, on the other hand, dramatically obstructs the speaker's expression.

Maintain eye contact. Natural, sustained eye contact improves communication by permitting speakers to determine listeners' receptiveness to them and their message.

Use smooth gestures. Recent research[23] suggests that it's usually best to avoid all angular body language, such as shaking your index finger, pounding your fist, or jabbing or whacking at the air with the side of your hand. This is irritating. Instead, emphasize smooth, natural gestures.

Avoid killer phrases. Kevin J. Murphy, author of *Effective Listening*, points out that the phrases "That's interesting" and "Is that right?" almost always indicate that you are only pretending to listen.[24] Be careful to notice the way you respond as you listen. Don't interrupt but do confirm that you are genuinely listening by interjecting "um-hmmms," nods, and occasional specific questions.

Stay cool. Remember from the outset that if you get angry, you lose. Alan Brown, a professor at Southern Methodist University, warns that your memory of key facts may well be impaired by the first rush of hot blood.[25] And Max Bazerman, a professor at Northwestern University's business school and an expert on negotiation, suggests considering the possibility that the other person could merely be using anger as a ploy to throw you off.[26] For the latest strategies on handling anger, see number 7, "Compliments, Anger, and Criticism," later in this chapter.

Practice active listening. Listening is a process that requires you to fully participate, not just sit there like a statue. So take a minute to clear your mind and put aside whatever else concerns you. Consciously slow down a bit and think of exactly what your goals are in having this conversation. Here are several guidelines for active listening:[27]

Acknowledge and paraphrase. This means stating in your own words what you think someone just said. It keeps you focused on understanding what the other person means. Paraphrasing lead-ins include "In other words . . . ," "What I hear you saying is . . . ," "So essentially what happened (or how you felt) was . . . ," and so forth. Paraphrasing helps avoid miscommunication and breaks down false assumptions, errors, and misrepresentations. It also helps you remember what was said and avoid comparing, judging, derailing, advising, and sparring.

Clarify and give reflective feedback. Clarifying, which often accompanies paraphrasing, means asking more reflective questions until you clearly understand the issue. After observing the speaker's tone of voice, facial expressions, gestures, and body language, you can check the congruency of the message (do the words say one thing and the eyes and body language another?).

You reflect feeling by identifying the emotional context transmitted in the message you heard. Verify your perceptions by creating a tentative description: "I want to understand your feelings (or this situation); is this (give your own description of the message you've received) the way you feel (or what really happened)?" You're not expressing your own feelings or approving or disapproving. You're simply checking to be certain your interpretation is correct.

Listen with empathy and explore the options. Listening with openness and empathy puts you on a heart-to-heart level with the speaker. It's difficult to listen when you're judging another person or finding fault. You need to hear the *whole* statement, the entire communiqué. You can compare what is being said — without judgment — to your own knowledge of life, people, history, and similar events. What are the options? In what way can you support the speaker or serve as a sounding board for possible next steps to take?

Respond — and take action. Your final responsibility as a tuned-in listener is to share your thoughts and feelings and to act on what you have heard. Otherwise, the speaker will often feel that the whole conversation ended up being a futile, manipulative exercise.

Receive and give feedback. "Giving feedback — criticizing and praising — is the most important tool of the managing trade," says Andrew S. Grove, president of Intel Corporation and author of *High Output Management.*[28]

To improve communication, you must ask for and encourage honest, constructive feedback. You can't take it for granted, since most people will tell you only *what they think you want to hear.* You might ask a close friend or relative to study with you, or you might tape yourself speaking so that you can listen to yourself as an outsider and make improvements. If you aren't comfortable taping or if the people you talk with aren't at ease being recorded, you can simply choose to be a keener conversational observer.

Feedback that helps co-workers and employees perform at top levels follows certain rules of thumb.[29] Meaningful feedback is (1) specific, (2) immediate, (3) something that the hearer can change, (4) given for the benefit of the receiver, not the giver, (5) more often positive rather than negative, and (6) verifiable — the giver can confirm that the receiver genuinely understands the true meaning of the message.

2. Language and Time Management

One of the most common complaints about people in leadership positions is the perception that they're rushing through interactions with employees, clients, and customers. This perception can be altered — and you can reduce hassles and increase the amount of valuable information you receive — by following three guidelines:

1. Listen effectively — with leadership posture. Beyond the basic listening habits presented in the preceding section, you can do two very important things right away to make time spent with you seem longer:

Sit down while you are interacting with other people.
Don't make any movements that seem to indicate you are concerned about how much time has passed.

"Nothing will shorten the perceived time for your client or subordinate more drastically than watching you stand at a door with your hand on it (or any other 'exit' position), poised to flee," warns communications expert Suzette Haden Elgin. "If you have only two minutes to spare, that posture will make those two minutes seem like only one to the person you're speaking with, and you have canceled out 50 percent of those precious minutes."[30]

It's a myth, say researchers, to assume that sitting down in a relaxed posture and not finding irritating ways to remind people about time constraints will prompt them to abuse their time privilege with you.

2. Choose your words carefully. In terms of leadership and the perception of time in human interactions, there are things you can say — and not say — that will help people feel that you have given them extra time.

First, when you state how much time you have, say it in a tone of voice that shows you're delighted to be so fortunate to have five minutes, or ten minutes, or half an hour. And be absolutely certain to eliminate the word "only" and any other negative presuppositions from your statement. Begin your announcement by saying "I have fifteen minutes to spend with you" instead of "I have only fifteen minutes." This subtle change makes a marked difference in the other person's perception of you.

Next, complete your statement by adding ". . . and if you need more time than that, just say so, and I will stay (or schedule another meeting)." Studies show that people usually won't take you up on the offer; in fact, they'll often be more effective in using the minutes they have with you. And, just as important, they'll feel that you always offer them ample time to communicate — and this is the perception that's so crucial for high-performance leaders to earn. The alternative is a relentless undercurrent of resentment, and even sabotage, which makes both sides stressed and less productive.

3. *Manage personal distance.* Another way to control the perception of time is to make choices related to *personal distance,* the space you put between yourself and others during a conversation. The best "talking distance" for each individual varies according to personal habits and cultural/subcultural traditions. But you can learn to tune in to the most comfortable and effective distance of the person you're speaking with by using three guidelines:[31]

Choose a location from which to talk, and begin.

If your partner moves toward you — or backs away from you — stand your ground until he or she stops.

Once the other person has chosen a location and is talking comfortably, you know that this is his or her preferred personal distance. Respect it.

3. Smart Questions

Gaining — or losing — the competitive advantage often depends on the type of questions you ask. Smart questions help you cut to the heart of difficult challenges, organize problems, and position yourself to seize opportunities most effectively. Whenever you reach a point where a situation looks snarled with complexity or you begin to feel stuck, ask yourself: *Am I asking the right questions?*

To identify readiness in your work team members, for example, ask on-target questions of the people who will be responsible and accountable for the success of the project. Most of us make the mistake of beginning with questions like "What do you think is causing the problem here"? or "What do you think it will take to solve it?" These queries encourage a shifting of responsibility and promote the tendency to point fingers at other people or outside conditions. So does the question "How can we achieve this goal?" In response, you'll often hear "We can't" or "Nobody knows."

In contrast, smart questions can shut off escape routes and zero in on results. For example: "Before we can accomplish (a goal), what specific things would have to happen?" Or, even more effective: "There are a number of ways to get started accomplishing a goal like this one. What specific steps do you think would be the smartest and easiest to take and will give us the greatest payoff in the shortest amount of time?" Or "What specific steps do you think you can carry out successfully, right away, with the resources and people you have in place right now?" *Then* build on these results.

Effective executives and managers who favor small breakthrough projects insist that each individual must begin accomplishing things right away — with whatever resources are at hand. It's time to wean employees away from comfortable rationalizations and excuses that encourage inertia or passing the buck.

Every time you hear a rejoinder that says "It just can't be done until . . ." or "But we need additional people, or resources, or equipment, or space, or systems, or measurements," immediately challenge it by asking: "Is there anything — *anything at all* — that can be done right now, by you or within your team or department, that can improve productivity or quality or service?" In almost every case, the response you'll receive is "Well, perhaps a few things." And then you can get going, directly toward an immediate result and improvement.

Choose Open Questions

There are two basic categories of questions. *Closed questions* — such as "Who's in charge of this assignment?" or "When is your scheduled completion date?" — can be answered with a simple yes or no or a statement of fact. In some situations, they're the query of choice when you need to save time, elicit information, or speed action.

However, closed questions like these tend to create an interrogation feeling and discourage further discussion. If used too often, they prompt feelings of resentment and powerlessness.

Open questions, when chosen with clear purpose and intent, stimulate thought and encourage discussion. They require more than a simple yes or no response, and they help the questioner clarify his or her thinking prior to asking the question.

Open questions can be extremely valuable in understanding the thoughts and emotions that influence other people's actions. Yet with all the advantages of open questions, researchers report that only one of every twenty questions asked by managers is phrased in an open style.[32]

"Open questions are vastly underused for two reasons," says communications expert Dorothy Leeds. "The first is sheer ignorance. Because questions are generally not part of the standard business communication repertoire, most people are unfamiliar with the technique and therefore don't know how to use it. The second reason is that it takes more effort to think up open questions and to pay the necessary close attention to the responses."[33]

You can easily turn a closed question into an open one by adding *What, Would, Could,* or *How.* Some examples:

What needs to be done next?
What results are you looking for, and *how* will you measure them?
What can I/we do to help you?
Would you please explain this idea/decision to me from your perspective?
How, specifically, can we improve this situation right away?
How do you feel about the new sales quotas (or production deadlines or scheduling commitments)?

What feedback are you receiving from your work team, and *what* suggestions make the most sense to you?

Choose Outcome-Focused Questions

When we ask *problem-focused questions* — usually beginning with *Why* — we usually receive lengthy justifications and excuses rather than clear information. In general, think twice before asking *Why* questions or other problem-focused queries like "What's wrong here?" or "What's the matter?" or "Who's to blame for this?" Instead, choose *outcome-focused questions* — frequently beginning with *How* or *What* or *Could* — since they tend to turn the attention toward solutions.

Compare "*Why* did you make the mistake that caused this big problem?" with "*How* can we do that (specific task) better from now on?" And contrast "What's *wrong* with you/me/them?" with "*What* are we trying to accomplish here?" or "*What* do you/we/ they need?" or "*How* did you come to your decision?" or "*What's* the best step to take right now to turn this around?"

Constructing Smart Questions

Asking insightful, on-target questions will help you gain the advantage in job interviews, leadership situations, performance evaluations, getting a promotion, asking for a raise, and working effectively with others. Here are some basic guidelines.

Prepare the groundwork. (a) Determine your purpose: Exactly what do you want to gain with each question? Information, cooperation, resources, support, commitment?

(b) Know your audience — to whom, exactly, are you asking this question and what do you know about their goals, interests, and views?

(c) Phrase the question carefully, in most cases using the open-question format. Is there a way to ask it so that everyone can benefit and no one gets hurt?

Deliver the question effectively. (a) Begin with the Instant Calming Sequence presented in Chapter 3.

(b) Speak calmly, clearly, and directly.

(c) Maintain a positive outlook and give the other person time to gather his or her thoughts before responding.

Listen carefully, assess the answer, explore the options, and respond. Listen carefully to the response and then nonjudgmentally evaluate what you hear, asking questions whenever necessary to clarify the exact meaning. Not every question requires direct action. Sometimes all that's needed is to listen and respond, acknowledging the issue at hand and confirming that you appreciate the other person's input. But in many cases you'll gain the respect of co-workers and employees only when you follow up on the feedback and information you receive.

Empowering Others

One of the best ways to motivate other people is to encourage them to identify and solve their own problems. When someone approaches you with an idea, instead of responding by saying something like "It will take too much time and cost too much," turn your thoughts into a question and say, "How much time and money do you think this would take to accomplish?" Then give the other person the chance to take a more careful look at the issue.

Another example: When you're ready to respond to someone by saying, "That's a poor idea and it's based on false assumptions," instead say, "In what ways does that approach seem profitable to you?" Without creating animosity, you have given the other person a way to assess the idea, to identify its strengths and weaknesses, and to make an independent judgment.

Problem Solving and Reducing Mistakes

When you're forced to deal with a problem, instead of asking "Why?" or saying something like "Tell me again about what caused this problem," listen carefully and then ask, "What solutions do you see?"

After explaining a task, a manager will often ask an employee,

"Do you understand?" Typically, the worker responds, "Yes," since saying no is an embarrassment. But in far too many cases, even when people *think* they understand what the manager wants, they actually don't.

Instead of saying "Do you understand?" you can generate feedback and reduce mistakes with a question like "To make sure we're on track with this project, would you please summarize the actions you're going to take as a result of this discussion/meeting/decision?" Listen carefully to the reply, correct any misunderstandings or faulty assumptions, and fill in any missing details. Then launch the project with a final question such as "Is there anything else I can do to clarify things before you begin?" or "Why don't you take a day to give some thought to our discussion and then get in touch with me tomorrow with any questions you have before you begin?"

Overcoming Objections, Easing Anger, and Reducing Conflict

Whenever you hear a string of objections, usually spearheaded by "Yes, *but* . . . ," it's pointless to go on responding with one option after another. Instead, turn the discussion around by asking a solution-oriented question, such as "What other choices do you see?" or "How, specifically, can I help you solve this?"

Asking the right questions also enables you to constructively confront people who are angry or upset. You ease defensiveness and encourage communication when, instead of saying "What's wrong?" you substitute "Can you tell me more about what you're thinking and feeling?"

Customer Service

Superior customer service is an essential characteristic of today's most successful, market-driven companies, and experts insist that there is "no such thing as paying too much attention to customers' ideas and opinions."[34]

When unexpected but unavoidable service errors or quality

breakdowns occur, top-flight organizations have their people trained to immediately swing into action, helping the customer with what is commonly referred to as "recovery." A recent National Consumer Survey conducted by Technical Assistance Research Programs Institute (TARP) for the U.S. Office of Consumer Affairs, confirmed that resolving customer problems quickly and efficiently had a strong, positive impact on customer loyalty. In fact, when handled well, complaints can be a corporate asset.

From a communications perspective, recovery involves at least five steps on the part of the company's front-line personnel:[35]

1. *A genuine acknowledgment of error,* followed by an apology delivered in the first person. The standard corporate "We're sorry" speech does little to make people feel that you care that they've been delayed, annoyed, or victimized in some way.
2. *An urgent reinstatement.* This action gives the customer a clear sense that the employee and the company are doing everything possible to quickly bring things back into a state of balance. If the customer has been victimized, rather than just annoyed, then the following ingredients are critical.
3. *Demonstration of empathy.* "Expressing compassion may be the mother lode of all service gold," writes researcher Ron Zemke. "Victimized customers are likely to insist that before you attempt to redress their views or feelings you first demonstrate that you understand them."[36]
4. *Symbolic atonement.* This consists of the gesture, statement, and actions that unequivocally demonstrate that "We want to make it up to you."
5. *Follow-up.* In cases in which the customer has been victimized in some way, this step is essential to provide a sense of closure, affirm the authenticity of the recovery actions, and provide feedback on its effectiveness.

4. Clear Perceptions

> People can seriously misunderstand what it is they're not say-
> ing to each other.
>
> — *Jack Rosenthal, "On Language,"* New York Times

Communication breakdowns in the workplace almost always result from *perception gaps* — sharp differences in the way people
perceive situations.

"Radically varying meanings for certain key words causes severe communication breakdowns over and over again," says language expert Suzette Haden Elgin, "leaving people baffled and
frustrated and wondering what could have caused the resulting
mess. Unless we have a way to construct bridges across these reality gaps, communication breakdowns will occur, and their consequences will be grave."[37]

In work conversations, certain traffic rules determine the outcome. Communication breaks down when

- you are unable to communicate with the clarity and vision to win
  and hold the listeners' attention;
- it's your turn to talk but you miss your cue;
- you stop listening because you think it's your turn to talk.

"Much of the confusion that arises in the course of bargaining,"
says a recent report in *The Royal Bank Letter* of Canada, "is the
result of one party missing the meaning of the other's words —
usually because the first party's mind is occupied rehearsing what
he or she will say when his or her turn comes. Successful negotia-
tors generally do more listening than talking."[38]

Clarify Your Perceptions Before You React

The only sure way to avoid communication mix-ups and misunderstandings is to clarify what you *think* you hear from other peo-

ple and to be certain that they actually understand both the intent and meaning of your own communications.

First, be alert for congruency in the messages you give and receive. *Body language* is the nonverbal statement made by your tone of voice, word emphasis, rate of speech, volume of speech, gestures, posture, breathing pattern, and facial expression. Is it consistent with the verbal statement or question you are giving or hearing? If not, gently but firmly determine why it isn't and seek out the correct meaning of the message.

Even if your words are clear and true, they can immediately be canceled by contradictory body language. The meaning — or semantic content — conveyed by your body language is a crucial communication factor, and each of us must take responsibility for it when we listen and speak. It is the single most powerful communication message we give, overshadowing or nullifying our words.

Second, avoid *killer phrases* such as "The problem with that idea is . . . ," "No way could that ever work here," "Get serious, this is the real world," and "You've got to be kidding! We tried something like that before and it didn't work." Statements like these shut down input and trigger negative responses.

Substitute *encourager phrases* such as "That's an interesting suggestion. What, specifically, would it take to make it profitable in our company?" or "I always welcome new ideas, and your enthusiasm makes me want to learn more about this."

Third, be alert for *"red flag" words* that have radically different meanings for different individuals and different cultures. Examples include *failure, defeat, cheat, lie, deceive, trick, fool, loss, mistake, blunder, responsibility, oversight, problem,* and *disaster.* Whenever possible, avoid using these words yourself, and immediately clarify what other people mean when they use them. For example, a recent article in *Inc.* magazine reviewed the word *failure* as it is interpreted by Japanese managers: "It is actually *fear* that moves those managers. There is no tolerance for failure. The penalty for failure is out, finished. It's a powerful motivation."[39]

Even in the American workplace, the word *failure* has a range of meanings — from a momentary disappointment to a corporate disaster or the end of an entire career. When you use *fail* or *failure* in a statement, be certain that the meaning you intend is the meaning your listener actually receives.

When you want to learn what another person's representation is for a certain word or phrase, use the following types of questions, inserting your own definition of meaning in each blank:

Do you feel that *failure* means to . . . ?
Do you agree that *failure* means to . . . ?
Some people use the word *failure* to mean. . . . Do you think that's accurate?

It's a waste of time and energy to proceed on a work project or discussion when another person thinks that your approach is wrong or feels that your opinion doesn't make sense. When you want to work *with* another person but you begin to detect disagreement in his or her voice, words, or body language, stop the conversation. Ask the following kinds of questions with a neutral tone of voice and unemotional body language:

- "I think it would be very helpful if you would give your view of the strategy or action plan we're discussing (or following) here. What are the best steps for us to take, as you understand them?" If the other person actually disagrees with you, he or she will explain that "As far as I'm concerned I don't think we even *have* a real strategy or effective procedure to deal with this problem."
- "If we really wanted to solve this problem as soon as possible, what we should be doing is. . . ." Here the individual will give a strategy opposed to your own or your team's: "Here's what we're doing [and the individual gives an accurate description of your strategy or procedure] — but I strongly disagree with it."

In each case, once you have some clarity, there's a chance to solve the problem. You can take steps to sort out the confusion, realign the team, redefine the goal, and get on with things.

Otherwise, these partly hidden, contradictory views will end up breaking down your performance. The individuals who disagree with you will often express their dissatisfaction through passive-aggressive behavior reactions such as work slowdowns, nods of agreement that aren't backed by appropriate action, deliberately missed deadlines (but always with some plausible excuse), or other forms of costly sabotage.

"The most important thing," says Deborah Tannen, professor of linguistics at Georgetown University, "is to be aware that misunderstandings can arise, and with them tempers, when no one is crazy and no one is mean and no one is intentionally dishonest. We can learn to stop and remind ourselves that others may not mean what we hear them say." [40]

Communicating What You Really Mean

> How well we communicate is determined not by how well we say things but by how well we are understood. As communicators, we *can* and *must* tailor our message so it's appropriate.
>
> — *Andrew S. Grove*, High Output Management

Our conversational style seems self-evidently natural to each of us; yet ingrained habits — involving our choice of words, voice level and tone, the use of questions and certain phrases, and how much or how little we talk — differ from person to person, far more than we're aware.

"Nothing is more deeply disquieting than a conversation gone awry," says Tannen. "To say something and see it taken to mean something else; to try to be helpful and be thought pushy; to try to be considerate and be called cold . . . such failure at talk undermines one's sense of competence and . . . can undermine one's feeling of psychological well-being." [41]

When it comes to communication skills, small things make a big difference. Most of us operate on the premise that everyone else understands what we *mean* to communicate whenever we speak. Yet there are countless ways that our messages get mixed up and, in spite of our best efforts, we fail to communicate clearly. You say what you mean — but the other person hears what he or she *thinks* you mean, which wasn't what you meant. It's terribly frustrating when you present an idea that you expect to win instant approval and it's dismissed out of hand. The value of your contribution is obvious *to you,* but for some reason it's not obvious to the other person.

You have several priorities here. First, pay careful attention to the next section of this chapter, which is devoted to cutting the fog, or imprecision, out of speech. Second, learn to pause at the first moment you sense a misunderstanding and remind yourself that others may not mean what you thought you just heard them say. Instead of immediately feeling that the other person must be illogical, wrong, or out to get you, assume that there's simply a perception gap and that the other person is bright, rational, and well meaning. Then clarify the message.

In business settings, most opinions and solutions are in some way incomplete — they have missing parts. But that doesn't make them worthless. The value is in *what's there*.

---

5. Precise Language

The limits of my language are the limits of my world.

— *Ludwig Wittgenstein, philosopher (1889–1951)*

Language precision — communicating with maximum clarity — deserves everyone's attention. The less distortion you have in your communication, the more your goals, feedback, and other messages will be received as they were intended.[42] Strong corporate communication networks reduce employee turnover,[43] whereas distortions, ambiguities, and incongruities all increase uncertainty in the workplace and lower job satisfaction.[44]

Choose your words carefully. Certain words and phrases create instant resistance and damage rapport and friendship. A classic example is the conjunction *but.* It is often used to negate everything said before it. While *but* and the similar word *however* are usually spoken unconsciously and automatically, they still irritate and alienate almost everyone. Notice how it feels to hear these statements: "I agree with you, but . . ."; "That's true, but . . ."; "I respect your opinion, but. . . ."

According to communications experts, one way to solve this dilemma is something called an *agreement frame*. Certain phrases can be used to establish rapport, to share honest feelings, and to minimize resistance to the opinions of others, thereby avoiding many conversational conflicts. You first point out something positive and specific about what the other person has done or said and then add your comments or ideas with the connection *and*.

Examples: "I agree with your basic idea (or a specific point you made), *and* here's another angle (thought/suggestion/resource) that might be helpful." Or "I respect your intense feelings about (a problem), *and* here are several of my thoughts." The process works just as effectively in self-talk: "I want to solve this conflict, *and* (not *but*) that looks very challenging to do." Or "I'm choosing not to get so upset over little things and (not *but*) it's taking me quite a while to learn how."

In each case, you're establishing rapport by acknowledging the communication rather than blocking, ignoring, or denigrating it with trap words like *but* or *however*. You are bringing attention to areas of mutual agreement, a process that tends to form a positive bond. And you are creating the opportunity to redirect the conversation by avoiding and overcoming resistance wherever possible.

The following are examples of imprecise word usage and suggestions for using precise language to prevent miscommunication.

Avoid Erroneous Limitations

Universal qualifiers. All, always, constantly, never, none, every, everybody, nobody. These words imply categorical truth and wind up in many dialogues to hide ignorance or add emotional emphasis. Rarely are they true. Cut through the fluff and get down to specifics by repeating the absolute as a question. "All?" "Always?" "Everybody?" "Never?" This helps the speaker become more aware of the problem and helps you be clearer about the actual message.

Restrictives/rules. Must, can't, ought to, shouldn't, have to, forced to, no choice, must not, unable to. These trap words imply impossibility or assume inevitability. It's easy for them to block change and to suggest that there is something wrong with the speaker or listener — you don't measure up. Step outside these words by posing simple consequence questions (in your mind or aloud), such as "What would happen if you did or didn't do that?" or "What causes or prevents you from doing that?" And begin substituting *choose to* in place of *have to, can't,* and *try to.*

Stop Errors in Information or Logic

Overloads. Too much, too many, too expensive, too complicated, too difficult. To cut through the fog, ask, "Compared with what?" Be specific.

Deletions. "I disagree." Get at the real message by asking, "With what, exactly, do you disagree?"

Unspecified nouns and verbs. "They don't *understand* me." "*It* always *gets me* down." If left unclarified, references to unspecificed nouns and use of vague verbs foster helplessness. Get an exact frame of reference. Ask, "*Who* doesn't seem to understand you, and *how* do they make you feel misunderstood?" "Exactly *what* happens to get you down, and in what ways does it make you feel unhappy?"

Speak from the first person — and collaborate with others. Expressing your thoughts and feelings with "I" statements ("I'd like to talk to you about something very important to me") bypasses the "you" comments ("You ignore me"; "You're never willing to hear what I say") that make listeners feel as if you are blaming them. And be sure to err on the side of inclusion — "we" statements make your co-workers, staff members, and employees feel part of the issues and activities at hand. Cooperative — not competitive — efforts are a key to success.

Judgments/comparatives/superlatives. Obviously, clearly, without a doubt, good, better, best, bad, worse, worst, more, less, least. To clarify, ask, "Compared with *what* is it (good/bad/better/ worse)?" "To *whom* is it clear or obvious?"

Because distorted thoughts twist our words and lead to conflict, one way to improve our communication is by improving our thinking. Chapter 7 focuses on identifying and correcting distorted thinking patterns that influence your communication and work performance.

6. Dealing with Difficult People

> Talking to you is like talking to the wall.
>
> — *Anonymous*

> You can send a message around the world in one-seventh of a
> second, yet it may take years to move a simple idea through a
> quarter-inch of human skull.
>
> — *Charles F. Kettering*

No matter how well you get along with people, every once in a while you run into someone with whom nothing seems to work, someone who seems to take pleasure in *not* getting along with you. As luck usually has it, you must regularly interact with this person — as a boss, co-worker, supplier, client, or customer.

Difficult people come in countless varieties, and each may provoke you in a different way. One may sit back and glower, never really telling you what he or she thinks or feels. Another may whine and complain for hours on end. Another may be loud and self-centered, unwilling to let you work together in any cooperative or productive way. Another might talk endlessly, getting little accomplished and interfering with your work. At times, you may be left fuming, yelling, or speechless.

Some of these people may get along just fine with your co-workers but antagonize or irritate you as an individual. Others can frustrate and demoralize an entire work team or department. Worst of all, many difficult people seem immune to the usual methods of communication.

But first, let's distinguish between *different* and *difficult*. Someone who is *periodically* hard to get along with usually isn't what would be defined as a difficult person. By recognizing this, you can become more empathetic to someone suffering temporary distress and take more effective action to deal with those people whose behavior *regularly* interferes with your ability to get your work done effectively and on time.

"Regardless of to whom a person appears difficult," says Donald H. Weiss, corporate training director and expert on interpersonal relations, "the difficulty results from the two of you trying to fulfill your desires or meet your needs in different ways, from holding different opinions, from acting on different attitudes, from having different goals and values. Both of you want conflicting payoffs from your relationship or from the work situation in which you're both engaged. What usually separates you from the other person is that he or she is *unwilling* to yield, or to accept feedback, or to confront issues — at least, so far. . . . Expect no more from other people than you expect from yourself — *a willingness to try to change their behavior* in relation to you, not to change their personalities."[45]

Sometimes the organizational climate is so stressful that it evokes the worst behavior in just about everyone. So it's important not only to deal with the people involved but also to clear up discordant areas of corporate culture, purpose, power, and psychopolitics. Even if changing the organizational climate is outside your current control, you can ease stress and increase productivity by encouraging as many people as possible to develop Performance Edge skills.

Beyond the other priorities in this chapter, effective communication depends on (a) acknowledging, appreciating, and productively utilizing human differences; and (b) developing a personal strategy for dealing effectively with those individuals who, for you, are truly difficult to work with. Here are several insights from researchers in this field.

Separate people from problems — and acknowledge and appreciate differences. No matter how perplexing it is to deal with difficult people, always remain aware that the problem is in the *relationship,* the way you interact with these other people, not in the people themselves. Moreover, many interpersonal conflicts arise simply because one individual is inflexible to another's viewpoint or work style.[46] And this stress diverts both people's energies in unplanned, low-priority directions.

Much of this mental inflexibility is habitual and unconscious. But it can be changed. We often get so caught up in our work that we become oversensitive about our personal viewpoints and fail to recognize that a differing opinion or approach isn't necessarily better or worse than our own — it's just different. Let's face it, every one of us is hard to get along with in some way, sometimes, with some people. And in most cases these natural, inherent differences become *difficulties* only when we let them.

"When trying to make sense of the nonsensical, look *first* for a thinking style difference," say communication researchers Marcia B. Cherney and Susan A. Tynan.

> Have you ever
> - Gone into a meeting with THE PERFECT IDEA only to have it bomb?
> - Walked away from a discussion in which, no matter how you put it, the other party couldn't understand your point?
> - Avoided asking someone a question because you knew the answer would get you nowhere?
>   The next time you get a "wrong" answer, ask yourself, "Is the answer really stupid, or could it be a smart reply from an opposite thinker?"[47]

According to Cherney and Tynan, there are two broad, basic thinking styles in the workplace:

Vertical thinkers detect and manipulate differences, methodically finding distinctions and making separations. They look at endpoints, identify the route, pinpoint problems, eliminate the unnecessary, and then break up the task into small, discrete, doable steps.

Horizontal thinkers detect and manipulate commonalities, methodically finding constants and making novel, unpredictable associations among unrelated items, ideas, or events. They focus on a common thread that all points share and organize their thoughts according to significance to an underlying purpose or theme.

Of course, neither style is superior, and most of us don't fall exclusively into any one pattern. But the useful point is that there are a variety of ways to approach job challenges — and, as discussed previously in this chapter, it's important to avoid getting trapped in perception gaps.

Many of us make the mistake of affixing negative labels to behavior that's unexpected or different from our own, and we're primed to condemn whatever doesn't fit with our personal thinking style at the moment. This shortsighted habit costs us dearly.

Every time you notice yourself beginning to label someone else or become upset, use the Instant Calming Sequence (Chapter 3) to help you remain in control of your thoughts and emotions. Pause for an extra few seconds to decode unexpected behaviors or responses to your requests. Ask yourself, Could this simply be a difference in thinking style? In many cases, it is. And if it is, find new ways to clarify things and work together toward results.

Be mentally flexible — and stay focused on outputs rather than positions, activities, or tasks. To be an outstanding achiever in today's business environment, it takes a variety of leadership skills. These include the ability to think creatively, invent options for mutual gain, and deal with competing demands and differing values among members of your department or work team.[48] "A master manager must be able to get free of his or her preferred way of seeing and behaving," says Robert E. Quinn, author of *Beyond Rational Management* and visiting professor at the University of Michigan School of Business.[49]

Quinn has developed a program that helps managers learn to assume various roles depending on the challenge at hand: producer, director, coordinator, monitor, facilitator, mentor, innovator, or broker. The key is to recognize your preferences and perspectives and then loosen their grip, increasing your openness to alternative viewpoints and methods.

It also pays to regularly remind ourselves that *outputs* — results or accomplishments — are what every organization needs to focus on. For the most part, positions, activities, tasks, and variations in method are not the determining factors; they are simply a means to the end, and their value is determined only by how much they help achieve the desired results.

Decide if the payoff is worth the effort. Coping with difficult people takes considerable amounts of effort and will. Before you plunge ahead with a plan to change behavior — your own or another person's — decide what it will probably take to accomplish the change, what it's worth to you, what kind of payoff you expect to receive, and the chances you'll receive it. Base your decision on three business factors that could be affected by the way you or the other person deals with the interaction: stress, interpersonal relations, and productivity. How will a positive or negative change in behavior influence these areas? What are the risks? The expected benefits?

Accept the fact that you can't turn everyone into a willing partner to create change. Some people are extremely stubborn about change. At times, their ultradifficult behavior is so disruptive that you need special self-defense tactics (effective ways to defuse anger, deliver criticism, and protect yourself against verbal attacks are covered in the next two sections of this chapter). You may even be forced to go over the antagonist's head to seek a solution. But be certain you have sufficient grounds for the person up the line to take action on your behalf.

When it's not worth this kind of effort, either find a way to remove yourself from the stressful situation or resign yourself — temporarily at least — to the status quo and improve your stress management skills. In either case, shift your attention away from the problem itself and onto those work areas where you can create progress.

---

7. Compliments, Anger, and Criticism

Compliments of . . .

In our age of computer databases and complex information exchanges, the simple compliment is one of the most powerful and motivating aspects of human conversation. By definition, a compliment is a positive evaluation, says Mark L. Knapp, professor of speech communication at the University of Texas at Austin.[50] Research confirms the value of compliments in all work settings — they are desired by everyone trying to perform well and should be given when earned.

One reason it's difficult for many businesspeople to stop emphasizing negative or judgmental statements is that most of us have years of practice with put-downs. In fact, some surveys project that the national average of parent-to-child criticisms is 12 to 1 — a dozen criticisms for every single compliment or positive comment. And in the average secondary school classroom, the ratio of criticisms to compliments from teacher to student is as high as 18 to 1.[51] Stanford University researchers report that in business situations the negative-to-positive ratios range from 4-to-1 to 8-to-1.[52]

"There are so many opportunities to compliment an individual's performance," says Jerald D. Hawkins, director of sports medicine services at Lander College in Greenwood, South Carolina, and a researcher who has studied compliments in both sports and business settings, "yet I have been struck with how management and coaches, in many regards very similar, see their role relative to feedback and reinforcement as one-dimensional. They use criticism almost exclusively. These people believe that complimentary praise leads to complacency."[53]

Research confirms Hawkins's statement. Beyond the motivational aspects, compliments — when appropriately given and received — generally make individuals work closer together and disclose more about themselves, and this sets up a positive motivational cycle between individuals. As a result, says psychologist Perry W. Buffington, "individuals who compliment each other tend to disagree less, cooperate more, and generally think that similarities exist between them. Individuals who use compliments also tend to utilize positive voice inflections more frequently."[54]

"It's amazing," adds Hawkins, "how such a simple action [appropriate praise] can create a 'complimentary cycle' which continues to increase performance on its own."[55] He recommends the following guidelines to guarantee that your compliments will be accepted and will prompt best performance:

1. Be honest.
2. Take the initiative — don't wait for someone else to do the complimenting. Compliments "should be paid to anyone who deserves them, regardless of his or her stature in any pecking order."
3. "Timing is everything" — when you observe behavior that merits praise, give it immediately.
4. Mean it. Be prepared to back up your praise with specific details that confirm why you mean what you say.
5. Move from general to specific. Both Hawkins and Knapp point

out that compliments that focus on the totality of the person are most readily accepted. Therefore, when possible, focus on this kind of positive comment first and then, as you get to know the other person, move from general to specific. This will help ensure that your compliments are valued.

6. Keep your compliments simple, clear, and to the point. Don't contaminate them with backfiring phrases such as "I really appreciated the way you did that, but. . . . "

Dealing with Anger

> People in corporations are going to have to find new ways to express anger . . . without scaring each other to death, offending anybody's professional dignity, or plunging the company into anarchy.
>
> — *Walter Kierchel III in* Fortune[56]

"Now we know that anger is a killer." With these words, CBS News medical correspondent Dr. Robert Arnot recently summarized research on the effects of mismanaged anger. When you lose your cool, you lose time, energy, your health, maybe even your life.

"If I were to take a poll," says Andy Grove, president of Intel Corporation and author of *High Output Management*, "I think it would show that one of the top complaints about bosses and managers has to do with their tendency to let their tempers fly."[57]

For years, researchers have known that anger contributes to high blood pressure, heart disease, and heart attack risk.[58] "Hostility, anger, and their biological consequences are the toxic part of Type A behavior," says Dr. Redford Williams, professor of psychiatry, associate professor of medicine, and director of the Behavioral Medicine Research Center at Duke University Medical Center. "In contrast, those aspects of Type A behavior concerned with rapid accomplishment of tasks and the achievement of lofty career goals are at least not toxic and even, when not associated with hostility and anger, confer some protection (against coronary heart disease)."[59]

A recent fifteen-year controlled study by the University of Michigan School of Public Health measured the effects of expression of anger, supression, and "cool reflection." The researchers discovered that ineffectively managed anger was linked to 2.5 times greater risk of death from all causes.[60]

The findings held true for both sexes and all age groups and education levels, regardless of whether the individuals smoked or had other common risk factors for heart disease. "The key issue," says Dr. Ernest Harburg, one of the researchers, "is not the amount or degree of your anger, but *how you cope with it.*"

There are three standard responses to anger:

1. *Anger-in* — suppressing your angry feelings altogether
2. *Anger-out* — explosively venting your anger immediately
3. *Reflective coping* — waiting until tempers have cooled to rationally discuss the conflict with the other person or sort things out on your own.

Reflective coping is by far the best choice because, as the research team discovered, it enables you to avoid hostility traps, restores a sense of control over the situation, and helps resolve it.

Those people who kept their cool — who acknowledged their anger but were not openly hostile, physically or verbally — felt better faster, solved problems more easily, and had superior health. While venting anger does relieve tension for some people, it can also ignite additional conflicts with others and contribute to guilt feelings, which become an added source of stress.

What conclusions can we draw from this? The events of life don't make us angry — our "hot thoughts" do. Anger is usually a defense against loss of self-esteem and comes from frustration and unmet expectations. In group discussions and decision-making efforts, innovative thinking patterns (see Chapters 7 and 16) can neutralize anger and increase effectiveness. Most thoughts that generate anger contain distortions (discussed in Chapter 7), and most anger can be quickly defused if you take a moment to see the world through the other person's eyes. Although we each have the *right* to get angry whenever we want, in almost every case it's not to our advantage to do so.

Each time you begin to feel a surge of anger, pause for a moment

— using the Instant Calming Sequence in Chapter 3 — and ask yourself, Is my anger useful? Does it support my integrity and help me achieve my goals, or does it just hurt others, waste my time, or defeat me?

Another way to head off hostility and anger is to develop a more trusting heart, advises Dr. Williams. His research suggests that when you begin to feel angry, it really pays to pause for an extra moment to reason with yourself, gently laugh at yourself, forgive others, put yourself in the other person's shoes, and, in short, find ways to keep things from getting blown out of proportion.

The true test of anger control often comes when you have to discipline someone or deliver a bad performance review or when a customer, co-worker, subordinate, or boss walks up to you blistering mad.

If the anger is targeted at you personally, in most cases the best approach is to immediately acknowledge that the issue needs attention and then — using reflective coping — schedule time to deal with it later that day or the next. Remind yourself that when anger is unmanaged or mismanaged, it can be a life-destroying emotion. However, during those times when the anger *isn't* directed at you personally, sometimes it pays to take a minute or two to see if there's some constructive way to support the other person or to respond right now.

According to John Kello, a Davidson College psychology professor and communications instructor for IBM and Chrysler, the way to deal with many of these unpleasant situations is to grab an agenda and stick to it.[61] You might try saying something like "I can see that you're very angry. Tell me exactly what happened." Then listen calmly and attentively.

Your objective, says Kello, is to let the other person talk himself or herself down, cooling out to a level where a clear-headed exchange can take place. Before long, you'll know you're succeeding when the other person begins to say things like "Look, I don't mean to dump all this on you." Then seize the moment to redirect the conversation in a constructive manner.

But if things don't simmer down quickly, you're best off breaking away from the fireworks and selecting another time and place to resume the discussion. Say, "Look, you're angry, and *I'm* becoming angry, and together we're getting nowhere. Why don't we sleep on it and talk in the morning?" Then *immediately* redirect your attention away from the volatile issue and onto the next priority task on your schedule.

Productive Criticism

Anger is frequently triggered by criticism. Shaming people, assigning blame, giving incomplete or inaccurate feedback, and over-emphasizing the negative aspects of a situation all make problems worse. In one study on criticism by Dr. Robert Baron at Rensselaer Polytechnic Institute, among 108 managers and supervisors the poor handling of criticism was one of the top five causes of work conflicts. And in this group of five causes, criticism ranked higher than mistrust, conflicting personalities, and disputes over power and pay.[62] Furthermore, studies show that even a single inept criticism can have a devastating effect on a person's morale and can directly impair his or her ability to think clearly and work effectively.

Make it a point to remind yourself often that your job is not to *criticize* your employees or co-workers but to help them by *critiquing* their work. One of the most common ways for both managers and employees to deal with performance problems is to avoid them and hope they go away. Yet it's to everyone's benefit to identify problems, discuss them constructively, and try to resolve them in their early stages before serious or extreme solutions are required.

"Stop listening to excuses," advises Andy Grove. "You must emphatically and energetically convince your employees that they are responsible for *results,* period." [63] How performance problems are managed can have a lasting effect on workplace productivity. Ideally, most organizations should evaluate their employees' work in two ways: first, in an ongoing, informal review process and, second, in a periodic formal performance appraisal. Be certain you tell people beforehand that you're going to honestly let them know how they are performing. To give criticism effectively and constructively,[64] first ask yourself:

Have I given the person every reasonable opportunity to succeed?
Am I certain this person understands what is expected of him or
  her?

Have I been accessible for questions, and have I removed obstacles
   for achievement?
Am I convinced that this person is deserving of whatever time and
   effort it may take to turn this situation around? (If not, you may
   want to seriously consider firing the person.)
Exactly what do I want to communicate? What do I want to change?
What are my motives for expressing this criticism? (Getting even
   with someone else is the worst possible motive for criticism.)
How can I communicate the information so that the other person
   will be most receptive to it?
What specific solutions or goals can I offer, and in what specific
   ways can I help the other person accomplish them?
What is a realistic time frame for these changes to occur?

If you can't answer each of these questions, then you're not yet
ready to offer productive criticism. Once you're prepared, wait for
the appropriate time and place. Focus your comments on the problem behavior, not on the person. When possible, use "I" and "we"
statements ("It was my understanding that we . . ." or "Let's talk
this over so we can . . .") instead of the accusatory "you." Be
certain that the behavior you are criticizing *can* be changed and
state it as your opinion, not fact, using neutral gestures and voice
tones that do not ridicule, accuse, or threaten. At all costs, avoid
absolutes and generalizations.

   "One way productive criticizers make criticism improvement-
oriented is to move the criticisms forward, into the future," says
psychologist Hendrie Weisinger, an expert on anger and criticism.
"They emphasize what the recipient is 'doing,' not what she 'did.'
Change becomes possible as the critic begins to stress how the
recipient can do it better 'next time.' This lets the recipient feel
secure in knowing that he or she will get another chance."[65]

   Make your comments as specific and as brief as possible. When
you prepare your message, some authorities suggest using the following three-part structure:

When you X, I feel Y, because Z.

   Beginning with "When" is more effective than beginning with
"If," which presupposes that an event has not happened. The fol-

lowing two parts of the message — "I feel . . ." and "because
. . ." — are directly observable and verifiable. Be absolutely certain that the third part — "because . . ." — refers to something
concrete. Saying things like "because no one should have to put
up with that" is not constructive and can trigger a backlash.

With practice, constructing these X-Y-Z statements will be easy,
and the specific details tell the other person *precisely* what he or
she does that you object to, the exact reaction it creates in the
victim, and the real-world justification you think you have for
making the complaint. Examples:

"When you scream and yell like that, I feel upset, because I get
so distracted I can't concentrate on my work."

"When someone keeps interrupting me with *Why* questions like
that, I feel irritated — and sometimes really angry — because I can't
seem to finish explaining my point of view before being cut off or
having my thoughts taken out of context or getting stuck arguing
about some minor detail."

Once you finish, pause for a few seconds of silence to let the
other person feel how you're feeling. And, finally, demonstrate
empathy for the other person's feelings and problems and, if appropriate, offer to help resolve them. Shake hands or pat the other
person on the back in some symbolic, acceptable way that genuinely communicates that you are on his or her side, that you value
him or her. Reaffirm that you think highly of the person — but
not his or her actions in this situation. Then let go. When the criticism is over, it's over.

"Criticism is much more likely to pay off," says Weisinger, "when
the recipient perceives the critic to be genuinely concerned with his
or her welfare. Positive criticizers act on this by demonstrating the
'helping spirit.'

"Showing the helping spirit means giving three important messages to the recipient: (1) I care about you and will prove it by
investing my time and energy in helping you; (2) I am confident
that you can improve, that you can do the task at hand; and (3) I
am committed to helping. You are not alone. I will support your
efforts."[66]

If you must go to the boss to discuss a co-worker's mistakes or
resistance, ask the boss for *what you need* (time, access to data,
additional personnel, specific support — whatever is required) rather

than presenting a case *against* the other person. This, says management consultant Pat Nickerson, "reduces the risk of your complaining, judging, or demanding. It keeps the boss's guilt to a minimum and helps the boss focus on the solution, not the complaint."[67]

Criticism is a two-way street; in addition to being given, it's also taken. Stonewalling ("I've always done it this way" or "That's just the way I am") and excuse making are common examples of inappropriate criticism taking.

To learn to take criticism more productively, use Performance Edge skills to keep yourself relaxed and under control. Pay special attention to your posture and breathing patterns. Ask yourself how important the criticism is, how objective the source is, and how emotional the climate is in which it arises. And then, if the comments seem the least bit valuable, take the point of view that constructive change can make you a healthier, more productive person — and welcome the ideas.

8. Verbal Self-Defense

In business, verbal attacks are commonplace — and costly. The toll can be high in terms of damage to teamwork, productivity, quality control, and customer service. In most cases, verbal onslaughts have nothing to do with what most of us imagine a verbal attack to be — blasts of anger, ranting and raving, and yelling obscenities. In reality, verbal attacks in the corporate world are usually far more sophisticated, subtle, and dangerous.

We've already identified many of the common communication mix-ups that create this damage. Now let's take a brief look at several other situations. In the following examples of verbal attack patterns, look beyond the words and notice the importance of the intonation or emphasis they are given:

• If you REALLY . . .

"If you REALLY cared about this company/department/team, you wouldn't DO that!"

"If you REALLY noticed how hard other people work around here, you wouldn't MAKE decisions like that!"

"If you REALLY wanted a promotion, you'd pay more attention to the goals of this company!"

This childlike verbal attack pattern begins with a presupposed attack — "If you REALLY . . ." — followed by the bait, the openly insulting or hurtful part of the sentence intended to grab your attention and lock you into a victimizing argument. Classic stabs here include: ". . . you wouldn't BE the way you are!" or ". . . you wouldn't DO the things you do!"

To beat this and most other kinds of verbal attack, first use the Instant Calming Sequence presented in Chapter 3 and keep your voice and body language neutral. Don't let your responses sound sarcastic or insolent.

Second, avoid the mistake of taking the bait and letting the presupposition escape, because then you're playing right into the attacker's hands *and* inadvertently admitting the truth of the presupposed attack by default. Instead, zero in on the presupposed attack that immediately follows the "If you REALLY. . . ." For example:

ATTACKER: "If you REALLY cared about this company/department/team, you wouldn't DO that!"

YOU: "When did you start thinking that I don't care about this company/department/team?"

ATTACKER: "If you REALLY noticed how hard other people work around here, you wouldn't MAKE decisions like that!"

YOU: "When did you start thinking that I don't notice how hard people work around here?"

ATTACKER: "If you REALLY wanted a promotion, you'd pay more attention to the goals of this company!"

YOU: "When did you start thinking that I didn't want a promotion?"

Instead of beginning your replies with "What makes you think that X . . ." or "Why do you think that X . . . ," the smartest choice is "When did you start thinking X." This is because *Why* and *What* questions give the attacker an invitation to blast you again, whereas *When* questions help defuse the confrontation by avoiding the presupposition that your attacker actually has a valid reason for the attack and instead presupposes that "At some time you began thinking X."

Researchers[68] have found that your attacker will usually be very surprised that you didn't take the bait and will drop the whole thing or will answer you with a specific incident — and then you'll know what the attack is actually about and can deal with it directly and in perspective.

An alternative, if you're especially pressed for time and don't want to enter into a discussion, is to respond firmly by saying, "Of COURSE I care about this company/department/team (or whatever the presupposed attack is), " and then immediately break eye contact and change the subject, directing everyone's attention to another area of interest.

Example: "Of COURSE I care about this company/department/team and, in fact, yesterday I called New York to learn more about a new option we have for solving this problem." By doing this, you are demonstrating that you refuse to be a victim for the verbal abuser.

• EVEN . . .

"Even a WOMan could handle THAT assignment!"

"Even an ELderly person could figure out how to use THAT computer!"

Again, skip the bait and respond to the presupposed attack:

ATTACKER: "Even a WOMan could handle THAT assignment!"

YOU: "The thought that women are somehow inferior or second rate is still common, and I'm surprised to hear it from you (*or* I'm sorry to hear that you feel that way)."

ATTACKER: "Even an ELderly person could figure out how to use THAT computer!"

YOU: "The idea that older people are somehow incapable of thinking clearly and performing well is common but inaccurate, and I'm sorry to hear that you feel that way (*or* but I'm surprised to hear it from you)."

• Innocuous Statements

"YOU'RE not the ONly customer I HAVE, you know!"

"SOME supervisors would FIRE an employee who fails to meet even ONE production/sales quota!"

Whenever a verbal attack presupposes some kind of irreproachable statement that is almost always true in the real world, the best strategy is usually to ignore the verbal barb and agree with the statement. This quick move surprises the attacker, gives the unmistakable message that you're not going to play the game, and forces him or her to choose some other move.

The Bottom Line of Communication

Good communication comes down to listening attentively and speaking clearly, congruently, honestly, compassionately, and with good timing (knowing when and where to communicate). Clarify what you don't understand, and ask for what you want and need. Presuppositions, hinting, and expectations put listeners in a cloud of confusion or create conflict.

Don't complain; request. Don't suspect; ask for what you need. Don't seek sympathizers for your resistance; seek support for your initiatives and proposals. This all takes regular practice and lots of attention to dialogue. Yet can you think of a better investment for your career and health?

Resources

For more on listening and communication skills, see Chapter 7 as well as the following books (listed alphabetically).

- *Anger: The Misunderstood Emotion* by Carol Tavris (Simon and Schuster, 1982). A fresh, well-researched look at understanding anger.
- *Communicoding* by Marcia B. Cherney and Susan A. Tynan (Donald I. Fine, 1989). Offers an innovative "decoding" system for dealing with difficult people at work.
- *The Critical Edge: How to Criticize Up and Down Your Organization and Make It Pay Off* by Hendrie Weisinger, Ph.D. (Little, Brown, 1989). A top-rate book on giving and receiving criticism.
- *Language of the Heart: The Body's Response to Human Dialogue* by James J. Lynch, Ph.D. (Basic Books, 1985). An important self-care book.
- *Smart Questions* by Dorothy Leeds (Berkley, 1988). This insight-filled business communications book zeroes in on the importance of questions — what works, what doesn't, and why.
- *Success with the Gentle Art of Verbal Self-Defense* by Suzette Haden Elgin (Prentice Hall, 1989). The best reference yet written for identifying and responding to verbal attacks.

- *You Just Don't Understand: Women and Men in Conversation* by Deborah Tannen, Ph.D. (Morrow, 1990). Why do so many women feel that men don't tell them anything, that they just lecture and criticize? Why do so many men feel that women nag them and never get to the point? A top sociolinguist offers answers to these and other questions that confound men's and women's attempts to communicate with each other.

7

Performance Turning Point #5: Decision-Making and Innovation Opportunities

Achieving — and Sustaining — the Mental Advantage

Chance favors the prepared mind.

— *Louis Pasteur*

IN TODAY's turbulent, high-velocity work world, mental fitness is imperative. Quick thinking under pressure is no longer just a boardroom priority — it's vital for everyone.

Contrary to common assumption, breakthrough ideas seldom happen as random flashes of cerebral good fortune or bolts out of the blue. Instead, they occur most often through what Louis Pasteur called "mental preparation" — which consists of establishing an energized, flexible state of mind that facilitates creative thinking and insightful decision making.

Brain scientists around the world are breaking down the barriers to our understanding of what it takes for each of us to create this kind of exceptionally alert, capable, and innovative mind. This chapter presents some of the most important recent discoveries.

Your Untapped Mental Potential

You may already be aware that the capabilities of the human brain to create, learn, and store are virtually unlimited. You might have also heard that most of us use only about 10 percent of our mental powers. But this calculation is way off. According to the most recent estimates, we actually only use about one-hundredth of 1 percent (1/10,000) of our potential brain power over the course of a lifetime.[1]

"Throughout our lives we only use a fraction of our thinking ability," writes the prominent Russian scholar Ivan Yefremov. "We could, without any difficulty whatever, learn 40 languages, memorize a set of encyclopedias from A to Z, and complete the required courses of dozens of colleges."[2]

In the no-holds-barred business environment of the twenty-first century, say neuroscientists, there will still remain one vast, largely unexplored frontier for establishing a decisive advantage: *the untapped mental potential of our work force.*

The future depends not so much on technological advances as on advances in unlocking the further reaches of the human brain and mind. Yet the latest discoveries in neuroscience and performance psychology receive scant attention in today's business school curricula and are seldom part of corporate training programs in Fortune 500 companies. In the years ahead, this oversight may well prove fatal.

The *brain* is the physical site and fluctuating physical-chemical state in which the body's nervous system activities originate, are moderated, or are controlled. To some scientists, this is all there is: no mind, only the brain. Other experts have thrown their formidable scientific weight behind the idea that the mind is far more than the brain organ.

The *mind* is an interpretive state, influenced by emergent properties of the brain, and represents the totality of all that makes us human, or as *Webster's* defines it, "the element or complex of elements in an individual that feels, perceives, thinks, wills, and especially reasons; the organized conscious and unconscious adaptive mental activity of an organism."

The brain processes information using special cells called *neu-*

rons. There are about 100 billion neurons in your brain, each making between 5,000 and 50,000 connections with surrounding nerve cells. Even using the most conservative estimates, there are 100 trillion neuron junctions in your brain.[3] And a growing number of scientists insist that these numbers are much too small.

By some estimates, the number of connections among the brain's nerve cells is 2 to the 100-*trillionth* power. According to Dr. Carl Sagan of Cornell University, this means that *there are more possible mental states in each human being's brain than there are atoms in the known universe.*[4]

As myths have been cast aside, we've learned that brain function is remarkably changeable and that we possess nearly unfathomable capacities for learning, achieving, and remembering. This quality is called neuroplasticity.[5]

"The brain is not a machine in which every element has a genetically assigned role; it is not a digital computer in which all the decisions have been made," explains neuroscientist Michael Merzenich of the University of California at San Francisco. "Anatomy lays down a crude topographic map of the body on the surface of the cortex [the upper brain's outer covering where the cerebral hemispheres are located], which is fixed and immutable in early life. But the *fine-grained* map is not fixed. Experience sketches in all the details, altering the map continually throughout life."[6]

Your *crystallized intelligence* — also called *verbal intelligence* — depends on well-established habits of judgment and experience to function well. But fewer and fewer business situations present themselves in a neat, orderly fashion. The new "routine" business environment — characterized by sudden, unexpected changes and complex, contradictory demands — cannot be mastered by this aspect of the mind.

Therefore, it has become a priority to develop what is known as *fluid intelligence.*[7] Also called *performance intelligence,* fluid intelligence involves the timing and integration of three areas:

1. Accurate, full-spectrum sensory assessments of each challenge
2. Rapid, creative thought processes that scan an entire range of possible options
3. On-target, appropriate responses

Fluid intelligence is called for in all business situations where reaction speed and quick, objective problem solving and decision making are imperative.

The Speed and Power of Thoughts

> Our life is what our thoughts make it.
> — *Marcus Aurelius*

Thoughts are brief electrical flashes in the brain. Although they happen so fast we often don't "hear" them, we *feel* their effect because our thoughts create or influence our perceptions, emotions, and behaviors.[8] In fact, there is evidence suggesting that *every one of your thoughts affects every cell in your body.*[9]

We each give acceptance and life to our thoughts. Accordingly, our perceptions, feelings, and behaviors are our own. They are not thrust on us by an outside force (other people, our job, or a particular situation).

When our emotions are positive, we feel optimistic, motivated, productive, and creative. Regardless of external events and stress pressures, when our mood is high we have a general sense of well-being and hope for the future. We are more helpful and generous toward others and experience improved cognitive processes such as judgment, problem solving, decision making, and creativity.[10] In essence, we have a higher psychological vantage point from which to view the challenges and conflicts that enter our work and our lives.

In contrast, negative feelings and emotions are a sharp signal that we are dropping into a lower psychological state of functioning, reverting into negative thinking. We start attacking ourselves with our thoughts and lose our ability to "go beyond the information given" to solve difficult work problems and make innovative breakthroughs. We may also feel insecure and emotionally fragile and become poorer in various intellectual functions.

Most of us have been led to believe that we can find solutions to our emotional distress if we think or talk about it enough. But that's often untrue. Thinking or talking about our difficulties and inadequacies — dwelling on them in our mind and conversations — is sometimes precisely what keeps them alive and growing.

Self-suggestion, or self-talk, magnifies the dilemma. We live with this inner mind chatter all day, every day. Research shows that much of it comes in the form of negative self-judgment, and we often have trouble being as compassionate or rational with ourselves as we would be with a co-worker, friend, or loved one. To succeed in the workplace of the future, each of us must learn ways to get rid of this widespread sabotage to personal effectiveness and breakthrough achievement.

Breaking Down Barriers to Creativity and Innovation

> If you want to go from here to there in business, no straight line will take you.
>
> — *William H. Ahmanson*

Innovation in business has little to do with random good ideas that turn out to be successful. Rather, it's an expression of the creative process — a productive attitude developed by individuals throughout an organization. It's distinctive for every person and idea. Each of us, say experts, possesses a nearly limitless, untapped inner creative resource. The challenge is to uncover it, develop it, and then apply it to the fullest extent in the workplace.

"The analytic approach to thinking can take us only so far," says Robert T. Davis, professor of marketing at the Stanford University Graduate School of Business. "Creativity is far more powerful than analysis and profoundly shapes the strategic decision. The need for creativity greatly adds to the complications of the job."[11]

Until a few years ago, standard management rhetoric claimed that creativity was unteachable. But as professors at some top business schools have discovered, exploring the creative process can be an experience of tremendous value in terms of corporate leadership and competitive advantage in the years ahead.

In business, creativity is the ability, the *personally developed skill,* to form something different, helpful, or new — a thought, emotion, perception, or behavior. Whether your task is to invent new products, develop new services, expand market share, streamline production, reach zero-defect quality control, bend over backward to serve customers, or provide leadership that ensures that all activities and departments in your company "add value," creative thinking is pivotal to your success now and in the days ahead.

"Someone who thinks that creativity is hard or impossible will never attempt to use the fabulous power of his or her own mind," says Roger C. Schank, professor of computer science and psychology at Yale University and chairman of Cognitive Systems, Inc., an artificial intelligence software company. "The creative attitude is, among other things, the desire to go against the mainstream. . . . The words *creative* and *unexpected* have a great deal in common in ordinary usage." [12]

It's important to recognize that creativity is more than simply generating new ideas. "Over the years I've become increasingly frustrated with the belief that more ideas alone mean better results," says James L. Adams, professor at Stanford University and author of *The Care and Feeding of Ideas: A Guide to Encouraging Creativity.* "If you're serious about encouraging creativity in yourself or others and if you want to deal with change effectively, then implementing ideas is at least as important as generating ideas. You need to understand the entire process — from concept to reality." [13]

Innovative thinking develops from personal explorations of the creative process — blending your "inner creative life and its application to the business world," says Michael L. Ray, professor at the Stanford University Graduate School of Business. There are, of course, many different ways to become more creative, and the most effective programs present a wide range of options. According to business researchers, the following are some potentially useful maxims for developing a more innovative attitude and stimulating and nurturing the creative process: [14]

Establish and maintain an open mind and spirit of inquiry. The more often you look at things in the same way, the more difficult it is to think about them in any other way. Break out of this "prison of familiarity" by venturing off the beaten paths of your mind. In their book *Creativity in Business*, Ray and co-author Rochelle Myers put it this way: "Destroy judgment, create curiosity." Creativity is inhibited by fear, negative personal judgment, and the chattering of your mind. The most powerful destructive force against creativity is what Ray and Myers call the Voice of Judgment (VOJ).

"If you lack the confidence to create," they explain, "you are undoubtedly tuned in to the Voice of Judgment that all of us have within. The VOJ is a criticism (and source of blame, shame, scolding, and sabotage). Its function is to close the door on further investigation or even curiosity. Even a slight decrease in judgment increases your ability to respond creatively to situations. The first step is to become more aware of the VOJ. You will probably be amazed at the number of negative and judgmental statements you make throughout the day."[15] Specific strategies for exposing and defeating the VOJ — and other distorted, self-destructive thoughts — are included later in this chapter.

Remove hidden obstacles to creative thinking. "It's a paradox," observes Rosabeth Moss Kanter, professor at Harvard Business School. "Creating change requires stability."[16] This principle can be extended to the entire creative process. Innovative thinking emerges from — and some say depends on — a healthy level of personal balance.

Most creativity programs fail to address the fact that "creative work takes enormous personal energy," says Thomas E. Backer, research professor at the UCLA School of Medicine.[17] "After working with approximately 20,000 individuals, I have no doubt that physical and emotional health are intricately connected with creative productivity.

"Poorly handled stress," Backer continues, "is one of the greatest impediments to creative productivity. . . . It depletes energy, creates anxiety that impedes or blocks altogether the process of creative inspiration, and generates interpersonal tensions that make team creativity more difficult."

The Performance Edge draws together a variety of discoveries that have a bearing on your ability to cope with change, think creatively, and make effective, insightful decisions under pressure.

New research suggests, for example, that the right kind of regular aerobic exercise (Chapter 10) is vital to a high energy level and consistent innovative thinking in the workplace. Poor sleep (Chapter 13), imbalanced posture (Chapter 9), and tension and pain syndromes (Chapter 4) must be corrected and prevented to head off such debilitating problems as mental fatigue, shortened attention span, and loss of creative energy.

Mismanaged stress (Chapter 3) and poor communication and inappropriately handled anger (Chapter 6) prompt rigid — rather than open and innovative — responses to workplace challenges. Evidence from MIT suggests that dietary imbalances — such as dehydration, overeating, skipping meals, or consuming high-fat foods — can dull the mind and block certain creative processes (Chapter 11). And frequent, carefully designed work breaks (Chapter 8) have been shown to be important for increasing alertness, productivity, and creative problem solving on the job.

Laugh more: Humor can increase creativity. Dr. Alice M. Isen, of the Department of Psychology and Johnson Graduate School of Management at Cornell University, has conducted a number of studies suggesting that laughter can increase creativity and mental flexibility.[18] So it may pay to loosen up a bit — and have more fun.

Look for anomalies and reject old explanations. This means learning to approach new challenges *and* routine experiences with sharpened inquisitiveness. "Be aware that your brain would like to follow a traditional pattern," says Professor Adams from Stanford. "It would like to simplify your life by applying solutions that have successfully worked before. Be grateful for that, but suspicious that the creativity you are looking for may not occur automatically."[19]

Develop the habit of wondering (or stop being afraid to wonder) why things work the way they do and whether they should actually work that way or could be improved. "Virtually nothing you do can't be done in a slightly different, slightly better way," says Dr. Ruth Richards, a psychiatrist and creativity researcher at McLean Hospital in Belmont, Massachusetts.[20]

It also pays to expect the unexpected. Columbus was looking for India when he discovered America. Alexander Graham Bell was experimenting with a hearing device for the deaf when he discovered the principles of the telephone. Reflect for a moment:

What are the five most unexpected things that might happen to the most important current projects you're working on? And in what ways might this knowledge modify your plans?

Ask creative questions. "Creativity and progress depend upon asking the right question at the right time," says Roger Schank of Yale University and Cognitive Systems. Implicitly or explicitly, adds Michael Ray, creativity begins with a question.[21] As discussed in Chapter 6, insight-seeking questions help establish a climate in which the creative process can flourish.

Listen carefully — and pay attention. Contrary to popular opinion — which contends that creative people *tell* other people their ideas and that they don't have to listen — creative businesspeople tend to ask searching questions, have well-developed concentration and observation skills (see "Mindfulness and Concentration" in Chapter 16), and are good active listeners (Chapter 6).

Continually expand and develop your work expertise. In spite of what most of us have been led to believe, expertise and intuition may be directly related, say a group of researchers including Nobel laureate Herbert Simon, professor of psychology and computer science at Carnegie-Mellon University.[22] Exceptional proficiency of field, say these psychologists, is what makes most abrupt flashes of intuitive thought possible.

Certain people seem to see straight into the heart of a problem, while the rest of us must plod step by step toward a solution. This is because expert knowledge not only is organized in the memory but is organized for *use,* and experts who combine this cognitive competence with the other principles of creative thinking have taught themselves to see deeply into problems. This enables them to frequently and automatically perceive the relevant pattern behind the details. With practice and a dedication to expanding and deepening our work expertise, says Simon, we can all develop this ability.

And the benefits extend beyond creativity. People who find a balance between the depth of their work skills and the stressful challenges they face are more likely to be highly productive, says Mihaly Csikszentmihalyi, professor and former chairman of the Department of Psychology at the University of Chicago.[23] He calls that balance *flow* and has found that high achievers spend more time than low achievers in periods of flow.

Be willing to be uncertain. "Of all the qualities in a manager conducive to innovation and initiative, a degree of *uncertainty* may be the most powerful," says Ellen J. Langer, a professor of psychology at Harvard University. "If a manager is confident but uncertain — confident that the job will get done but without being certain of exactly the best way of doing it — employees are likely to have more room to be creative, alert, and self-starting. When we are working for confident but uncertain leaders, we are less likely to feign knowledge or hide mistakes, practices that can be very costly to a company."[24]

Gather data. In general, the more you know, the more you can create. Get in the habit of noticing what's happening around you, and then ask a deeper question: What's *really* happening?

"Changing of contexts generates imagination and creativity as well as new energy," says Professor Langer. "Innovation can be dampened by too narrow an image of the task."[25] Reversing how you look at a situation can dislodge assumptions and open up new possibilities. If you are a man, try describing your job challenge from a female point of view — and vice versa. The creative mind needs facts to draw from, so it pays to be assiduous in collecting them. Other people will gladly provide much of this data — and it's up to you to let them.

Be goal-guided, not goal-governed. While there is strong evidence that setting explicit and challenging goals is essential to top productivity, be careful not to carry this too far. Blind pursuit of any one goal may hinder creativity and limit the overall level or quality of your achievement.[26] This is because the initial course you set may not turn out to be the wisest or most fruitful.

The Mental Edge: Rapid, Strategic Decision Making Under Stress

> Problems are reflections of states of mind.
>
> — *Gerald Nadler and Shozo Hibino*

In every field of endeavor, making difficult decisions under pressure is the mark of a leader. In fact, in decentralized, customer-driven companies, the ability to make decisions at all levels in an organization is an emerging priority, and it enables these corporations to respond far more rapidly to opportunities to upgrade quality, beat performance deadlines, and capture new advantages in the marketplace.

Yet few of us have systematic training in expanding our creativity or mastering the decision-making process.

Practical recommendations in this field have emerged from pioneering academic research by scholars such as Daniel Kahneman and Amos Tversky[27] and from studies on how people process information by Herbert Simon,[28] the 1978 Nobel laureate in economics. Recent research has examined how top-rate thinkers cope with complexity, how people in numerous fields tend to make the same basic kinds of decision-making mistakes, and how any of us can become excellent decision makers.[29]

Of course, in most simple daily decisions, such as whether to return a phone call or delegate a routine job task, few of us need to be concerned about the science of decision making. Often what we need is better time management. But in all of the bigger decisions — the stream of challenges and problems that determine the quality and productivity of our work — nearly all of us can benefit from new scientific insights.

Research indicates that as workplace stress rises, so does the tendency to jump to conclusions and make narrow, faulty decisions.[30] "In any organization," says Allan R. Cohen, professor of management at Babson College and author of *Effective Behaviors in Organizations,* "there are daily occurrences of managers leaping before looking, causing unforeseen consequences they later regret. Even worse, managers can cultivate a mountainous problem where a mere molehill previously existed."[31]

A primary goal of the Performance Edge is *clear-minded, innovative thinking under pressure* — learning to stay exceptionally alert and mentally flexible in difficult situations, thereby having the greatest opportunities to recognize and seize the competitive advantage.

According to new studies by business and management professors in Europe and America, "In the days and years ahead, companies will remain viable only if their managers and top executives can manage continuously changing, complex, and sometimes surprising situations — the unpredicted or unanalyzed phenomenon, the chaotic environment, the unprogrammed event, the unforeseen occurrence, the random catastrophe — situations *not* treatable with standard textbook solutions."[32]

Many managers contend that decision making is simply and primarily a matter of dealing with categories of circumstances that repeat themselves. Correspondingly, these so-called type 1 business situations can often be analyzed in advance, planned for, and decided on before they actually happen. This kind of management science is the core of most M.B.A. programs and relies on the crystalized intelligence described at the beginning of this chapter.

And yet, more often than ever, managers, supervisors, sales professionals, and service representatives are confronted with problems beyond the scope of business school curricula and traditional corporate training programs. These type 2 circumstances cannot be adequately planned for. They are complex and chaotic, and solutions can be unpredictable or unforeseeable.

Type 2 business situations are increasing dramatically, in part because of accelerating social, political, and technological change in the work world.[33] Responsive, prosperous organizations must now be led by individuals and teams adept at handling these tough situations that cannot be planned for.

When it comes to increasing these skills, there are many options — and no hard and fast rules. With this in mind, it can often prove helpful to have access to opinions from various experts in the form of *heuristics* — which are, by definition, incomplete guidelines or rules of thumb that may improve performance or lead to learning, discovery, or problem solving.

Five Key Mental Turning Point Questions

> Flawless execution cannot compensate for implementing the wrong solution.
>
> — *Daryl Conner, president, ODR, Inc., Atlanta*

Whenever things begin to heat up, unexpectedly change directions, or start to come apart in some way, trigger the Instant Calming

Sequence (Chapter 3) and then immediately shift into your most effective personal mental focus by asking yourself the following heuristic questions.

Five Key Mental Turning Point Questions

1. What is the *heart* of this issue or problem?
2. Is what I'm seeing/hearing/thinking/feeling accurate?
3. How important is this going to be in the long run?
4. What can I *do* about it right now?
5. What's the best way to express my thoughts or feelings?

Intuitively, you may already be applying some of these principles in your approach to problems and challenges. But it's much less likely that you are applying all of them, consistently and in coordination. Let's look at each of these questions in turn.

1. What Is the *Heart* of This Issue or Problem?

This is a primary element in decision making. Scientists refer to it as *framing*,[34] or structuring, the question and then gathering intelligence and data. The more pressure you must handle on the job, the more essential it becomes to have perceptual flexibility.

The danger is that past experience can become a trap, a rigid way of seeing and interpreting work situations. Typically, under stress, the brain retreats to old habits, doing "more of the same" — only harder — and becomes strongly resistant to creative insights and innovation. There's an immediate, almost irresistible temptation to categorize, define, subdivide, and analyze each new challenge or problem in comparison with previous experiences. But, as noted earlier, this restricts vision and blocks you from making innovative, effective decisions in type 2 situations.

To avoid this problem, it's necessary to control the focus of your mind, remaining exceptionally alert and mentally flexible at the first instant of a challenge. One of the most pervasive and persistent mental mistakes is to assume that new problems are in some way identical with old ones. The reality, of course, is that every challenge is unique, and the most effective business leaders immediately direct their minds toward identifying these distinctive features rather than getting stuck looking for similarities with other situations.

In high-stress Performance Turning Points, an excellent first mental response is to *pause* — just for a split second, long enough to sidestep old habits and reach a level of *deliberate mental clarity,* an open-mindedness that promotes a *creative skill in thinking.* Before plunging in, ask yourself, What is the *purpose* of solving this problem? and Is this even a problem that I/we should be working on? How, specifically, does it fit into the greater picture of my/our priorities and vision? Is it ethical? In what ways will this affect other people? Is the price that I — and others — will have to pay worth it?

Peter F. Drucker observed that in Japanese corporations that seem especially adept at making big decisions, "the important element in decision-making is *defining the question.* The crucial steps are to decide whether there is a need for a decision and what the decision is about. And it is in this step that the Japanese aim at getting a consensus."[35]

"Tackling a difficult problem," explains Peter M. Senge, director of Systems Thinking and Organizational Learning at MIT's Sloan School of Management, "is often a matter of seeing where the high leverage lies, a change which — with minimum effort — would lead to lasting, significant improvement."

When you train your mind to approach new challenges from this perspective, it's easier to grasp the crux of the problem and focus on its novel aspects. This erases much of the doubt — or even dread — that comes from habitually dwelling on what's wrong with difficult situations. Just as important, in teamwork tasks, focusing on purposes turns attention away from points of controversy and toward common goals.

Instead of getting trapped in your own biases or tangled up in surface information or the faulty mental framework of other people around you, use the split-second pause to choose a higher than usual vantage point. Ask, "Are we (Am I) doing the right thing?" rather than, "Are we (Am I) doing things right?"

Research[36] confirms that only when you first remain open-minded and identify your *purpose* in solving a problem can you then accurately, objectively zero in on the depth and range of available facts, identify and close any knowledge gaps, and scan for productive solutions.

---

2. Is What I'm Seeing/Hearing/Thinking/Feeling Accurate?

> Men are disturbed not by things, but by the view which they take of them.
>
> — *Epictetus*

> The test of a first-rate intelligence is the ability to hold two opposite ideas in mind at the same time and still retain the ability to function.
>
> — *F. Scott Fitzgerald*

Whenever you're poised to start accusing, blaming, or feeling victimized, stop for a moment to step into the other person's shoes and perspective. What's the view from that side? Is there a logical alternative explanation for the problem or situation? Is what you're seeing, hearing, thinking, and feeling accurate?

Most of us implicitly assume that the information that is most readily available to us is also the most relevant. But it's important to avoid overconfidence in your own judgment and to develop the self-discipline to seek information that might disconfirm your initial opinions.

"Managers become increasingly effective as they develop a wider range of perspective for viewing the world they live in," says Robert E. Quinn, professor of organization studies at the State University of New York, Albany, and a visiting professor at the University of Michigan School of Business. "Ineffective managers have great difficulty balancing competing philosophies and roles. They become stuck in their biases."[37]

Through extensive research, Quinn has found that "the key to becoming a master manager is seeing past your own blinders and the blinders imposed by the expectations of others. You begin to do this by obtaining an awareness of your own style, learning what your own strengths and blind spots are."[38]

There's little doubt that intuition can be a valuable aid when you are dealing with difficult issues, but misreading this "inner sense" or "gut reaction" is a common pitfall in decision making. Without realizing it, we fail to apply penetrating objective observation to challenging situations. Instead, we jump to conclusions, solve the wrong problems, and get trapped in predetermined perspectives. We lose control and inadvertently block ourselves from taking a clear-eyed view of the problem and solving it in the best possible manner.

Your brain uses neurochemicals, electrical impulses, and trillions of special receptors to spread the influence of your thoughts and decisions to every cell in your body. Every job pressure triggers a host of questions: Am I right about my thoughts and feelings on this? Can I handle the stress? What happens if I can't? What are my options?

Each negative thought encourages and amplifies others. It's easy to end up trapped in a labyrinth of pessimism, and it takes dedication to break out. The word *cognitive,* derived from the Latin word for "thinking," refers to the ways in which people make judgments and decisions and the ways in which they interpret — or misinterpret — one another's words and actions.

Because automatic thoughts flash by so rapidly, we are often aware only of feeling angered or offended and, perhaps, capture some fleeting, irksome image of the other person or task at hand. Our daily conversations and mental dialogues are filled with these bombshells but, amazingly, most of us are unaware of them. Automatic thoughts may take the form of words or images or both. As distress mounts in work relationships, the twists and turns of each person's thoughts tend to expand and spread.

One of the keys to taking charge of your mind and mood is to identify distorted thinking patterns and replace them with clear, constructive alternatives.[39] No matter how irrational they are, distorted, automatic thoughts are almost always believed, and they often appear in incomplete sentences — several key words or a visual image flash.

With practice, automatic, twisted thoughts can be straightened out. To sharpen your awareness and thought-correcting actions, consider these typical examples of distorted thinking (listed alphabetically):

Being right. You need to always prove that your statements and actions are right. You are quick to launch into defensive rationalizations whenever your "rightness" seems in question.

Blaming. Your problems are either *never* your fault (other people and situations cause whatever goes wrong) or *always* your fault.

Change illusion. Your happiness and success depend on other people changing their bad habits — "bad" from your perspective of reality — and you believe they will make these changes if you keep pressuring them enough.

Control illusion. You feel either externally controlled — and therefore victimized — by other people and circumstances or internally controlled, which leaves you feeling that you cause everyone else's unhappiness.

Disqualifying the positive. You reject positive experiences on the grounds that they somehow "don't count" when compared with the endless list of problems at your job and in your life.

Either/or thinking. There is no middle ground — things are either good or they're bad. Either you perform perfectly or you're a total failure.

Emotional reasoning. You automatically assume that your feelings are facts and therefore must reflect the way things really are. If you *feel* incompetent or indecisive, then you must *be* incompetent or indecisive.

Fairness illusion. You think you know exactly what's fair in all situations but feel victimized when other people often don't agree with you.

Filtering. You find negative details in any situation and dwell on them so exclusively — ignoring the positive — that no matter how bright an experience may initially be, it soon looks bleak.

Jumping to conclusions. You quickly leap to negative interpretations of statements and situations even though you usually lack the facts to support your conclusion. This includes *mind reading* — without checking to find out the truth, you assume that you know precisely why other people are thinking, feeling, and acting the way they are — and *fortune telling* — you anticipate that a future event will turn out badly and act as if this is a predetermined fact.

Labeling and mislabeling. This is an extreme version of overgeneralization. When you make an error or become irritated with others, you emotionally assign a label to yourself ("I'm a loser"; "I'm an idiot"), another person ("He's a quitter"; "She's a liar"), or situation ("It's a lost cause").

Magnification (catastrophizing) and minimization. You exaggerate risks, anticipating disaster; you overplay your mistakes or the importance of someone else's achievements; or you erroneously shrink your positive attributes or another person's imperfections until they appear insignificant.

Overgeneralization. You make a sweeping assumption based on only a shred of evidence — a single negative event becomes a never-ending pattern of defeat.

Personalization. You see yourself as the cause of some negative work occurrence for which you were not primarily responsible. You think that everything other people say or do is a reaction to you. You keep comparing yourself to others, wondering who's smarter, more successful, better looking, and so on.

"Shoulds." You try to motivate yourself and others with guilt, using statements filled with *should*s and *shouldn't*s, *must*s, and *ought*s. When you or others break your rules you feel anger, resentment, and frustration.

Ultimate reward illusion. You talk and act as if monumental daily sacrifices and self-denial are what will ultimately bring you great rewards. You feel resentful when the rewards don't seem to come.

Distorted thinking is contagious — the habit spreads. "If you consistently respond to events pessimistically," says Martin E. P. Seligman, professor of psychology at the University of Pennsylvania, "that negative style can actually *amplify* your feelings of helplessness and spread to other areas of your life."[40]

Resist the natural tendency to accept distorted thoughts as true simply because they seem reasonable or "feel right." Begin paying closer attention to the way you explain unpleasant situations and outcomes to yourself and others.

Catch negative, stressful thoughts and examine them clearly and carefully, looking for supporting evidence, contradictory evidence, alternative explanations, and more logical inferences. Derail the temptation to resort to habitual, self-defeating reactions, such as defensiveness, retaliation, or withdrawal. In short, it's necessary to begin building somme new habits of mind.

3. How Important Is This Going to Be in the Long Run?

Contemporary brain researchers are discovering the important relationship between our sense of mental vision and our ability to cope with pressure and handle complex tasks. Recent studies[41] on the decision-making styles of fifty of America's top CEOs revealed two key elements:

1. *Focusing on the long term* — the ability and habit of examining the long-term implications of decisions
2. *Acknowledging the "big picture"* — maintaining an awareness of the range of factors affecting major decisions.

Whenever you're faced with a difficult challenge, be careful to avoid typical decision traps such as plunging right in. Instead, take a moment to establish a broad perspective and acknowledge the sphere of larger issues that are linked in some way with the immediate concern. You can thereby avoid solving the wrong problem, overlooking the best options, or losing sight of important objectives.

According to recent European neuroscience research by Dr. David Ingvar and colleagues, directing your mind at the initial stage of decision making is more crucial than most of us realize. Using positron emission tomography (PET scan), Ingvar studied computer-generated pictures of the neocortex during different states of mind, concluding that the brain seems to "turn off" — and problem-solving efforts fail — when people cannot anticipate a possible positive outcome or future.[42]

All problems have implications extending into the future, say decision science researchers Gerald Nadler and Shozo Hibino. "By being able to mentally put yourself at a point in the future when you might have to re-solve your problem, you can save yourself a lot of headaches. The insight you gain will improve your immediate solution and help you incorporate adaptations into your solution to meet future needs. . . . This elevates your thinking beyond any obvious first solution."[43]

When facing a decision or beginning to solve a problem, first stretch your mind, asking, What is likely or possible to be needed next, and then after that? What boundaries have I set on the problem? What reference points am I using to define and measure success? These are some of the simplest, most effective ways to keep today's actions linked with long-range planning.

Your Time Horizon

Evidence is growing that the further into the future your brain can see itself functioning, the more competent you'll become right now in handling complexity, managing myriad responsibilities, and integrating tasks. Your *time horizon* is the maximum cognitive period in which you can plan and execute specific, ongoing, goal-directed activities. The forebrain, or frontal lobe region of your brain, is the area that handles this task.

Soviet neurosurgeon A. R. Luria, a leading forebrain researcher, has discovered that the frontal lobes are involved in a "program which ensures not only that the subject reacts to actual stimuli, but within certain limits foresees the future, foretells the probability that a particular event may happen, will be prepared if it does happen, and, as a result, prepares a program of behavior."[44] Many of us — even most of us — fall short of optimal forebrain development, and we end up struggling to move ahead with our lives. In essence, we're captives of our past. But, with practice, we can change this pattern.

The brain's "time window" is of great significance in human achievement, says Elliott Jaques, a leading professor of sociology in Great Britain. After three decades studying the relationship between time and job competence, Jaques concludes that if you can determine what a person thinks about time, you can determine the extent of his or her work capacity.

In terms of personal vision building, Jaques adds that "the maximum time span an individual can work with — that person's maximum achieved time span — measures and defines that person's level of cognitive power. I call this measure a person's *time horizon*."[45]

A growing consensus among brain researchers — neuroscientists, neurosurgeons, mathematicians, psychologists, physicists, chronobiologists, and sociologists — is that we humans are time-binding beings. Each of us places limits on what we will allow ourselves to do with time, and within these limits we choose our level of work performance. Jaques and other scientists have traced the emergence of this key factor in the coping behavior of successful people.

With a limited time horizon — less than a year, for example — the brain appears to be rigid and rule-anchored. The individual tends to overreact to minor problems and has difficulty seeing the long-term consequences of current behavior. In contrast, with a time horizon of five to ten years, a person's ability to handle complexity, ambiguity, change, and paradox is dramatically enhanced.

Time horizons are different from what many of us in business have come to call "strategic thinking" or "strategic planning." Jaques determined that, with regular practice (even as little as a few minutes a week), time horizons can be expanded and extended, and the individual is then more capable of[46]

- Viewing uncertainty as a resource
- Thinking outside the rules
- Being willing to generate new theories
- Using contradictory knowledge or data
- Being open to all sources of information
- Paying attention to what's left unsaid
- Looking for more than one answer to problems.

To create your own ten-year time horizon, begin by developing a personal vision of the time ahead — a "future autobiography"[47] — in which you vividly see yourself functioning a decade from now (the forebrain is stimulated whether or not your mental images are logically attainable or possible). Schedule some weekly time to sit in a quiet place, relax, and look intently into your personal, family, and work future, using mental imagery and language that is

- Clear, specific, comprehensive, and detailed
- Stated in the future perfect tense ("This is how I/we will have achieved this goal . . . and this goal . . .")
- Stated proactively (placing your focus on envisioning what *is* possible, rather than on worrying about fixing what's wrong)
- Powerful and compelling enough to draw your full personal commitment.

4. What Can I *Do* About It Right Now?

One of the surest ways to avoid getting stuck in difficult work situations is to first clearly and quickly acknowledge current reality and then direct your mind away from the problem or task itself and toward specific outputs and possible solutions — staying mentally flexible, exploring the issue from every direction and perspective.

Ask yourself, What can be accomplished here? and What's the most effective role for me in this *specific* situation — innovator? mentor? friend? team player? facilitator? negotiator? monitor? coordinator? leader?

Studies indicate that by stretching your mind and senses in this way, you can increase your ability to handle pressure and deal with complexity, unfamiliar problems, competing demands, and contradictory objectives and approaches.[48]

As discussed in Chapter 6, in fast-paced business situations, effective decision making depends on asking the right kind of questions. In most cases, one key subquestion here is *What next?* rather than *Why?* or *What's wrong?*

Whatever has happened, has happened. If an opportunity has been missed, then it's gone. Thinking about what went wrong and why it went wrong is the quicksand of emotion. It leads to indecision and inaction — giving up and giving in. Switching the mental focus to what can be put right, what action can be taken now, what new opportunities can be developed, leads to a winning attitude and an acceptance of change.

5. What's the Best Way to Express My Thoughts or Feelings?

This is the final mental checkpoint. It pays to remember that no matter what the work situation, the best solutions and sharpest insights amount to very little if they're poorly expressed or misunderstood. In addition to the communication skills presented in Chapter 6, the following discoveries may help you express your thoughts and feelings in the most effective way.

First, do your best to *avoid making statements or decisions when you're fatigued or distracted.* Decision making and communication are affected not only by the evidence that *should* affect your choice and by the appropriateness of your message and its delivery but also by such factors as mental or physical fatigue, tension, pain, anger, or anxiety. Every aspect of the Performance Edge has some bearing here in helping you prevent and correct these stressful conditions. In the meantime, it makes sense whenever possible to delay making important decisions or statements when you temporarily find yourself tense, tired, or down.

Another way the mind affects work performance is through *explanatory style* — the way we describe our experiences to ourselves and others. Evidence shows that when we consistently make certain assumptions about the cause of bad things that happen to us, we fuel emotional turmoil and undercut our health and performance.[49]

According to the results of more than one hundred experiments involving nearly 15,000 subjects, people with negative explanatory style tend to explain the bad things that happen to them in terms that are *internal* ("It's all my fault"), *stable* ("It's going to last forever"), and *global* ("It's going to spoil everything I do"). These individuals are at the greatest risk for depression, repeated mistakes, and illness.

If, like many of us, you tend to be hard on yourself whenever you make a mistake or miss an objective on your daily schedule, get into the habit of pausing for a split second at the moment you start berating yourself and ask, *Is it worth dying for?* This final-straw question is particularly crucial whenever you feel a flash of anger. If you're about to become very upset or explode, remember that toxic emotions always come with a price.

By reacting inappropriately or overreacting — with anger, anxiety, accusing, blaming, and so on — you can damage your own body and mind, and even trigger a heart attack.[50] In peak pressure situations, head off anger right away, using the Instant Calming Sequence (Chapter 3) and reflective coping skills (Chapter 6).

To improve your explanatory style, begin with awareness. Pay closer attention to the way you explain mistakes and unpleasant situations to yourself and others. Use the strategies in the preceding section of this chapter to begin catching distorted thoughts and replacing them with constructive attributions. Be specific, honest, and positive. And be gentle with yourself. Work is challenging enough without letting your own mind stack the odds against you.

To further ease mental stress and upgrade decision making, it also pays to *clarify statements to include an accuracy range and level of confidence* when presenting your ideas and soliciting opinions from your co-workers and employees. This helps reduce the chances of taking shortsighted shortcuts or being unclear about your viewpoints or estimates.

Ask that statements — by yourself and others in your organization or team — be in a form that allows everyone to evaluate accuracy. One of the best ways to do this is to provide a range and level of confidence for every opinion and estimate instead of permitting dangerous single-point predictions.[51]

All kinds of misinterpretations and misunderstandings result when people say that they're "reasonably sure" that in a given time period they, their department, or work team can produce X products, increase quality measures to Y, reduce defects to Z, sell X units, perform Y services, or generate Z creative ideas. A more effective alternative is to estimate a specific range of numbers and add a level of confidence ("I'm 50 percent sure" is very different from "I'm 90 percent sure").

By requiring that statements like these be straightforward, individuals learn to place their reputation behind calculations. With some practice and feedback, everyone will begin to make better calibrations. In turn, fewer offhanded estimates will be issued because the accountability factor encourages everyone to gather more complete and accurate data.

Why "Positive Thinking" Isn't Enough

Over the years, some popular motivational speakers have suggested that all we really need to master job stress and be in great mental health is the right self-talk. That's a myth. As you can see by reading this chapter, positive thinking by itself just isn't enough.

Moreover, it's all but impossible to think truly positive thoughts (you can recite empty mental jingles perhaps, but not thoughts with meaning) when stress hits and you've halted your breathing, frowned, collapsed your posture, tensed your muscles, closed your mind, and opened the floodgates to negative emotions — all about as fast as you can blink your eyes.

Another widely held myth suggests that "positive thinking" is simply a matter of filling your mind with "good" thoughts and blocking out the "bad." Many of my business clients are surprised to learn that "positive thinking" can backfire and actually be negative when, instead of choosing exactly what you *do* want, you focus on preventing and inadvertently magnifying what you *don't* want — mistakes, fatigue, forgetfulness, or interpersonal conflicts, for example. By doing that, you actually *help* things go wrong because the brain is not only extremely fast but also extraordinarily precise in its interpretation of, and response to, incoming messages.

For some reason, the mind does not respond as well to words such as *prevent* and *avoid* as it does to the image of the problem, which is thereby made even more formidable. Therefore, to clear the way for progress in your chosen direction, select a description — or place a picture in your mind — that creates a positive image of exactly what you *do* want to achieve.

The recommendations in this chapter are designed to help you increase your ability to handle mental stress, think more innovatively, expand your performance capabilities, and make effective, insightful decisions under pressure. But remember that mental health and well-being also depend on the other Performance Edge factors throughout this book. Only with all the pieces of this puzzle can you form an inner environment in which constructive, creative thoughts and images gain the clarity and power to propel you toward your dreams.

Resources

To learn more ways to explore the creative process, sharpen innovative thinking, and increase your mental powers, see Chapter 16. To expand your knowledge of performance psychology and work-related mental development in the 1990s and beyond, refer to the following publications (listed alphabetically).

- *Beyond Rational Management: Mastering the Paradoxes and Competing Demands of High Performance* by Robert E. Quinn (Jossey-Bass, 1988). Discusses effective ways to deal with contradictory objectives and approaches in today's changing workplace.
- *Breakthrough Thinking* by Gerald Nadler and Shozo Hibino (Prima, 1990). A Japanese-American collaborative effort reporting the results of studies on effective problem solving.
- *The Care and Feeding of Ideas: A Guide to Encouraging Creativity* by James L. Adams (Addison-Wesley, 1986). Adams is chairman of the Values, Technology, Science, and Society Department at Stanford University.
- *The Creative Attitude: Learning to Ask and Answer the Right Questions* by Roger C. Schank (Macmillan, 1988). Reaches into some deeper realms of creative inquiry. Schank is a professor of computer science and psychology at Yale University and chairman of Cognitive Systems, Inc., an artificial intelligence software company.
- *The Creative Quest* by Lorna Catford and Michael L. Ray (J. P. Tarcher, 1991).
- *Creativity in Business* by Michael L. Ray and Rochelle Myers (Doubleday, 1986). An entertaining and inspiring book, written by two Stanford University business professors.
- *Decision Traps* by J. Edward Russo and Paul J. H. Shoemaker (Doubleday, 1989). Insights on identifying and avoiding common barriers to effective decision making.
- *The Feeling Good Handbook* by Dr. David D. Burns (Morrow, 1989). An in-depth review of cognitive distortions and how to correct them.
- *The Fifth Discipline: The Art and Practice of the Learning Organization* by Peter M. Senge (Doubleday, 1990). A practical look at systems thinking and related issues by the director of Systems Thinking and Organizational Learning at MIT's Sloan School of Management.

- *Flow: The Psychology of Optimal Experience* by Mihaly Csikszentmihalyi (Harper and Row, 1990).
- *Lateral Thinking: Creativity Step by Step* by Edward de Bono (Harper Colophon, 1973). A classic.
- *Software for the Mind: How to Program Your Own Mind for Optimum Health and Performance* by Emmett E. Miller, M.D. (Celestial Arts, 1987). A collection of scientific insights and practical guidelines from a leading authority on optimal performance under pressure.
- *A Whack on the Side of the Head* by Roger Van Oech (revised edition, Simon and Schuster, 1990). Combines humor, paradox, ancient philosophy, and scientific facts to help jolt the reader into getting rid of some common mental blocks that stifle innovation.

8

Performance Turning Point #6:
Mental and Physical Stamina

Beating Fatigue and Increasing Your
Effectiveness on the Job
with 60-Second Work Breaks

DAILY WORK BREAKS. How often you take them and exactly what you do during these free minutes on the job is one of the most decisive but overlooked factors in gaining — and keeping — the Performance Edge.

"Research has shown that rest breaks are an effective way to fight the effects of fatigue in both physical and cognitive tasks," say the editors of *Industrial Management*. "Although this is generally recognized by managers, rest breaks are not designed or scheduled with an eye toward maximizing productivity."[1]

Most of us think of work breaks as chances to escape from pressure. To stretch our legs, daydream, drink coffee, avoid the phone, or just plain stop rushing and sit still, wrapped for a few minutes in a kind of job recovery blanket.

Some of us seem to barely make it from this break to the next and the next. We survive one hour at a time, checking off the days on the calendar. In contrast, a growing number of us are giving up on breaks entirely — we never seem to stop working at all.

Take a moment to look back at the work breaks you have taken in recent months. What do you think an ideal work break should include? And how many minutes do you think it actually takes — and how often — to revitalize your body and mind and keep your energy and performance levels high throughout the day and well into the evening?

Based on extensive research, the Performance Edge Workbreak system presents an advanced 60-second action plan to quickly and easily release tight muscles and balance your posture; send a wave of relaxation through your body; replace nutrients and replenish fluids; rejuvenate your vision; lift your mood; and clear and refocus your mind.

Fatigue Cripples Performance

Work fatigue attacks the heart of productivity, customer responsiveness, and quality control, and it may be the single greatest barrier to consistent breakthrough achievement.

Study after study reveals that capital investments in sophisticated computer systems and other technological advances can take work performance only so far. Then it's *human* productivity — output per hours worked — that tells the story. As the joint Toyota–General Motors project at the NUMMI plant in Fremont, California, illustrates so well, high-tech, automated production fails to produce breakthroughs when managers at work stations and workers on the assembly line become fatigued and error-prone.[2]

At the NUMMI plant, there is "constant pressure to work harder and faster, not just smarter."[3] Expert observers at this automobile assembly facility report that "as the line goes faster and the whole system is stressed, it becomes harder and harder to keep up. Since tasks have been so painstakingly charted, refined, and recharted, management assumes any glitch is the worker's (or his supervisor's) fault. The chimes and lights of the *andon* board immediately identify the person who is not keeping up . . . and the rules mandate discipline — including firing — for 'failure to maintain satisfactory production levels.' . . . In reality, the only solution is to keep up, no matter what it takes. Some NUMMI workers use break time or come in early to 'build stock' or get ready. Thus,

NUMMI's high productivity figures result at least in part from pushing managers and employees to work overtime for free."[4]

While there's no doubt that profits can be increased using this new "management by stress" approach, it occurs at great cost to a humane work environment. Fatigue not only is an ongoing threat to peak productivity, it also stifles innovation and promotes job burnout.

"Individuals and organizations are discovering that just learning how to have more good ideas is not enough," says Dr. Thomas E. Backer, research professor at the UCLA School of Medicine and professor in the Department of Management at California State University. "Innovative, creative work takes enormous personal energy. Especially for companies battling to keep a competitive edge, even a temporary energy drain can spell disaster."[5]

Worldwide research in brain science, biochemistry, occupational medicine, and ergonomics indicates that the most serious causes of work fatigue fall into four broad categories:

1. *Biochemical:* Including dehydration; hypoxia (not enough circulation of oxygen); dietary (skipping meals, overeating at main meals, or consuming high-fat foods and snacks); and lack of the right type of regular fitness activities to build stamina and endurance.
2. *Biomechanical:* Repetitive-motion injuries; muscle tension and pain-generating "trigger points" that cause headaches, back pain, stiff neck, and tired shoulders; poor posture; and lack of regular physical movement through the day.
3. *Mental:* Mismanaged stress; arguments and communication mix-ups; breakdowns in teamwork; cynicism and hostility; time urgency; scheduling conflicts; mishandled anger; criticism; negative self-defeating thoughts; unclear work purpose; unrealistic expectations; lack of empowerment to make important decisions; and unresolved personal and family concerns.
4. *Environmental:* "Techno-stress"; eyestrain (due to prolonged close work, poor lighting or glare); indoor air pollution; stressful work station design; and background noise.

Repetitive-Motion Injuries:
Hottest Hazard of the Information Age

Over the past decade, new technologies and competitive pressures have combined to create some debilitating occupational hazards. Many of today's jobs — from typing at a computer work station to advanced assembly line tasks — involve constant repetition of motion for prolonged periods of time without a break. Over time, this stresses and then strains muscles and tendons, irritating or damaging nerves in the hand, wrist, shoulder, neck, or back.

These ailments have been labeled *cumulative trauma disorders* (CTDs), and they currently afflict some 5 million Americans, according to the National Institute of Occupational Safety and Health.[6] By the year 2000, experts predict that half the work force will be vulnerable. CTD is already the most frequently cited on-the-job ailment, accounting for nearly 50 percent of all occupational illness since 1988.

The American Academy of Orthopaedic Surgeons estimates that CTD-related injuries cost $27 billion a year in medical bills and lost days. Without changes in the workplace and in the design of work procedures, warns OSHA ergonomist Roger Stephens, "it won't be uncommon to see 50 cents on the dollar going to treat [such] disorders."[7]

The Productive Capacity of the Individual

Soviet researchers in the Department of Engineering Psychology and Work Psychology at Moscow State University report that work fatigue has a measurable impact on short-term memory, communication clarity, and information transfer.[8]

"Under the influence of fatigue," say Drs. V. P. Zinchenko, A. B. Leonova, and Y. K. Strelkov, "performance indices . . . fall off considerably, especially accuracy. . . . Fatigue also disturbs the performance of those operations which call for maximum mobilization of attention."[9] In short, *mental and physical fatigue, re-*

gardless of its cause, results in a decrease in the productive capacity of the individual.[10]

One of the simplest and most effective ways to counteract fatigue is through scheduling and design of work breaks. American, European, and Japanese research substantiates the need for short daily work breaks to revitalize the body and mind, measurably increasing job satisfaction, productivity, and quality control.[11]

Studies indicate that people at work take rest pauses of various kinds and under varying circumstances.[12] There are four general types of rest:

1. *Spontaneous pauses:* the obvious pauses, usually brief, that workers take on their own initiative to relieve fatigue.
2. *Disguised pauses:* pauses that take place when the individual switches focus to some easier, routine task to relax from concentrating on the primary job. Examples include looking out the window or away from the work site; sorting through files, rearranging office materials on top of the desk or work station, or cleaning equipment; shifting into a different sitting or standing position; and even leaving the work site on the pretext of consulting someone in another department.
3. *Work-conditioned pauses:* the interruptions that are caused by the operation of equipment or organization of the work effort. Examples include waiting for customers or orders in sales and service industries; waiting for the office photocopier to make a dozen copies or for the facsimile to transmit a memo; waiting for machines to warm up, cool down, be repaired, or complete a work cycle in manufacturing industries; and assembly line pauses waiting for the conveyor belt to move the next assembly piece along.
4. *Prescribed pauses, as directed by management:* pauses such as traditional midday breaks and snack breaks (coffee breaks).

Contrary to popular management opinion, spontaneous and disguised pauses are not always counterproductive. In fact, when there are an optimal number of prescribed work breaks to help prevent mental and physical fatigue, spontaneous and disguised pauses decrease in number. In addition, when they do appear during the workday, they tend to change from costly lapses in concentration into useful moments of posture shifting, deep breathing, muscular tension release, or mental refocusing.

Although some managers still feel that breaks are not necessary in cognitive work, it's well documented that when work breaks are not authorized and scheduled, workers will adjust their performance and work rate to compensate for mental fatigue — and then, as errors increase, productivity and quality control deteriorate. In companies striving toward total customer responsiveness and zero defects (not just in manufacturing flawless products but throughout the entire organization), work breaks become a key issue.[13]

According to Alan D. Swain, senior scientist at Argonne National Laboratory in Albuquerque, New Mexico, certain factors such as routine, fatigue, stress, and distraction — notably noise — are associated with high error rates. Chief among these so-called error factors is routine, a finding that holds true even for those whose job is to find errors. *No one,* says Swain, *should be assigned to intensive work* — such as quality inspection tasks — *for longer than a half hour at a time.*[14]

Many investigations into work productivity conclude that "introducing rest pauses actually speeds up the work," observes Dr. Etienne Grandjean, an international expert on work productivity and director of the Department of Ergonomics at the Swiss Federal Institute of Technology in Zurich, "and this more than compensates for the time lost during prescribed pauses, as well as leading to fewer disguised and spontaneous pauses.

"The hourly output of work usually declines towards the middle and end of the morning shift," explains Dr. Grandjean, "and even more towards evening, as the rate of working slows down. Various studies have shown that if prescribed pauses are introduced the appearance of fatigue symptoms is postponed and the loss of production through fatigue is less . . . rest pauses tend to increase output."[15]

Another high-priority benefit from frequent, short work breaks is to interrupt the constant job-related stress to muscles and tendons that can lead to repetitive-motion injuries known as CTDs.

There's also a payoff for work skills development: When corporate training sessions are regularly interrupted for short breaks, new skills can be acquired more quickly than if training is delivered in the traditional, more continuous manner.[16]

Solving Persistent Problems

As the hours wear on during the workday, it becomes more and more difficult to remain in complete control of our thoughts, feelings, speech, and actions. The more tension you pick up, and the more anxious or fatigued you become, the harder it is to feel enthusiastic and to work effectively. Everything turns into more of a struggle. And things may get so hectic that you're lucky to find more than a free minute or two here and there.

But even if you do have the time to spend 20 minutes in the middle of the morning and afternoon meditating or listening to a relaxation tape, scientists have discovered that while these techniques relieve muscle tension and provide other benefits, they can also reportedly *have a detrimental effect on attention span, reaction time, and other aspects of performance and productivity.*[17]

This is not to suggest that practicing meditation and deep relaxation aren't valuable. But by themselves, these self-improvement techniques aren't enough to make the best use of your work breaks even if you do have the time for them. And neither is aerobic exercise, a power snack, weight training, listening to a motivational tape, or any other factor, by itself.

The Performance Edge Workbreak includes the Instant Calming Sequence (ICS) and goes beyond it, combining key priorities in a commanding 60-second technique that can be (a) used successfully on its own or (b) added before or after your favorite relaxation, meditation, lunch, or exercise session. Either way, you have a winning formula.

The Basic 60-Second
Performance Edge Workbreak

The basic 60-second Performance Edge Workbreak combines the latest scientific discoveries into a comprehensive four-step approach:

1. Instant Calming Sequence (ICS)
2. Physical moves

3. Mental moves
4. Replenishment of nutrients

---

1. The Instant Calming Sequence (ICS)

Time required: 1 second or less.

The ICS is a five-step technique to help keep you calm and in control whenever bad stresses strike or you walk into a high-pressure situation. In a Performance Edge Workbreak, the ICS gives you a unique "safety valve" to release any accumulated stress, disengage from your current work task, and shift your mind and senses into a state of calm, attentive, *present-moment awareness* so that you can take fullest advantage of every second in your upcoming break.

Once learned (see Chapter 3), the five steps of the ICS — uninterrupted breathing, positive face, balanced posture, release muscle tension, and mental control — refocus you in an instant and make what follows more effective.

---

2. Physical Moves

Time required: 25–30 seconds (more if you have it).
Get up, walk, and unstress by moving. Your posture contributes to — or reduces — mental and physical fatigue. Work breaks provide an ideal time to release any accrued muscle tension and invigorate your mind.

It's important to change your physical position often throughout the day since nutrients reach the spinal column only when you shift your posture, whereby a muscular pumplike mechanism uses the movement to exchange fluids in the spinal disks.[18] "No matter how good the chair," says David Thompson, Stanford University ergonomist, "human beings weren't designed to sit in one position for extended periods."[19]

"Even the most ideal posture can lead to musculoskeletal 'loading' if it is maintained too long," warn occupational health experts

Jeanne Stellman and Mary Sue Henifin, "because the human body is designed to move. Static positions are contrary to biology."[20]

For best posture, follow the guidelines in Chapter 9. Take a physical break at least once every hour, advises Thompson, and if you're working at a desk or computer, "make it a habit to stop and stretch your arms and do a couple of shoulder or head rolls every couple of pages."[21]

Make a quick assessment: What part of your body is in greatest need of attention right now? Choose a range of motion exercise to fit that need — such as gentle head nods or neck ovals; shoulder shrugs; pelvic-leveling exercise, range of motion exercises for your wrists, hands, and fingers; or other choices (see Chapter 10).

Shift your visual focus to relieve eyestrain and sharpen your vision. One recent study of 2,330 people from fifteen different workplaces reported that 77 percent of the users of VDTs (computer terminals) and 56 percent of all other workers reported a problem with eyestrain at work.[22] In addition to making changes in lighting and reducing air pollution sources (Chapter 12), you can ease eyestrain and revitalize your vision with several simple guidelines.

First, if you've been doing close work, take a few moments to blink your eyes and look at more distant objects. If you've been scanning faraway scenery, switch to focusing on something nearby.

Second, if you wear contact lenses you should know that you blink less when you concentrate, and your eyes can get very dry at work. Take frequent breaks, advises Thompson, "and allow your blink rate to come back to normal."[23]

Relieve tension or pain by treating neuromuscular "trigger points." Take a moment to reach up and press the muscle areas of the base of the skull, neck, jaw, shoulders, or lower back. If you notice any sensitive areas — trigger points — apply moderate pressure for six seconds and release. This fast, easy method (presented in Chapter 4) is a safe, medically sound way to eliminate the causes of many headaches, backaches, and other pain-tension syndromes that are common in the workplace. If you pick up muscle tension at work, using this technique several times a day is also one of the quickest ways to increase your comfort and stamina.

3. Mental Moves

Time required: 20–25 seconds (more if you have it).

To a surprising extent, we often unintentionally create our own mental and physical exhaustion. When we automatically expect a task to be stressful or tiring, that mental picture alone can lower productivity,[24] and such unquestioned expectations can even dictate when our energy will run out.

Taking regular, brief work breaks to change your mental focus can increase your alertness and help prevent this problem. Research by Harvard psychology professor Ellen J. Langer indicates that staggering different kinds of work, shifting the mental work focus throughout the day, and taking short breaks all help prevent fatigue and boost energy "by shaking free of the mindset of exhaustion."[25]

If you're struggling with a problem or concern, use the Performance Edge Workbreak as a quick way to clear your mind, change your mental focus, step back for a moment from the issue at hand, and ask the five mental turning point questions presented in Chapter 7:

1. What is the *heart* of this issue or *problem?*
2. Is what I'm seeing/hearing/thinking/feeling accurate?
3. How important is this going to be in the long run?
4. What can I *do* about it right now?
5. What's the best way to express my thoughts or feelings?

It takes regular practice to change automatic thoughts and deeply ingrained imagery habits. One of the best ways to do this is to take advantage of each Performance Edge Workbreak throughout the day as an opportunity to replace old, ineffective patterns of thinking with new, more productive ones.

---

4. Replenishment of Nutrients

Time required: 10–15 seconds (more if you have it).
Drink some cool pure water. Water is a forgotten nutrient for mental and physical health in the workplace. Without realizing it, nearly all of us experience job performance limitations because we're dehydrated.

Loss of water during the workday contributes to fatigue and muscular discomfort. It also reduces blood volume, creating thicker, more concentrated blood, which may stress the heart and is less capable of providing muscles with oxygen and nutrients and eliminating accumulated wastes.[26]

In addition, "because a deficiency of water can alter the concentration of electrolytes such as sodium, potassium, and chloride, water has a profound effect on brain function," explains Dr. Vernon H. Mark, author of *Brain Power: A Neurosurgeon's Complete Program to Maintain and Enhance Brain Fitness Throughout Your Life.*[27] "Even a slightly dehydrated body can produce a small but critical shrinkage of the brain," add sports medicine authorities Dr. Bob Goldman and Robert M. Hackman, "thereby impairing neuromuscular coordination, concentration, and thinking."[28]

Dehydration stresses are particularly high in modern office buildings and during air travel. It takes surprisingly little fluid loss — 1 to 2 percent — for your body to become dehydrated, and you can't depend on thirst to tell you that it's happening. "Even a tiny shortage of water disrupts your biochemistry," says Michael Colgan, nutritional researcher and recent visiting scholar at Rockefeller University. "Dehydrate a muscle by only 3% and you lose 10% of contractile strength and 8% of speed. Water balance is the single most important variable in top performance."

Few of us realize that we don't have to be perspiring profusely or urinating frequently to lose water. We're losing it all the time. If you work in a stuffy office, you lose large amounts of fluid by invisible evaporation from the skin and lungs. If you're a frequent business traveler, the rapid circulation of dry airplane air can cause your body to lose as much as two pounds of water in a three-to-four-hour flight.[29] And alcohol and caffeine, both diuretics, increase the body's fluid loss. So does stress.

How much water do you need to drink? It depends on many variables, including the foods in your diet, metabolic rate, weather, temperature, climate, physical activity level, and job stress factors. But, in general, *we each need to drink more water than our thirst calls for.*

Every day the average worker loses at least 2 cups of water through breathing, another 2 cups through invisible perspiration, and 6 cups through urination and bowel movements. That's *10 cups a day* without taking into account fluids lost through perspiration in exercise or hard physical work.[30]

In general, drink between 6 and 8 cups of pure water every day. Develop new water-drinking habits by ensuring that water is readily accessible in your work area — and monitor how much you consume. Keep a glass or cup of water next to you throughout your work hours. *Cool water* (40–50 degrees Fahrenheit) is more quickly absorbed than warm and, contrary to popular opinion, won't cause cramping.[31]

If you're like most of us who've spent years underhydrated, all this may have you wondering why you haven't dried up and blown away before now. But like suboptimal breathing habits (from which it's easy to grow accustomed to being tired) and chronic tension (from which the slightest easing of muscle tightness can trick you into thinking you're relaxed), persistent dehydration, however slight it may be, covertly cuts your quality of work and life. The solution takes some getting used to, but it's well worth the effort.

Every two to three hours, eat several bites of a carefully selected snack. First of all, as described in Chapter 11, "small snack" means just that — small. Second, "carefully selected" means taking full advantage of the latest discoveries of nutritional science. Make it a point to find a way to keep a variety of snacks on hand at work, in a portable cooler pack or the office refrigerator.

Eating food five times daily — three moderate meals and a mid-morning and midafternoon snack — is highly recommended "for both health and work efficiency," says Dr. Grandjean.[32] Recent research published in the *New England Journal of Medicine* indicates that this eating pattern can also lower blood cholesterol levels, increase metabolism, and boost energy.[33]

But be aware that eating *high-fat foods causes fatigue*.[34] There-fore, the best general advice is to choose wholesome, fresh foods that, overall, are high in complex carbohydrates and fiber, mod-erate in protein, and low in fat, cholesterol, and salt.

With these basic guidelines in hand, you're ready for a key de-cision. Researchers have discovered that food choices can influ-ence the production of brain messenger chemicals called neuro-transmitters, which in turn affect mental alertness, concentration, attitude, mood, and performance. There's increasing evidence that you can help *manage your mind and mood through food*.[35] Here's a quick summary of the best foods.

- *Foods for increased alertness:* Snacks that are low in fat and in-clude a small amount of protein-rich food can reportedly pro-mote faster thinking, greater energy, increased attention to detail, and quicker reaction speed.

  Options include baked or broiled skinless chicken breast, tur-key breast, or fish; a bean or lentil salad, soup, or casserole; low-fat or nonfat yogurt or cottage cheese with fruit; or a glass of skim milk with a piece of fruit. In addition to the high-protein food, balance the meal or snack by including vegetables or fruit and some complex carbohydrates such as a piece of low-fat, whole-grain bread, a bagel, muffin, baked pita chips, rye crackers, or a whole-grain side dish.
- *Foods for increased calmness:* Snacks that are low in fat and pro-tein as well as high in complex carbohydrates can reportedly help produce a calm, focused state of mind and relaxed emotions (al-though in late afternoon these snacks make some people drowsy, so be certain to experiment to find which snacks are best for you).

  Options include cooked whole grains (rice, wheat, oatmeal, corn, buckwheat, barley, and so on) eaten with fruit or a sweetener but without milk; low-fat pasta salad with fruit or vegetables; or some low-fat, whole-grain bread, a bagel, muffin, baked pita chips, or rye crackers topped with your favorite all-fruit preserve.

For more on the mind-mood-food connection, see Chapter 11. *Note:* Bring a glass or container of pure water (and the rest of your snack if possible) back to your desk — or the vehicle seat next to you if you're traveling. Then you'll have a chance to sip some extra water (and eat the remaining bites of food) to further boost your performance until the next break.

Observations

To accomplish these four work break steps in 60 seconds, it's obvious that you need to make advance arrangements to have the water and snack nearby (a lunch box and quick-pour Thermos work just fine). After some practice, try combining steps 2 and 3, going through the mind moves while your body is in motion. This gives you an extra 25–30 seconds of physical movement time.

I'm the first to admit that you need to be well organized and move at a calm but quick pace to complete this routine in one minute. But the bottom line is that it works. And if you have 60 seconds, you may often actually have two or three minutes. Most of us could arrange for at least one 60-second break every half hour throughout our work shift. You can even do these routines while on a commuter train or airline flight.

Sample Work Break Schedules*

How often should you take time out for a Performance Edge Workbreak? It depends on your job demands and varies from company to company and work team to work team. In most cases, once every half hour would be ideal, but begin with whatever you can. Whenever possible, it's advisable to encourage personal control of the timing of work breaks.

A number of studies confirm that a series of short breaks during a work shift is superior to one or two longer, less frequent breaks, even when the total amount of break time over the course of the day is the same.[36] Some studies suggest that work breaks may be more effective if scheduled more often during the early hours of

---

* These work break scheduling examples are for illustrative purposes only. The possible variations are endless. Assess your own work situation and scheduling priorities as you begin to implement a work break strategy. Remember: Even just one extra work break during the day can produce benefits.

the work period (this is called *front loading*, shown in example B below) than when evenly spaced.[37] The small snack from step 4 is included once every two to three hours. The other steps are included every time.

Example A
6:00 A.M. Arise
7:00 A.M. Breakfast
8:00 A.M. Arrive at work
8:45 A.M. Work break
9:30 A.M. Work break with snack
10:15 A.M. Work break
11 A.M. Work break
12:00 Noon Lunch break

1:00 P.M. Return to work
1:45 P.M. Work break
2:30 P.M. Work break with snack
3:15 P.M. Work break
4:00 P.M. Work break
5:00 P.M. Leave work
6:30 P.M. Evening meal

Example B
6:00 A.M. Arise
7:00 A.M. Breakfast
8:00 A.M. Arrive at work
8:30 A.M. Work break
9:00 A.M. Work break
9:30 A.M. Work break
10:00 A.M. Work break with snack
10:45 A.M. Work break
11:30 A.M. Work break

12:00 Noon Lunch break
1:00 P.M. Return to work
1:30 P.M. Work break
2:00 P.M. Work break
2:45 P.M. Work break with snack
3:30 P.M. Work break
4:15 P.M. Work break
5:00 P.M. Leave work
6:30 P.M. Evening meal

2-Minute to 5-Minute Work Breaks

You can expand the 60-second work break routine into 2-minute or 5-minute versions. Some management experts recommend creating your own personal agenda for each individual break.[38] Possible priorities include the following.

• *Health and fitness:* Take several additional bites of your small snack; walk outside for fresh air and a moment of sunshine; add a breathing exercise or several "transpyramid" abdominal exercises (Chapter 10), a flexibility and posture exercise, a balance and agility exercise, or some resistance exercises; release tension with some quick postural shifts (Chapter 9); or relieve pain by treating irritated trigger point areas of the neck, back, and shoulders using the 6-second NeuroMuscular Technique (Chapter 4).

- *Self-renewal and social support:* Look over your to-do list to make sure you're on track with priorities; go through a mental exercise to boost creativity or problem-solving skills (Chapters 7 and 16); take a quick look at ways you might take better care of yourself over the next hour, improve performance, or support your co-workers; read an inspiring quote or look at a beautiful photograph or painting; vividly visualize — rather than just count — your blessings; read something humorous or tell a joke; take a minute to learn more about the specific needs of your fellow workers, and find ways for you or your company to help meet them; begin a postcard- or letter-writing campaign to communicate with your political representatives, correct a social problem, improve the environment, or otherwise make your community a better place to live; or send a silent lighted thought or prayer to a person or group in need.

- *Work effectiveness:* Jot down brainstorming notes on specific ways your company or department could do a better job in the hours or days ahead; prepare several smart questions (Chapter 6) to clear up important issues you want to discuss with your boss, co-workers, employees, clients, or customers; take a minute to expand your "time horizon" (Chapter 7); pause to think of something funny or lighthearted; look over your schedule and prepare for upcoming appointments or tasks (Chapter 5); think creatively about a new income-generating project; listen to an audiotape to improve some facet of your work knowledge or performance; call or write a key customer or colleague; conduct a one-minute "personal think tank" aimed at finding innovative ways to improve quality, penetrate a new market, serve customers, or boost company morale.

- *Work relations:* Walk over to someone who's been doing a good job and give him or her a pat on the back and a genuine word of appreciation; team up with a co-worker or friend for a quick seated massage to relieve tense, painful areas of the neck, back, shoulders, and arms (Chapter 4); jot out a note of praise or make plans for a thoughtful face-to-face reprimand to catch small errors before they turn into big problems; or write or call someone special for a brief "thinking of you" greeting.

Why Small Steps Beat Big Leaps

Performance Edge Workbreaks are a natural complement to productivity habits that the Japanese call *kaizen* — living your life with full awareness so that not a day goes by without one, and usually many, small improvements.

Kaizen is "the single most important concept in Japanese management" and an underlying reason for Japan's economic growth in recent decades, says management consultant Masaaki Imai.[39] Rather than focusing on colossal breakthroughs and breathtaking leaps — with the crash landings that characterize so many American efforts — *kaizen* aims at "constant revision and upgrading" in one's personal and work life.

Kaizen relies on open, clear communication and a deep sense of responsibility to notice opportunities and eliminate problems. A problem is defined as anything that inconveniences someone downstream from you, in your work, family, anywhere. Individuals resolve to notice opportunities for improvement and to identify problems, which are solved immediately and corrected right where and as they are found.

That's the *philosophy* of *kaizen* — yet in reality it's difficult even for the best organizations to apply it successfully on a company-wide basis day in and day out, hour after hour. Why? In part because making these continuous improvements requires an exceptional level of alertness and stamina. What's missing is the Performance Edge — including the optimal work breaks presented in this chapter.

PART II

The Other Pieces of the Performance Puzzle

9

Posture: Up, Relaxed, and Energized

IN BUSINESS, excellent posture is a universal sign of competence and power. Yet few of us realize the importance of posture to our health and performance.

To most of us, "good posture" simply means sitting and standing up straight. But that's a myth — and a costly one. Of the 680 muscles in your body, only a few are specially designed to hold your body upright and relaxed. And most of us tense dozens — sometimes hundreds — of the *wrong* muscles when we sit, stand, and move. Over the course of a typical workday, this results in an enormous waste of personal energy.

But, you may be wondering, when my posture's out of balance, won't I notice it? Not necessarily. You'll always feel the *effects* of postural stresses and strains, in tension, mental and physical fatigue, eyestrain, difficulty concentrating, and so on. But because these symptoms are so common and have a variety of causes, most of us just assume they're the result of working hard and therefore don't relate them to their actual cause.

With poor posture, just as with dehydration or shallow breathing, your body adapts to the imbalance. Over time, all you may notice about your posture is the great sense of relief you feel whenever you collapse into an easy chair after work.

What Price Are You Paying for Poor Posture?

Poor posture distorts the alignment of bones, chronically tenses muscles, and contributes to stressful conditions such as loss of vital lung capacity (by as much as 30 percent or more);[1] increased fatigue;[2] reduced blood and oxygen to the brain and senses; limited range of motion, stiffness of joints, and pain syndromes (headaches, jaw pain, muscular aches);[3] reduced mental alertness and work productivity;[4] premature aging of body tissues;[5] faulty digestion[6] and constipation;[7] back pain (perhaps 80 percent of all cases);[8] and a tendency toward cynicism, pessimism, drowsiness, and poor concentration.[9]

In addition, poor posture can diminish blood flow to the brain and cause impairments in creative thinking and emotional control, slow reaction time, magnify feelings of panic and helplessness, and may even *cause* depression.[10]

By definition, *posture* is the relative position and alignment of the various masses of the human body. But what comes to mind when most businesspeople think of "good posture"? A stiff, military-like, square-shouldered stance. But that position actually makes posture problems worse instead of better.

With optimal posture there's no tension or stiffness. You have an exhilarating sense of ease in your work, of moving buoyantly, fluidly, comfortably in space. The chest is open and "floats" upward; the head is up, with neck long and chin slightly in; jaw and tongue are relaxed; shoulders are broad and loose; pelvis and hips are level; the back is comfortably straight; and the abdomen is free of tension. You are "resting in motion" — with the feeling of an imaginary sky hook gently lifting your whole spinal column upward from a central point on top of your head.

Every movement you make depends on the split-second tensing and relaxing of muscles that keep the bones of the body aligned. *How* you use those muscles in your body can make the difference between feeling stiff, irritable, and out of balance or fluid, energized, and productive.

Turning Things Around — It Begins with Awareness

Many people assume that good posture is instinctive or automatic. It isn't. "We're not born knowing how to do it right," says Dr. Wilfred Barlow, medical director of the Alexander Institute in Great Britain. "No reflex system sets up good posture. We have to learn it." [11]

"*Use*," explains Dr. Barlow, "means the way we use our bodies as we live from moment to moment. Not only when we are moving, but when we are keeping still. Not only when we are speaking, but when we are thinking. Not only when we are communicating by gestures and attitudes, but when, unknown to ourselves, our bodily mood and disposition tell people what we are like and keep us that way whether we like it or not." [12]

Right now, you are sitting somewhere reading this book. Exactly *how* are you sitting? Direct your attention to various areas of your body as you read these pages. Are your knees open or crossed? Is one shoulder higher or more forward than the other? Where are your shoulder blades? Is the weight of your body more on one buttock than the other?

Where is your neck positioned? Do you feel any tightness in the muscles there? Where are your elbows? Which of your upper arms is more relaxed? Is your chest "open" or collapsed? How does your lower back feel — is it straight or swayed forward or backward? Are your ankles and feet relaxed or cramped? Is your abdomen tight or knotted up? How about your jaw and tongue?

It's easy to keep these areas needlessly tense. Are you aware of how each of your hands is holding the book? Direct your attention to your wrists, palms, and fingers for a moment. Notice the pressure on your palm or fingers where they take the weight of the book. As you run your eyes over the page, does your head move from side to side to shift your eye position or do just your eyes move? If you expand your awareness, you can lift your posture.

Postural State, Mental State

"Posture is not solely the manifestation of physical balance," writes occupational medicine specialist Dr. David Imrie. "It's also an expression of mental balance. Think about the way you stand when you are depressed or tired: you stand with your shoulders rounded and drooping. Your body represents your emotions by giving up the fight against gravity, sagging just as low as you feel. . . . It's also notable that the term 'well-balanced' is used to describe someone who 'won't go over the edge' and whose emotions are 'on an even keel.' "[13]

A recent series of studies report that, compared with subjects in a good postural position, subjects with a slumped posture had a greater tendency toward feelings of helplessness and frustration during work tasks and perceived themselves to be under greater stress.[14] Other researchers have reported that poor posture decreases mental alertness and increases work errors.[15]

In Chapter 3, we discussed the fact that your "facial posture" is linked to mental attitude, mood, and performance. A positive facial expression — even if it's only a slight smile and even if you don't *feel* like smiling — increases blood flow to the brain and appears to predispose your brain chemistry toward nondestructive emotions.[16] Studies also show that posture influences your voice quality and ease of speaking in high-stress business situations: Good posture contributes to what experts call a "compelling, natural voice image."[17]

Posture Improvement Techniques

The priority areas that follow are the quickest and simplest place to begin to improve your posture.

1. Head and Neck Position

Poor posture often causes headaches and neck pain. "It's extremely difficult to work in a technological society and not develop a forward head," says Dr. Rene Cailliet, director of physical medicine and rehabilitation at Santa Monica Hospital Medical Center and clinical professor at the University of Southern California School of Medicine.

"If you're sitting at a typewriter or a computer, or working on an assembly line, chances are that you have one. Even cooking and cleaning can produce one. Any activity that requires you to look down for protracted periods, even reading or simple desk work, can produce a chronic forward head position."[18] And this postural stress causes or contributes to tension headaches, vision problems, and jaw and neck pain.[19]

"Jaw joint pain is so widespread today," adds Dr. Cailliet, "that a majority of adults have experienced it. This type of discomfort was once considered to be exclusively a dental problem . . . but we now know that it is just as often caused or aggravated by faulty posture."[20]

For years, physical education instructors have admonished Americans to "stand up straight" — shoulders broad and pulled back, buttocks tucked, back ramrod straight, stomach sucked in. Pure military. The advice is well intended, but it doesn't work. The muscular bracing looks artificial, feels stressful, and causes fatigue. Even worse, you need to keep reminding yourself to maintain this stiff, unnatural position. Whenever it slips from your awareness, your tired body gratefully collapses back into old patterns.

Best posture isn't forced; it's unlocked. The most important part of the change comes in your head and neck position. Your head weighs between 10 and 15 pounds. To avoid stress on the neck, shoulders, and spine, the head must be poised precisely at the crest of the spine.

The best way to ease strain in the spine is to lengthen your neck and let your head move upward, chin slightly in, shoulders broadening, lower back flattening. Now gently lean your head to the left and then to the right, coming back to the most central, most balanced spot you can sense. Next, move slightly forward and then back, finding the precise center once again.

Here's another picture: "If you put a five-pound weight on your head, and you do nothing more than push up against the resistance, you will straighten out your spinal curves without so much as a thought," says Dr. Cailliet. "It is the weight that's doing the work by giving you feedback, telling you to push up toward the ceiling, and to stand tall. To your body, any other response is intolerable."[21]

Begin right now to think taller, to encourage your head to float upward. Don't push or strain your neck; simply bring your head back over your shoulders, with your chin slightly in. You'll sense the difference — and see it in the mirror. For a simple exercise to strengthen your neck muscles for better posture, see Chapter 10.

It's important to realize that the head does more than simply rest atop your neck. Whenever possible, your head should lead your body motions: *As you begin any movement or act, move your whole head upward and away from your whole body, and let your whole body lengthen by following that upward direction.*[22] The process is based on learning a new way to use your body, with smoothness and ease. Nothing is forced.

Here's an interesting note: Cornell University researchers discovered that when a businessperson's shirt collar was snugged a mere 1.27 centimeters smaller than that person's relaxed neck size, it restricted blood flow in the pulsing veins in the back of the eyes.[23] This appears to harm visual perception, slowing the ability of the brain to process visual information and convert it into a physical response.

Among businesspeople tested, two-thirds wore shirt collars and ties that were too tight, and nearly one in every seven had a tightness of at least 1.27 centimeters. This finding has particularly important implications for people in occupations where eye-body coordination is critical — airline pilots, computer operators, athletes, artists, motor vehicle drivers of all kinds, accountants, and so on.

2. Sitting

The way you sit influences your energy level and productivity. Most chairs create excessive stress on the spine, back, and neck. "Aside from causing discomfort and possibly ill health," warn occupational health experts Jeanne Stellman and Mary Sue Henifin, "poorly designed chairs impede work efficiency. Research has shown that *at least 40 minutes of productive time are lost each day* because of poor workplace design, some attributable to the chair."[24]

There are nine common faults with most chairs, writes rehabilitative medicine authority Dr. J. G. Travell: "No support for your low back; armrests too low or too high; too scooped a backrest in its upper-portion; backrest nearly vertical; backrest short, failing to support your upper back; jackknifing effect at hips and knees; high front edge of the seat, shutting down the circulation in your legs; seat bottom soft in the center, creating a bucket effect which places the load on the outer side of your thighs, rather than on the bony points in the buttocks; and an otherwise excellent chair may be the wrong size for you." [25]

Especially for use during prolonged hours of work, choose chairs that are fully adjustable. For best support and comfort, your chair must fit the length, size, and contours of your body. If you sit in various chairs at work during the day or if another person uses your chair, adjust it each time you use it, just as you adjust your car seat, steering wheel, and mirrors after someone else has driven your car.

The height of the chair seat should be adjusted to precisely match the position of the desk, drafting table, or countertop where you work. This enables you to sit with your feet flat on the floor, thighs approximately parallel to the floor, and knees slightly higher than hips and to work at about elbow height. Ideal chairs have adjustable seat height, and the exact height you choose should generally be two inches less than the distance from the floor to the crease behind your knees when you are standing up. [26]

The chair seat should be lightly padded and have fabric upholstery (wool or rayon are considered best) to allow perspiration to dissipate and to help prevent slipping and sliding. Seat size is important. The best-designed seat should end about five inches behind the crease at the back of your knee when you are sitting up straight and using the backrest. A chair seat that is too long from front to back will force you to lean forward, putting unnecessary strain on your lower back and thighs.

The chair backrest should provide firm back support, especially for the lower back. The best backrests arch forward to support the natural curve of the lower spine. Some people may need a chair with a full back, providing support all the way up to the shoulders.

Your chair should also allow you to sit up straight without bending your spinal column. To make this possible, the back of the chair should make firm contact with your back 4 to 6 inches above the seat. The shape of the backrest will depend on the type of job you do.

"For the desk worker who writes, reads, or sits, and does not operate a machine, a firm, straight-backed chair that allows the body to assume an unstrained position is appropriate," explain Stellman and Henifin. "For the VDT operator who works sitting with hands extended, the best backrest will be small and kidney-shaped, fitting snugly into the small of the back. . . . In general, it is better not to have casters on your chair, since these can cause strain on the calf muscles as you continually try to anchor yourself in place. . . . If casters are absolutely necessary to accomplish your tasks, you should be able to secure the chair by locking the wheels in place. For the chair to be stable, it should have a five-pronged base rather than the common four-pronged type."[27]

In the final analysis, your type of work determines the best way to adjust your chair. If your job requires reading, telephoning, using a calculator, or writing at a desk, it's important to be able to comfortably lean forward — so the "seat pan" of your chair should be tilted forward 10 to 15 degrees so that your thighs can be angled downward to minimize back strain. When the seat is adjusted correctly, your elbows or forearms should be able to rest comfortably on your work surface.

If you operate a VDT with a keyboard, the seat pan can be tilted backward slightly so that you assume a position much like that of a car driver. Adjust the height of the VDT so that, when you are seated, your eyes are 16 to 24 inches from the screen and your line of sight to the center of the VDT readout is 10 to 20 degrees below the horizontal.

An adjustable document holder can be used to allow typing from copy without neck strain. Your forearms should generally be held at a 70-to-90-degree angle to your upper arms. If you are using a typewriter, your forearms may be angled even higher (50 to 60 degrees). When a desk is a bit too high for keyboarding, an attachable drawer with a padded wrist rest can be used to place the keyboard lower so as to keep your wrists flat and prevent strain.

If your job requires leaning forward a lot, you may want to use a chair with a spring-loaded back support to move as you move. In this case, a 10 percent rearward incline of the chair back is ideal, says Dr. Cailliet,[28] and a short, stable footrest (a stool or hassock that is angled 5 to 15 degrees upward toward the toes and is comfortably wide with a nonskid surface) can help keep your thighs slightly elevated.

To minimize eyestrain, be certain you have good lighting (see Chapter 12), and keep your work between midchest and face height whenever possible. This can be accomplished by using an adjustable work surface such as a drafting table or slanting desktop or a tiltable screen on a VDT. In general, your desk is the proper height when it allows your hands and forearms to be at comfortable right angles to your body while you are sitting upright and using the desk surface.

Seat yourself squarely; don't slump. Slouching or hunching over not only restricts breathing but also impedes circulation and may put pressure on the heart[29] — and it creates *10 to 15 times* as much pressure on your lower back as does sitting up straight.[30]

Leaning to one side or becoming off-center in any other way shifts the line of gravity and causes problems if you stay in that unbalanced position for very long. Armrests on a chair can relieve about 25 percent of the load on the lower back[31] and help provide stability and support when you are changing to various sitting positions during work time.

It's also a priority to avoid sitting on your wallet, car keys, pens, comb, or checkbook. Several years ago, the *New England Journal of Medicine* published a study showing that, in a number of cases, chronic back pain was completely alleviated for male patients once they simply stopped carrying fat wallets in their back pockets.[32]

After your buttocks and upper legs are centered on the seat, simply let your upper body bend at the thigh/hip joints (*not* the lower spine) as you settle your properly aligned back (and neck if the chair is tall enough) against the seat back.

If you must cross your legs, do it at the ankles. Crossing at the knees misaligns the pelvis and can lead to back tension and pain if you don't change positions frequently enough. Whenever possible, place your feet flat on the floor. Another good option is keeping one foot elevated on a chair rung or placing it slightly forward of the other foot on a small stool.[33]

To find your most centered, unstressed sitting position, first repeat the instructions for balancing the neck: gently lean your head to the left and then to the right; then return to center. Next, lean slightly forward and then back, returning to the spot you sense as the exact central position. To balance your torso, repeat these instructions bending at the hips/thighs.

Perhaps most important of all: Once you've found a chair you really love, leave it. Often.

That's because sitting down all day is stressful, no matter how ideal the chair and work surface design. Make it a priority to get up from your desk at least once every 15 to 30 minutes to take a short work break lasting at least a minute or two (see Chapter 8).

One final factor to consider here is *work station design*. Beyond choosing an adjustable work surface and taking regular work breaks and in addition to dealing with environmental concerns such as noise, lighting, and indoor pollution (addressed in Chapter 12), it's important to create what experts call an *easy-reach circle*. Desk clutter not only is unpleasant to look at but can lead to postural strains as you contort your body searching for, and reaching for, needed items. The materials you must have ready access to throughout the day should be placed within an imaginary arm's reach half-circle to the front of your body when you're seated at your work station or desk.

3. Reading, Writing, and Telephoning

Select positions for these activities with care. When you read — at your desk, on the commuter train, or during air travel — watch out for a retracted or extended head position, protruding or dipped chin, distended neck, tight shirt collars, drooping shoulders, and sunken chest. These imbalances create tension, cut circulation to the eyes and brain, and decrease reading speed and comprehension.

Heighten your sensory awareness to find your own best reading posture. By adjusting your seating arrangement, you may be able to bring reading material up to your field of vision and avoid the strain of dropping your head down to it. Try a bookstand to hold books at a comfortable slant and consider buying a small reading light that clips on to the book (available at bookstores).

When talking on the telephone, bring the handset up to your ear and mouth; *don't* bend your head and neck down to the phone or cradle it between your ear and shoulder by forcing your neck to the side. Use an adjustable shoulder support, hands-free headset, or desktop speaker-phone when you want best posture or need both hands free for desk work during conversations.

4. *Standing*

In the workplace, most of us find it difficult to stand for an extended period of time. Standing fatigue occurs when you remain in a stiff, motionless position, losing energy from tension and blocked circulation in the legs.

For best upright posture, first stand in a relaxed manner, with your feet side by side about shoulder width apart. Slowly shift your weight left and right from your ankles. Notice the precise central point where your weight feels perfectly, evenly balanced between the ball and heel of each foot — carried through the center of your ankles. Once you have found that comfortable, stable position, bend your knees (just enough so that they're unlocked).

Some experts recommend standing in a slight step position, with one foot several inches ahead of the other.[34] Then slowly, gently shift some of your weight from foot to foot, keeping your pelvis level. This keeps leg circulation moving and reduces standing fatigue.

The image of a sky hook may help you keep your chin from pointing forward and thereby retracting your head and tensing your neck. Imagine that the crown of your head is attached to a strong cord extending up in the air to a large balloon. By releasing tension — rather than using force — you allow your head to gently float upward at the crown, with your neck lengthening.

Here are several basic standing position guidelines:

- Let your neck lengthen and become vertical, head floating on top (gently buoyed by an imaginary sky hook), chin slightly in.
- Breathe diaphragmatically — with the lower ribs expanding outward to the sides on each inhalation.
- Feel your spine lengthening, your back widening and flattening, abdomen trim, buttocks tucked in slightly, upper body floating upward from a level pelvis, not tipped forward (with pot belly

and sway back) or backward (with too much buttocks tuck, which keeps the legs off balance).
- Keep your knees slightly unlocked, floating your weight over the center of your ankles and evenly between toes and heels.
- Vary your stance often.

Certain working positions require special attention. For example, whenever you're working at a counter for a long period of time, bend one knee and place that foot up on a short stool or box. This helps reduce strain to the lower back area.[35] Remember not to try to force your body into a better postural position since this overtaxes muscles and quickly tires you out. Instead, use awareness and mental imagery suggestions.

5. Reaching, Bending, and Turning

Here's a cardinal rule for everyday work movements: Whenever you turn to reach for something, take a step in that direction. This helps coordinate and focus your power, integrating the body as it moves, taking strain off back muscles by better using the legs and trunk. When you're reaching, bending, or turning, lead the movement with your head floating upward, followed by your whole body.

6. In the Car

Although they feel comfortable when you slide behind the wheel in the auto dealer's showroom, most car seats force the driver and passengers into a pressured, flexed position with inadequate back support. In fact, automobile seating is so important that the type of car you drive correlates to back pain, says Dr. Jennifer Kelsey, professor of public health at Columbia University.[36]

Motorists commuting to and from work in cars with poor-quality seats faced three times the risk of developing lower-back problems over drivers of many Swedish and Japanese cars. A growing number of automobile manufacturers are offering seats with dozens of easy adjustments for supporting all areas of the back. In terms of comfort and reaction speed when driving, this is an important factor.

Of course, it's rarely worth selling your car just because the seats aren't ideal. In many cases, a small pillow or two can help back support. During long trips, you can incorporate a variety of techniques to avoid postural distress.

Adjust the seat and pillows so that you have the best visibility and easiest access to gauges, mirrors, and controls. For many people it's helpful to move the car seat forward so that the knees are moderately bent. Develop the ability to tense only those muscles necessary for driving control, leaving your shoulders, neck, and back relaxed. And keep revitalizing your posture by taking frequent, brief rest break stops.

7. *Pushing, Pulling, Lifting, Carrying*

Ease in pushing, pulling, lifting, and carrying objects depends on the alignment of your bones so that force can be applied in a balanced way. In pushing and pulling, the center of the height and weight of an object determines how much bend is necessary in the hip, knee, and ankle joints. If you apply power too high or low on the object, the lower back is strained.

When lifting objects you can comfortably manage, avoid unnecessary tension, especially in the neck and jaw, and don't hold your breath. Grasp the object securely, keeping it close to your body's center of gravity, with your feet on either side of it whenever possible. Keep your back straight and lift with your legs.

When carrying objects for a distance, it's also best to hold them near your center of gravity. Keep briefcases, purses, and luggage as light as possible and be sure to switch carrying sides periodically to ease stress. When racing through airport or train terminals, use a cart to move your travel bags without strain.

Posture can be seen as a metaphor for your response to business challenges. With balanced posture, physical activities are more pleasurable, emotions are calmer, thinking becomes clearer, and problems seem more manageable. No matter how you view it, good posture is an essential part of the Performance Edge.

10

Exercise: How to Do It Smarter to Save Time and Increase Benefits

Those who think they have not time for bodily exercise will sooner or later have to find time for illness.

— *Edward Stanley, Earl of Derby, 1873*

CARDIOVASCULAR DISEASE kills virtually half of the people in the United States. If it doesn't take your life, it will probably claim that of the person who works next to you. This year alone, 1.5 million Americans will suffer a heart attack, and 500,000 will die. Strokes will kill another 150,000.

Most of these fatalities are preventable. Part of the answer is an active lifestyle that includes regular, moderate exercise. But there's a problem: Most exercise routines are based on erroneous, obsolete, or incomplete information. Even top corporate executives, who demand high levels of accurate information to run their businesses, generally do not have the same quality of information when it comes to their personal health and fitness programs.[1]

Without realizing it, most businesspeople who exercise are wasting time and missing some — perhaps many — of the benefits. Even in moderate amounts, and without any pomp and ceremony, increased physical activity and exercise will improve the way you look, feel, think, and perform, if you know the right way — the *scientific* way — to do it. In this chapter you'll learn the latest proven strategies for exercising smarter — how to save time, cut injury risks, and increase benefits.

The "Corporate Fitness Explosion": Why the Payoff Has Fallen Short

In recent years, billions of dollars have been spent on corporate fitness programs, and there is a greater awareness of health at work than ever before. Although evidence shows that company-sponsored wellness and fitness programs offer some long-term financial gains,[2] in terms of performance enhancement and increased productivity the payoff has generally been disappointing. Why?

"A number of firms we know of have installed the most expensive state of the art gymnasiums/health centers imaginable," write Warren Bennis and Burt Nanus in *Leaders: The Strategies for Taking Charge.* "At the same time, these companies induce an unbearable amount of stress through prodigious work loads, unhealthy plant conditions, heavy travel schedules, and anxiety-laden situations, all of which nullify the presumed benefits of their formal 'health programs.' "[3]

No matter how well equipped or luxurious the company fitness center is, it's difficult to get even a modest percentage of managers and employees to stick to a serious exercise routine day after day. Instead of overemphasizing fitness *facilities,* companies must begin to offer their employees a wide range of new options for developing day-in, day-out fitness *capabilities.*

"Corporate fitness is not a monolith that requires a multimillion-dollar investment," says Dr. James M. Rippe, a cardiologist who has extensively researched corporate fitness programs. "In a matter of a few weeks, at relatively little cost, innovative practices and programs can be put in place that will have a long-term, positive impact on the health and fitness of employees."[4]

Beyond Toned Muscles and Stamina:
A Long List of Benefits

Good health on the job requires much more than just regular physical activity. Stress management, nutrition, a pollution-free working environment, balanced posture, and a positive mental outlook are among the other pieces of the puzzle.

But aside from those other elements, you can reap many rewards from an exercise program. In fact, fitness is so important to health that a recent national health report warned that physical inactivity should now be considered a major health hazard similar in magnitude to such primary heart disease risk factors as uncontrolled hypertension (high blood pressure), high blood cholesterol, and cigarette smoking.[5]

Physical activity and regular, moderate exercise increase circulation, tone muscles, build stamina, reduce resting heart rate and blood pressure, strengthen the heart, increase lung capacity and transport/utilization of oxygen, improve blood cholesterol ratios, increase protection against heart attack and stroke, and may decrease the risk of certain cancers.[6]

Research at New York University Medical School and other centers suggests that more than 80 percent of all lower back pain may be due to lack of exercise rather than pathology,[7] and fitness routines can increase bone density and help prevent osteoporosis.[8]

Regular exercise, especially aerobics, is one of the keys to losing excess body fat and can provide a powerful antidote to fatigue, says Dr. Per-Olof Åstrand, a top exercise physiologist from Sweden.[9] Other documented benefits include increases in mental alertness, self-esteem, cognitive abilities, sensory awareness, reaction speed, and physical coordination[10] and a slowing down of the aging process.[11] One recent major study, published in the *Journal of the American Medical Association,* reports that men and women with low physical fitness levels are more than twice as likely to die prematurely as are people with moderate physical fitness levels.[12]

Increased Creativity and Mental "Toughening"

The right kind of regular exercise may increase your work performance in some surprising new ways. Research indicates that in many cases the greater your level of aerobic fitness, the greater your nervous system's ability to handle emotional stress.[13] Regular aerobic exercise also results in an increased ability to rapidly recover from stress, creating a kind of "mental toughening" that promotes increased competence in staying on top of pressure situations.[14] This discovery comes from a series of studies directed by Richard Dienstbier, professor of psychology at the University of Nebraska and recent visiting scholar at Cambridge University in England.

Dienstbier theorizes that regular aerobic exercise increases the amount of glucose available to the brain, enabling you to respond more energetically and appropriately to challenges. Another reason for a connection between fitness and stress management, according to cardiologist Robert S. Eliot, is that "exercise appears to burn up excess stress chemicals by using them for energy expressed outwardly (rather than harming the body internally)."[15]

In addition, regular exercise increases mental creativity in the workplace,[16] says Thomas E. Backer, research professor at the UCLA School of Medicine. "In working with thousands of creative people, I now recommend a regular exercise program as the single best way both to increase resistance to stress and to facilitate personal creativity."[17]

When to Seek Medical Advice About Exercise

Do you need a medical examination and exercise tolerance test (ETT) before beginning a fitness program? The answer, say the experts, is maybe. It depends on which medical authority you listen to and on the common sense and balance of the program you choose.

The National Heart, Lung, and Blood Institute advises that if a person is at low risk for heart disease and has no symptoms, he or she does not need to see a physician before starting a moderate exercise routine.[18] The American Heart Association simply states that "older sedentary individuals may . . . wish to seek medical advice."[19]

According to the American College of Sports Medicine, apparently healthy individuals under age forty-five with no major coronary risk factors — family history of high blood pressure, heart attack, or premature cardiovascular disease (prior to age fifty); history of high blood pressure above 145/95; elevated total cholesterol/HDL cholesterol ratio above 5 for males or 4.5 for females; abnormal electrocardiogram; cigarette smoking; or diabetes mellitus — can usually start an exercise program without undergoing an ETT "as long as the exercise program begins and proceeds gradually and as long as the individual is alert to the development of unusual signs or symptoms."[20] Individuals at higher risk (above age forty with two or more coronary risk factors) or individuals at any age with symptoms suggestive of metabolic, pulmonary, or coronary heart disease should undergo a physician-supervised exercise tolerance test.

"People often ask, 'Should I have a medical check-up before I start training?' " says Dr. Åstrand. "The answer must be that people who are in doubt about the condition of their health should consult their physician. But as a general rule, moderate activity is less harmful to the health than inactivity. You could also put it this way: a medical examination is more urgent for those who plan to remain inactive than for those who intend to get into good physical shape!"[21]

Certainly you should consult your physician if you have any medical symptoms, are undergoing treatment for any ailment, or have one or more major coronary risk factors.

Listen to Your Body

Perhaps more than any other guideline for physical activity, "Listen to your body" is a cardinal rule. The best guide to safety in fitness is your self-awareness. Listening to your body takes practice — you have to sharpen your senses and think about how you feel. Appropriate exercise shouldn't make you feel unusually fatigued or sick in any way. If it does, pay attention to the feelings and stop exercising until you can determine that nothing is wrong with your health.

The All-or-Nothing Myth

Let me be clear in stating that fitness comes from more than formal exercise. *The fact is that just being more active brings rewards too.* A wide range of informal activities provide cumulative fitness benefits:[22]

> Taking the stairs instead of an elevator; choosing distant parking spots over close ones; walking or cycling to and from work or on errands; actively gardening with hand tools; cutting, splitting, carrying, or stacking firewood; doing household chores; getting out of your chair and moving around on work breaks; taking early morning or evening strolls; doing light, impromptu calisthenics while talking on the phone; playing half-court basketball games; taking weekend hikes; and so on.

An active lifestyle is a cornerstone of lifelong good health *and* highly productive work. There's little value in spending your money and time doing a formal regimen you detest. Therefore, the goal of this chapter is to offer a variety of insights on fitness and to provide you with a collection of "scientific shortcuts" to increase your exercise benefits.

Exercising Smarter: Five Priorities

An excellent, enjoyable physical fitness program takes an average of only 25 to 35 minutes a day and includes five types of exercise:

1. Breathing enhancement
2. Abdominal fitness
3. Flexibility and posture exercises

4. Aerobics
5. Muscular strength and endurance training

In my recent book *Health & Fitness Excellence: The Comprehensive Action Plan* (Houghton Mifflin, 1990), I present a detailed, illustrated program. Here are the five Performance Edge strategies for all of us who want the best possible results in minimum time.

1. Breathing Enhancement

We each breathe about 20,000 times every day, and we assume that we take in plenty of oxygen. But the fact is that most of us breathe just deeply enough to keep from falling over unconscious. Although we remain technically "alive," we don't supply our brain with optimal levels of oxygen.[23]

Why is the problem so widespread? Because of a common habit — shallow, upper-chest breathing. Here's a startling estimate: Blood is flowing at the comparative rate of about one tablespoon a minute at the top area of your lungs, about one pint a minute in the middle area of your lungs, and about one quart a minute at the bottom of your lungs.[24] Upper-chest breathing automatically leaves you underoxygenated.

At least one-fourth of the oxygen in every breath you take is needed to fuel the central nervous system.[25] With shallow breathing, you silently strangle yourself. Poor posture, tense muscles, and lack of fitness make things even worse, further restricting blood flow to the brain.

Poor breathing also contributes to high blood pressure. "If we don't take in enough oxygen by breathing, our blood has to circulate more rapidly to compensate and carry the same amount of oxygen," reports James J. Lynch of the Center for the Study of Human Psychophysiology at the University of Maryland School of Medicine, after studying more than a thousand people over a five-year period. "This can result in an increase in blood pressure, because our blood has to move faster to maintain the oxygen supply."[26]

Here's a fast, simple exercise to improve your breathing: Sit or stand with good posture — your head up, neck long and relaxed, chin slightly in, shoulders broad and loose, and back straight. Place your hands lightly around the sides of your lower ribs with the fingertips pointing in toward the front centerline of the body, and with your thumbs to the rear. Slowly inhale.

As the abdomen expands slightly downward and forward (with the lower back staying flat), feel your lower ribs move out to the sides. Then, as you complete the breath in, feel your chest expand comfortably. Exhale slowly, releasing muscle tension. Repeat the exercise several times a day.

2. Scientific Shortcuts to a Slim, Toned Abdomen

You may be surprised to learn that the two most popular abdominal exercises, traditional sit-ups and leg-lifts, don't slim the waistline, no matter how many you do. In fact, they often cause or aggravate lower back pain.[27] Sit-ups and leg-lifts pull on the front of the lower spine, causing pelvic tilt — with your back swayed in and the lower abdomen pushing out — and contributing to a "pot belly" appearance.

The *transpyramid exercise* is one example of the abdominal exercises that are overlooked by popular fitness programs but are far better and easier than sit-ups and leg-lifts if you want a strong, slim, toned waist.[28] Here's how to do the transpyramid exercise:

Sit or stand with balanced posture. Place your hands on your hips, thumbs pointing to the back. Slowly exhale and, as you reach the place where you normally finish breathing out, smoothly and forcefully breathe out more, lifting up with the lower abdominal muscles. Use your hands to help gently push up on the abdomen. You can feel the transversalis and pyramidalis muscles working — this is the only way to exercise them and strengthen your lower abdomen.

Now relax and take several normal breaths. Then repeat the transpyramid exercise. Be careful not to hyperventilate and become dizzy. Do this exercise two to five times twice a day.

One other tip: If you're doing other abdominal exercises (such as abdominal roll-ups and reverse trunk rotations), don't do them every day. You'll get better, faster results by doing them *less* often;

5 to 25 repetitions of each exercise two or three times a week is a good goal.

3. Flexibility and Posture Exercises

The simplest key to increased flexibility is to pay attention to relaxing and balancing your posture during each fitness activity. This also helps reduce the risk of injury. In terms of specific guidelines, here are three priorities:

1. *Warm up without stretches.* You may be shocked to learn that it's inadvisable to warm up using stretches of any kind. Stretching cold muscles causes tiny tears in connective tissue and damages your muscles and joints.[29] Instead, mimic your sport or activity with smooth movements to warm the muscles and bring up your heart rate. Examples: spend several minutes going through a relaxed rowing motion, jogging slowly, swimming several easy laps, or cycling at reduced speed.
2. *Keep joints loose and flexible throughout the workday.* It's a good idea to take 20 to 30 seconds several times every hour or so to go through some dynamic flexibility exercises — moving your fingers, wrists, elbows, shoulders, neck, hips, knees, ankles, and feet. To remain flexible and healthy, these joints must be used every day.
3. *Strengthen your neck posture.* To improve your neck posture at work, perform a simple head nod exercise every morning and afternoon. A little-known muscle called the rectus capitus anterior is attached to the top of the spine and base of the skull. It flexes and rotates the head. Perhaps most important, it helps you maintain the buoyant, relaxed neck posture that is essential for best blood flow to the brain and senses.

    You can perform this simple exercise in a comfortable sitting or standing position: Place your hands — thumbs facing to the rear — on the rear base of the skull just behind and above your earlobes. (Once you've had some practice, you can skip using your hands to assist in the exercise and do it inconspicuously at work.) Let your neck lengthen, gently extending upward as if lifted by an imaginary sky hook attached to the top of your skull. With your neck in this slightly up position, nod your head as if in agreement, bringing the forehead a little forward and chin slightly in. Repeat this nodding motion several times. Then take an extra moment to become more aware of your neck alignment (discussed in Chapter 9). Do this simple neck-strengthening exercise five or six times during the day.

4. Aerobic Exercise: Seven Maxims

Aerobic exercise tops the list in terms of importance to your heart and lungs — and for burning excess body fat. Outdoor aerobic exercise options include walking, cross-country skiing, cycling, jogging, running, rowing, roller skating, ice skating, canoeing, and kayaking. Indoor choices include cross-country ski machines, stair climbers, stationary cycles, rowing machines, aerobic dance, roller skating, jumping rope, walking or jogging on a treadmill, and so on.

Aerobic means "with oxygen." Aerobic exercises increase your body's ability to deliver maximum amounts of oxygenated blood to exercising muscles and increase the ability of muscles to extract oxygen from the blood to make energy.

It's interesting to note that one of the first signs of improved aerobic fitness is a lowered *resting heart rate*. Elite athletes in endurance sports can become so well conditioned that they have resting heart rates between 30 and 45 beats per minute. People who have developed good cardiovascular fitness from regular aerobic exercise will generally have a heart that beats 45 to 50 times a minute when at rest, pumping at least the same amount of blood as does an unconditioned person's heart beating 75 to 80 times a minute. Result: Over the course of a day, the unconditioned person's heart must beat 50,000 times more than a conditioned person's heart.[30] In a year, that's a workload of 17 million extra beats that an unfit person's heart must provide!

More than 90 percent of Americans don't do aerobic exercise — and the majority of the other 10 percent don't do it correctly and can end up missing many of the benefits. Effective aerobic exercise is based on seven simple scientific maxims:

Principle #1. Exercise at a *steady, rhythmic, very comfortable pace.*

Begin gradually. Listen to your body. Stop at the first sign of any serious discomfort or pain.

Principle #2. Choose an exercise intensity that allows you to work steadily while still being able to talk without gasping for breath. This is known as the "talk test" and will help you stay within your "target heart rate zone," the intensity at which you receive greatest benefits.

During aerobic exercise sessions, it can be helpful to know your *pulse rate range* — the precise number of heartbeats per minute where you're most likely to be in the benefit zone. A sensible aerobic intensity level for many of us is 65 to 75 percent of our predicted maximal heart rate (PMHR).

To calculate your PMHR, subtract your age from 220 (Dr. Kenneth Cooper at the Institute for Aerobics Research recommends that people already in moderately good physical condition should subtract half their age from 205). Then multiply your PMHR once by .65 and once by .75 to find the lower and upper limits of your central target heart rate zone. These figures fall within the latest guidelines from the American College of Sports Medicine, the Institute for Aerobics Research, and the American Heart Association.

Take your pulse at the radial artery of the wrist shortly after beginning to exercise, again at a midway point in the aerobic session, and once more when cooling down. Count for 15 seconds (starting with the first beat as zero, not one) and then multiply by 4. This gives you an estimate of your heart rate per minute. You can quickly learn to ease off or work harder during aerobic exercise sessions so that you keep your heart rate "in the training zone" for greatest benefits.

You may want to invest in an electronic heart rate monitor. While not essential, these high-tech devices can prove helpful. The best pulse monitors have sensing mechanisms that attach with a comfortable elasticized strap directly to your chest and feature a remote, wristwatch-type monitor. They are accurate and can be easily programmed to monitor your upper and lower target heart rate zone limits, sounding a warning beep when you drop below the lower threshold or exceed the upper.

Principle #3. Whenever possible, perform aerobic exercise either three times a week for 30 minutes each session or four times a week for 20 minutes each session. But *don't* get stuck counting minutes. If on some days you can get in only a few 5-minute mini-walks or slip off to climb several flights of nearby stairs once in the morning and again after lunch, then by all means do it. Increased overall physical *activity* — not a rigid exercise regimen — is the foundation of lifelong fitness.

Moreover, new studies suggest that for body fat control one of the smartest exercise strategies is to simply increase your physical activity level for 2 to 5 minutes after every meal and snack (see Chapter 11 for nutritional guidelines). This brief after-meal break to walk, climb a flight of stairs, do some light calisthenics, or pedal on a stationary cycle boosts your body's metabolism and helps burn fat calories.

Principle #4. Precede each aerobic session with a *warm-up* that mimics your activity or sport, moving around at an easy pace.[31] Spend at least 3 minutes — and remember not to do stretches.[32]

Then follow each aerobic session with a 3-to-5-minute *cool-down.* Keep moving, and let your heart rate gradually return to normal. Dr. Kenneth Cooper's research team suggests that if your heart rate isn't below 120 beats per minute (or less than 100 if you're over fifty years old) after 5 minutes of cool-down, then your workout was too strenuous.

The cool-down period, brief though it is, is critical for health safety because it allows the body to return gradually to its pre-exercise state. The basic guiding principle is never to stop exercising suddenly. The drop in blood pressure that occurs during the cool-down period should take place gradually, so keep moving, swiftly at first and then at a slower pace.

Don't stand still, sit down, start talking to a friend, or get distracted in any other way from a sensible cool-down period of up to 5 minutes — longer if you end your aerobic workout with a final burst of speed. When you take your pulse, learn to check it while moving rather than standing motionless.

Principle #5. Avoid competitive thoughts. When you exercise, don't use competitive words like *harder, faster,* or *better.* A recent study shows that such terms can increase hormone stress on the heart[33] and reduce benefits to your blood cholesterol profile.[34] Instead, use words like *calm, steady,* and *relaxed.* This will also help you enjoy the exercise more and may protect benefits to your HDL (good) cholesterol level.

Principle #6. Replace fluids. Drink plenty of extra water before and after your exercise sessions. Losses of only 1 percent of body fluid from sweating can cut strength, speed, endurance, and the heart's output capabilities.[35] Studies recommend cool water, since it enters the digestive tract faster than tepid or warm liquids.

Principle #7. Cross train. Pick several different aerobic activities you enjoy and alternate them. For example, walk, swim, or cross-country ski on one day, and then cycle or row on the next. This variety is rewarding for both the body *and* the mind.

5. Muscular Strength and Endurance Training

Muscular strength and endurance exercises are increasingly popular in corporate fitness programs — and for good reason. More than 400 muscles keep your body firm or let it sag. If those muscles aren't made strong and balanced in relation to each other — and kept that way through an active lifestyle and some regular exercises — they become flabby and slowly wither away as time goes by.

Abdominal exercises and posture exercises strengthen certain key muscles. Aerobic fitness programs build strength and endurance, too, sometimes in isolated body areas (such as the legs in cycling, running, skating, or walking) and sometimes in several muscle groups (such as the arms, shoulders, back, and legs in cross-country skiing or rowing).

But for overall fitness, we each need to take additional steps to make certain that we're shaping and toning the majority of our 400 skeletal muscles, not just a handful, and doing it as quickly and enjoyably as possible.

The dividends are many. With healthy, well-toned muscles, your body is balanced and better coordinated. Since muscle is the chief energy burner in the body, toned muscles will help you burn more excess body fat 24 hours a day. You will have an increased ability to resist work fatigue, and your joints will become well protected against common strains and pains that debilitate millions of businessmen and businesswomen.

To achieve balanced results, without any weak points, first take a look at what strength and endurance benefits you're already receiving from other parts of your lifestyle activities and fitness program. Then choose the fastest, easiest ways to take care of those muscles not yet being toned.

Option 1: The minimum. This is the best strategy if you feel especially pressed for time. Step back and survey your weekly fitness schedule.

Select activities and aerobic exercises that build strength and endurance in the greatest number of body areas. Cross-training — choosing several different aerobic activities every week — is better than sticking with one type of exercise. Some combined upper body–lower body aerobic sports are (alphabetically): aerobic dance with hand or wrist weights; cross-country skiing or indoor cross-country ski machines; jumping rope with a weighted rope; outdoor rowing or indoor rowing machines; integrated stationary cycling (on special cycles where you pedal with your legs and push-pull with your arms using resistance levers); swimming; or walking or jogging with light hand or wrist weights.

In addition, wisely choose recreational activities that strengthen whichever major muscle areas (shoulders, chest, upper arms, forearms, back, abdomen, thighs, and lower legs) you don't catch with your regular fitness activities.

For example, if your favorite aerobics choice is legs-only cycling or walking, select complementary formal or informal recreational activities — such as tennis, racquetball, squash, handball, canoeing or kayaking (on peaceful waters), softball, or basketball (using both hands and both arms to paddle, hit, catch, or throw), golf (as long as you carry your own clubs), or splitting and stacking firewood. In other words, choose activities in which you use your muscles to reach, lift, rotate, push, and pull in different ways from your daily activities and aerobic exercise sessions.

Option 2: More comprehensive strength and endurance training. For best overall fitness, at some point you'll want to take strength and endurance training at least one step further. That means scheduling some weekly time — a lot less than most of us think — for specific resistance exercises. These may be performed without equipment (body weight resistance or dynamic isometrics) or with equipment (rubber tubing, dumbbells, barbells, or machine weights). An illustrated, step-by-step program is included in my book *Health & Fitness Excellence: The Comprehensive Action Plan* (Houghton Mifflin, 1990).

For tips on exercising while on business trips, see Chapter 15.

When all is said and done, the most important basic fitness principle is *Get up and move more*. Build strength and aerobic endurance first and foremost by finding ways to incorporate a greater variety of pleasurable physical activities into your daily life. Think of it as a special personal and family priority and as a means to increase your health and stamina on the job. And when it comes to formal types of exercise, learn the facts and then choose those that you enjoy and need the most.

11

Nutrition: Healthful, High-Stamina Eating

Tell me what you eat, and I will tell you what you are.
— *Anthelm Brillat-Savarin (1755–1826)*

YOUR DIET has a major effect on your work performance. Until recently, a statement like this seemed little more than trite speculation. A passing fad, perhaps. But a number of new research studies confirm that what, when, and how much you eat not only affects your health[1] but exerts a powerful influence on your mental and physical alertness, energy, stamina, and productivity.[2]

Seven Dietary Priorities

By scientific standards, the average American diet still falls short. In *Health & Fitness Excellence: The Comprehensive Action Plan,* I have written extensively about optimal nutrition. In terms of fueling top-level work performance, a healthful diet is founded on the following seven basic principles.

1. Eat an Exceptionally Varied Diet

An optimal diet consists of wholesome, fresh foods — high in complex carbohydrates and fiber, moderate in protein, and low in fat, cholesterol, and salt.

Leading researchers and health organizations now advise[3] moving toward a vegetarian diet (including whole grains, beans and legumes, fruits, vegetables, and low-fat or nonfat dairy products) or semivegetarian diet (a vegetarian diet plus limited amounts of skinless poultry or fish and little, if any, beef or pork). In addition, you should limit the amount of refined carbohydrates (simple sugars), alcohol, and caffeine that you consume.

Despite increased awareness about the basic principles of a good diet, a recent Gallup poll sponsored by the American Dietetic Association indicates that only 5 to 8 percent of people are actually eating more whole grains, legumes, fruits, and vegetables.[4]

An exceptionally varied diet — this means real *biological* variety, not a dozen different snack foods — improves your digestion, expands and pleases your food tastes, increases availability of nutrients, and aids in controlling excess body fat. A healthful diet includes an assortment of different whole grains (eaten as breads, pasta, side dishes, and in soups or casseroles), a variety of legumes (beans, peas, and lentils), and a diverse mixture of your favorite fruits and vegetables.

2. Eat Smaller Amounts of Food More Often

For best health and performance, eat frequent small meals and light snacks five or six times a day. Of course, this doesn't mean eating large main meals and then adding snacks or junk food treats. Rather, you should improve the quality — and cut back on the size — of breakfast, lunch, and dinner and *then* add some light between-meal snacks.

Recent research published in the *New England Journal of Medicine* indicates that such an eating pattern can lower blood cholesterol levels, lessen the risk of heart disease, increase metabolism, and boost energy.[5] With this plan, the body's digestion, absorption, and metabolism function more efficiently, contributing to a steady supply of energy and improved mind power, emotional control, and physical effectiveness.

"Millions of Americans have fallen into a pattern of too-late-for-breakfast, grab-something-for-lunch, eat-a-big-dinner, and nib-ble-nonstop-until-bedtime," writes *New York Times* health columnist Jane Brody. "They starve their bodies when they most need fuel and stuff them when they'll be doing nothing more strenuous than flipping the TV dial or pages of a book. When you think about it, the pattern makes no biological sense."[6]

Large meals swamp your digestive system and interfere with absorption of nutrients. It's easier for the gastrointestinal tract to absorb nutrients from small amounts of food every two to three hours during the day.

When you eat too much at a sitting, you experience what is called a postprandial dumping syndrome — lots of blood is drawn to the digestive tract. When this happens after a large business meal, for example, there's not enough blood flowing to your brain or muscles to supply energy, and you experience a kind of after-meal stupor that can severely limit your effectiveness. Even worse, when the meal is high in fat and refined foods, it can cause fatigue that lasts for hours, sabotaging your thoughts, feelings, and productivity.[7]

Skipping meals — such as breakfast or lunch — hurts your productivity and, contrary to popular opinion, triggers biochemical and hormonal changes in the body that make it more difficult (rather than easier) to lose excess body fat and control your weight. And skipped or delayed meals often cause blood sugar levels to drop below normal, resulting in fatigue, loss of concentration, headaches, weakness, hunger, and added stress.[8]

According to experts, eating frequent, small, low-fat meals and light snacks not only boosts job performance (as noted in Chapter 8) but also is one of the most powerful strategies for winning the war against excess body fat.[9] "Guard against generation of new fat cells by avoiding large intakes of food at one time," says Dr. Peter D. Vash, endocrinologist, eating disorders specialist, and faculty member at the UCLA Medical Center. "Space smaller meals throughout the day. This tactic reduces the hormonal signal that causes fat cells to divide and multiply."[10]

Overall, daily caloric intake should be adequate to maintain your desired body weight. For a rough estimate of daily calorie needs for a generally healthy adult, multiply body weight in pounds times 12 for sedentary people, times 12 to 15 for low-to-moderate-activity people, times 15 to 18 for moderately to very active people, and times 18 or more for extremely active people and serious athletes. Compare this figure with your normal daily calorie intake.

3. Control the Fat in Your Diet

Today, the average American diet still includes more than 40 percent of its total calories from fat — nearly twice the amount recommended by many experts. Even if you are cutting back on salad dressings, butter, and margarine, you probably still eat far more fat than you realize because it's hidden in so many foods.

In the average diet, margarine, butter, mayonnaise, salad oils, frying oils, and shortening make up about 10 to 20 percent of fat intake. Fats in red meat, poultry, and fish account for about 30 to 40 percent of average dietary fat. Real and imitation dairy products constitute another 15 to 25 percent, and most of the remainder of fat comes from eggs, nuts, seeds, and other sources.

High-fat diets are linked to cancers of the breast, colon, prostate, endometrium (uterus lining), ovary, pancreas, and lung;[11] autoimmune disorders;[12] cardiovascular diseases including atherosclerosis (buildup of plaque in the arteries) and hypertension.[13] High-fat diets have also been associated with poor calcium absorption.[14]

Overall, one of your most important nutritional decisions is to control the amount of dietary fat you consume. By eliminating excess fat from your diet, you can improve your health and performance and halt unnecessary body fat gain. Futhermore, the fear that all carbohydrates — especially "starches" such as potatoes, rice, and whole-grain breads — can turn quickly into fat is unfounded. "We don't make fat from carbohydrate," says Dr. Elliot Danforth, director of clinical research at the University of Vermont, Burlington. "We make body fat from ingested fat."[15]

There are no panaceas when it comes to dietary fat — the truth is that most of us still need to cut back on fat intake in general.

But "cut back" doesn't mean "cut out." *Some* dietary fat is essential, although a small but growing number of experts recommend a mere 10 to 15 percent of total daily calories from fat.

In general, a reasonable goal seems to be an average for adults of between 20 and 25 percent of average total daily calories from fat, including about one-third as polyunsaturates, one-third or less as saturates, and the balance as monounsaturates.[16]* To calculate 25 percent of total daily calories in grams of fat per day, multiply your total daily caloric intake by .25 and divide the result by 9. Examples: At 2,000 total calories per day, fat intake should not exceed 55.5 grams; at 2,500 total daily calories, fat should not top 69.4 grams.

Reduce dietary fat intake by reading labels, using a food scale to weigh portions and a cookbook that lists the fat content in each recipe, cooking and sautéing with vegetable broths instead of fat, using nonstick sprays and pans, adding garlic, onions, and a variety of spices to enhance the flavor of low-fat recipes, choosing low-fat or nonfat dairy products instead of whole milk, cream, or high-fat cheeses, and so on.

Note: Beware of snacks and other packaged foods listing "pure vegetable oil" as an ingredient. Coconut, palm kernel, and palm oils are 86, 81, and 49 percent saturated, respectively.[17] The first two are even more saturated than beef fat and lard. And don't be misled by the "cholesterol-free" claim. While these three vegetable oils don't contain cholesterol, they do raise cholesterol levels in the blood.

4. Reduce the Cholesterol in Your Diet

If you don't smoke, elevated blood cholesterol is the greatest threat to your health because it can clog arteries and cause heart attacks. The cholesterol in the blood — measured in milligrams per deciliter (mg/dL) — is characterized by three major types of lipopro-

---

* More than 90 percent of dietary fat is composed of complex molecules consisting of three fatty acids — saturated, monounsaturated, and polyunsaturated. Animal fats usually contain a high percentage of saturated fatty acids, while most vegetable fats (which include many vegetables, grains, legumes, nuts, and seeds) contain mainly unsaturated (mono- or polyunsaturated) fatty acids.

teins, the compounds that transport the cholesterol around the body: high-density lipoproteins (HDL), low-density lipoproteins (LDL), and very-low-density lipoproteins (VLDL). The total cholesterol content in the blood — referred to as *total serum cholesterol* — is the sum of all three types of lipoproteins.

LDL cholesterol is generally regarded as the predominant culprit in heart disease.[18] Some LDLs are of great benefit to the body, delivered via receptors to the cells for productive work in cell growth. But other LDLs, teamed with a villainous chemical called apolipoprotein B, adhere to the artery walls specifically in the coronary arteries next to the heart, as part of the formation of a complex substance called plaque. The higher the LDL level in the blood, the greater the risk of heart disease.

VLDL cholesterol is manufactured by the liver and transports various fatty substances such as triglycerides and LDLs. The higher the VLDL level, the more LDL the liver can produce.

HDL cholesterol, often referred to as "good cholesterol," is the protective type. It actually draws cholesterol away from the coronary arteries. In general, therefore, the higher your HDL level, the greater your protection against heart disease.

As a good total serum cholesterol reading, 200 mg/dL has been the target advised by both the American Heart Association and National Institutes of Health in recent years.[19] However, the results of a major new study, published in the *Journal of the American Medical Association,* suggest that a lower level is better. The best total cholesterol level for the average adult may be in the range of 180 to 190 mg/dL or lower, and recommended total cholesterol-to-HDL ratio (which many health organizations now consider the most important cholesterol number) should generally be below 4.6 for males and below 4.0 for females.[20] In addition to providing protection against coronary heart disease, reducing elevated levels of serum cholesterol also reportedly reduces the risks of colorectal cancer.[21]

When you have your blood tested, be certain that your doctor or laboratory is using the reference standard established by the Centers for Disease Control. That is the most stringent standard for accuracy. To be assured that you are receiving a true reading, you may also want to have your cholesterol checked two or three times, at least one month apart, and then average the results.[22]

What are the best ways to control your cholesterol level? According to researchers, LDL production is decreased by regular aerobic exercise (which, as noted in Chapter 10, provides the additional benefit of raising protective HDL levels); effective stress management; and a widely varied vegetarian or semivegetarian diet that is low in fat (especially saturated fat) and refined sugar[23] and includes soluble fiber-rich foods such as vegetables, beans and legumes, grains, and fruits.[24]

The U.S. Senate Select Committee on Nutrition and Human Needs recommends limiting dietary cholesterol intake to less than 100 milligrams (mg) per 1,000 calories, not to exceed 300 mg per day. But a number of authorities now recommend lower limits — in certain cases a total of 100 mg per day or less.[25]

5. Eat Slowly and Relax Before, During, and After Each Meal or Snack

In the midst of the workday when you grab a quick lunch or sit down for an important business meal, do you "hold tension in your stomach"? Most of us do. This muscular tightness restricts circulation and can contribute to digestive disorders, fatigue, cramping, lower back pain, headaches, and other conditions.[26]

Eating speed is another concern. Millions of us "eat on the run" at almost every meal. Even when our schedule doesn't demand it, we hurry. In response to stress, the entire digestive tract experiences a type of shutdown, explains stress researcher Dr. Peter G. Hanson. "People who eat on the run under stress do themselves a lot of harm by forcing food at high speed into their inactive stomachs. Stomach bloating, nausea, discomfort, cramps, and even diarrhea can result."[27] Eating too quickly also contributes to overeating and excess body fat.

6. Drink Plenty of Extra Water Between Meals and Snacks

Water is a forgotten nutrient in most dietary programs and is an important factor in work performance. As discussed in Chapter 8, dehydration causes fatigue, harms physical coordination, and interferes with thinking abilities. And the dehydration problem becomes even worse when we drink beverages with alcohol or caffeine. The easiest way to prevent this problem is to keep a glass or cup of water next to you when you work and make it a new habit to keep drinking some throughout the work shift — a total of six to eight glasses per day is a reasonable goal.

7. It's What You Eat Most of the Time . . .

Of course, by itself, the most ideal diet in the world won't produce maximum work performance. That requires a balanced effort incorporating all of the Performance Edge factors. So it makes little sense to become fanatical about any single piece of the puzzle, such as diet or exercise. By all means choose high day-to-day dietary standards, but build in some flexibility. Dietary "cheating" — eating not-great foods — is usually acceptable on occasion (unless it violates your religious beliefs or the treatment advice of your physician).

Don't abandon social contacts just because meals or snacks offered at friendly gatherings are not ideal. Calmly change whatever you can whenever you can. Holiday recipes, for example, may not always be made from exemplary ingredients, but the love and camaraderie surrounding them provide vital nourishment of their own. As discussed in Chapter 14, family bonds, friendship, laughter, recreation, and other benefits of social get-togethers contribute to self-renewal and good health.

Strategies for Dining Out

Our health is not only in our own hands but in the pots, pans, and buffets controlled by chefs in America's 620,000 restaurants. Chances are that your tight schedule and workplace pressures often make it necessary for you to eat meals and snacks away from home. But there's no reason why dining out has to be a dietary disaster. While many menu items are still loaded with fat and cholesterol, making healthy choices is becoming easier.

Restaurants are adding more fresh salads, seafood, baked potatoes, grain-legume casseroles and side dishes, whole-grain breads, and lower-fat pasta recipes to their menus. Nonetheless, you still need to watch out for hidden fats, especially in prepared cookies, muffins, pie crusts, cream sauces and soups, and cheeses.

High-quality, low-fat dining begins with your selection of restaurant. Skip all-you-can-eat buffets and smorgasbords. Order à la carte since full-course bargain dinners encourage overeating and tend to be too high in fat and protein. If possible, look over the menu in advance or call ahead to ask about featured recipes and daily specials.

Don't be shy about making requests over the phone or in person to the waiter, waitress, or chef — many restaurants will eliminate salt, cook with half the amount of fat (or no added fat at all), and cut back on cheese, eggs, and whole-milk dairy products. Regional offices of the American Heart Association (7300 Greenville Ave., Dallas, TX 75231) print lists of local restaurants serving low-fat meals. Write for details.

Choose entrées that are steamed, poached, broiled, roasted, baked, or cooked in their own juices. Pass up anything fried or sautéed. Good restaurants will broil seafood or poultry dry (without fat) and unsalted and have or will create a special low-fat sauce to your liking. Salads and salad bars can be good choices if the vegetables are actually *fresh,* but steer clear of prepared salads with a cream or heavy oil base since they are usually high in fat. Instead, choose a variety of fresh raw vegetables or fruits, legumes, and whole-grain bread. As a salad dressing, use a very small amount of olive oil with vinegar or lemon added.

The best restaurant soups are vegetable-based since cream- and meat-based soups are usually high in fat. Pasta can be a good choice if served with tomato, wine, or other low-fat sauces. Whole-grain breads, rolls, bagels, and low-fat muffins are delicious sources of fiber and complex carbohydrates, but skip the nut spreads, mayonnaise, butter, and margarine. Hot cereals such as oatmeal and multigrain varieties and whole-grain dry cereals can be a good breakfast choice when served with skim milk and fruit.

When you choose to have dessert, make the portion small. A slice of home-baked pie or cake is all right as a once-a-month option, but on a more frequent basis fresh fruit tops the list, followed by fruit-based frozen sorbet, nonfat frozen yogurt, and low-fat or nonfat puddings.

If you eat out often, you run the risk of consuming excessive fat and protein. Watch quantities — many eateries serve extra-large portions of food. If you're dining with other people, consider having a fresh salad, vegetable/grain/legume side dish, and a piece of whole-grain bread and then splitting a main dish with another person.

Many ethnic restaurants offer exquisite-tasting cuisine featuring whole grains, legumes, vegetables, and fruit and recipes supplemented with fish or poultry. Here are several insights about ethnic specialties.

Italian. Delicious, low-fat foods with a pleasing array of tastes make Italian restaurants a good choice for dining away from home. Pasta with meatless marinara (tomato-based), vegetable, red clam, or wine sauce is first-rate. Shrimp al vino blanco (sautéed in white wine) gets high marks, too, for its low fat content. Pollo cacciatore (boneless chicken breast served in a tomato and mushroom sauce) is another option. The list also includes nonmeat (vegetable) lasagne, and cioppino — fisherman's stew with a variety of seafood and vegetables in a tomato-based stock (make certain it's low in fat). If you enjoy pizza, order it vegetarian (go very light on the olives) with extra vegetables and half or one-third the normal amount of cheese. Onions, green peppers, and mushrooms are standard fare, but try fresh spinach, garlic, tomatoes, artichoke hearts, beans, seafood, skinless turkey or chicken breast, and other ingredients for an inviting change of pace.

Mexican. When chosen with care, Mexican food is inexpensive, delicious, high in complex carbohydrates, and low in fat. Beans, rice, unfried corn tortillas, fish, and salads are common staples. Vegetable-bean burritos, fresh fish marinated in lime sauce, and beans with rice are low-fat specialties. A good practice when selecting a new Mexican-style restaurant is to call ahead and ask if the chef uses lard, coconut oil, or other oils in the refried beans. Many establishments have switched to small amounts of soybean oil or, ideally, no added fat at all. Skip the sour cream, guacamole, meat and egg dishes, and fried foods, and request no more than half the usual amount of cheese.

French. Traditional French restaurants offer rich, delicious foods that are high in fat, calories, and cholesterol. Fortunately, more and more French chefs are preparing nouvelle cuisine, including a special variety called cuisine minceur ("cuisine of slimness"). Cuisine minceur uses culinary techniques such as steaming or poaching seafood or poultry in vegetable juices and wine and serving side dishes of fresh vegetables, potatoes, and grains. For desert, skip the usual fare and request fresh fruit or fruit (usually peaches or pears) poached in a light wine sauce, which gives a delightful taste with few calories.

Indian. The recipes used in Indian restaurants often include vegetables, legumes, yogurt, and lots of spices. Avoid the dishes soaked in coconut oil or ghee (clarified butter). One popular recipe is murg jalfraize — chicken or legumes flavored with fresh spices and sautéed (request no butter or oil) with onions, tomatoes, and bell peppers.

Chinese. Some menu items at Chinese restaurants are good choices because of the emphasis on rice and vegetables with only small amounts of seafood or poultry. Bypass the fried appetizer dishes such as egg rolls and spring rolls. And don't choose duck — three and a half ounces of Peking duck has 30 grams of fat. Stir-fried dishes like moo goo gai pan — a combination of mushrooms, bamboo shoots, water chestnuts, and chicken, seafood, or tofu served over rice — generally get good ratings. At Chinese restaurants, stir-fried dishes tend to be cooked quickly in a lightly oiled, very hot wok, and the vegetables retain more vitamins than those cooked the traditional American way. The oil is usually peanut, which is high in monounsaturates.

Japanese. Generally low in fat, Japanese cuisine is based on protein-rich soybean products (such as tofu and tempeh), seafood, vegetables, noodles, and rice. The seaweed used in Japanese soups and stews is high in minerals. One top entrée choice is yosenabe, a vegetable dish with seafood.

American. Traditional American restaurants have contributed some healthful dishes to the array of dining options, including New England and West Coast seafoods, fresh salad bars, Cajun gumbos, and a variety of new "California cuisine" specialties.

Vegetarian. Although vegetarian restaurants serve nonmeat and even nondairy meals, many dishes tend to be high in fat. Limit your intake of cheeses and avoid items heavy with oil, butter, or cream. Choose fresh whole-grain breads, cooked grain-legume casseroles and side dishes, and rice or pasta with low-fat sauces and a variety of vegetables.

On the Road. When you have to be out of town for a few days, consider bringing along some basics, such as dry cereals, fruit, and nonfat yogurt for breakfasts and whatever you favor for light snacks. Brown-bagging can save you time, money, and needless calories. A small cooler in your car or a hotel room refrigerator can help keep perishables fresh.

If you travel by plane, call ahead to order a special meal for your flight. You can often choose from seafood, vegetarian, kosher, and other options. Some major carriers now offer a seafood platter with vegetables, whole-grain bread, and tomato cocktail sauce; low-fat meals with broiled chicken or fish, vegetables, whole-grain bread, and fruit; or vegetarian platters with vegetables over rice or legumes, a salad, whole-grain bread, and a piece of cheese or fruit; and even a fresh fruit plate.

Remember to drink plenty of water during the flight since aircraft cabin air rapidly dehydrates your body. In general, skip alcoholic beverages, coffee, and tea, since they exacerbate the water loss. A number of air carriers now offer a variety of complimentary bottled spring waters. For more on business travel, see Chapter 15.

Gaining Greater Control of Your Mind and Emotions with Food

One nutrition discovery in particular has tremendous potential implications for business performance. Compelling new research suggests that the foods you choose for meals and snacks may influence production of brain messenger chemicals called neurotransmitters, which in turn affect your mental energy, concentration, attitude, mood, behavior, and performance.

Recent studies at Harvard, MIT, the National Institutes of Health, and other research centers have been published in specialized scientific and medical journals.[28] The results of these studies were recently brought to the public's attention by Judith J. Wurtman, nutritional research scientist at the Massachusetts Institute of Technology.[29] Continued research has shed further light on this exciting subject.[30]

The emerging picture on the mind-mood-food connection suggests the following.

- The wrong personal choices and timing of foods for light meals and snacks may create or contribute to loss of enthusiasm, mental and physical fatigue, and poor performance or tension, anxiety, and irritability.
- The right personal choices and timing of foods for light meals and snacks may create or contribute to a more alert, faster-reacting, more focused, more productive mind or the calm composure for clearest thinking, problem solving, and relaxed emotions.

According to Wurtman and other researchers, mental behavior can be modified, often within 30 to 45 minutes, when the right kind of light snack or small meal is eaten. Neurotransmitters are manufactured by the brain from or in response to constituents of the food we eat.

Before we go any further, one point needs to be made absolutely clear: It would be an egregious oversimplification of human behavior to suggest that mental and emotional states can be controlled by the manipulation of a single aspect of life — *any* aspect. Food is an important consideration, but only one of many. Chapters throughout *The Performance Edge* provide you with scientifically based ways to manage stress and improve your brain/mind power and emotional/attitudinal control. So by all means test the following mind-mood-food principles, but be certain not to overlook the many other aspects of best health and performance.

Foods for increased alertness. Meals and snacks that are low in fat and relatively high in protein may help promote *faster thinking, greater energy, increased attention to detail,* and *quicker reaction speed.* Options for this type of meal or snack include baked or broiled skinless chicken breast, turkey breast, or fish; a bean or lentil salad, soup, or casserole; low-fat or nonfat yogurt or cottage cheese with fruit; or a glass of skim milk with a piece of fruit. In addition to the high-protein food, balance the meal or snack by including vegetables or fruit and some complex carbohydrates such as a piece of low-fat, whole-grain bread, a bagel, muffin, baked pita chips, rye crackers, or a whole-grain side dish.

At all times, avoid high-fat meals and snacks because they cause fatigue. "Fat seems to slow other processes, like thought or movement," says Wurtman. "It makes people very lethargic. During the long digestive process that follows a high-fat meal, more blood is diverted to the stomach and intestines and away from the brain."[31]

The quantities of protein-rich foods necessary to help many people increase mental alertness are very small — 2 to 4 ounces are usually enough, and that is generally consistent with the nutritional recommendations of leading health organizations.

Foods for increased calmness. Meals and snacks that are low in fat and low in protein but high in complex carbohydrates may help produce a *calm, focused state of mind* and *relaxed emotions.* Options for such meals or snacks include cooked whole grains (rice, wheat, oatmeal, corn, buckwheat, barley, and so on) eaten with fruit or a sweetener but without milk; low-fat pasta salad with fruit or vegetables or low-fat, whole-grain bread, a bagel, muffin, baked pita chips, or crackers topped with your favorite all-fruit preserve. Very small amounts of sweets and starches — 1 to 1½ ounces for most people — are usually enough for a calming, focusing effect. Exceptions include people 20 percent or more overweight and women in the days just preceding menstruation, when between 2 and 2½ ounces of carbohydrate-rich food may be required.

Note: A few people have a biological craving for carbohydrates and, rather than being calmed by them, find them energizing. For this small group of individuals, the "sugar buzz" is real. But contrary to popular belief, carbohydrates do not generally cause hyperactivity or increased energy or aggressiveness in normal, healthy people.[32]

Fruits (including the sweetener fructose) and vegetables (except potatoes and corn) appear to be mind-mood *neutral,* say researchers. That is, these foods don't directly affect neurotransmitter production for alertness or calmness and therefore can generally be eaten with either protein-rich or carbohydrate-rich foods.[33]

Test It Yourself

Your success in choosing the right foods and combinations of foods that help you manage your emotions and mind depends on careful observation of your body's responses and habits. Over the next few weeks, take notes on your state of mind and mood 10 to 15 minutes before meals and snacks. Do you feel alert and motivated? Calm and focused? Tense and irritable? One hour after eating, reassess your state of mind and emotions and quickly and honestly write down your observations.

Review your appraisals to create a list of the food choices that seem best for you and use it as a helpful tool in monitoring your day-to-day eating patterns.

The questions surrounding the mind-mood-food connection are complex. The preliminary answers are intriguing and the number of supportive studies is growing. To learn more, see *Managing Your Mind and Mood Through Food* by Judith J. Wurtman (Harper and Row, 1988).

Resources

You don't have to become a biochemist or registered dietitian to select food wisely and use nutrition to help improve your job performance. Nonetheless, it's important to understand the basic principles of nutritional science, especially in light of recent discoveries. In addition to my *Health & Fitness Excellence: The Comprehensive Action Plan* (Houghton Mifflin, 1990), consult the following (listed alphabetically).

- *Controlling Cholesterol* by Kenneth H. Cooper, M.D. (Bantam, 1988). The best book to date about the important issue of cholesterol.
- *America's New Low-Fat Cuisine: Quick and Easy Menus for Health & Fitness Excellence* by Leslie L. Cooper (Houghton Mifflin, 1991). Offers practical suggestions for meal planning and food preparation that match the recommendations given in *Health & Fitness Excellence* and *The Performance Edge*. Features unique 28 meal and snack menus for cool weather and 28 meal and snack menus for warm weather and gives a complete nutritional analysis (including percentages and grams of fat, cholesterol, protein, carbohydrate, fiber, calcium, and sodium) for each

recipe, meal, and snack. Preparation times are given, and an index notes the recipes that can be prepared in 5 to 30 minutes.

- *Jane Brody's Nutrition Book* by Jane E. Brody, rev. ed. (Bantam, 1987). This nutrition fact book by the award-winning *New York Times* health columnist is filled with good, sensible information.
- *Nutrition Wizard* (Center for Science in the Public Interest, 1501 16th St., NW, Washington, DC 20036; 202-332-9110), 1987. Computer software designed by Michael F. Jacobson, a microbiologist from MIT. Nutrition Wizard is intended as a comprehensive program to help people eat a more healthful diet. The first part gives a standard analysis of dietary needs based on age, body size, and activity level. The second part uses a databank with more than 1,700 food items (which can be expanded by the user) to analyze recipes, meals, and an entire day's diet for twenty-five nutritional components, including protein, carbohydrate, soluble and insoluble fiber, fat (polyunsaturates, monounsaturates, and saturates), cholesterol, sodium, and many other minerals and vitamins. Easy to use. Good, clear instructions.

12

Healthy Environments: Simple Steps to Create a More Pollution-Free, Revitalizing Work Space

It is safer and healthier to work in an office than it is to dig in a coal mine or labor in a steel mill. The air is cleaner and the work less strenuous. The noise is less deafening and the temperature more bearable. But the merit of the comparison ends there, for simply being safer and cleaner than a coal mine doesn't make the office clean or safe.

— *Jeanne Stellman, Ph.D., and Mary Sue Henifin, M.P.H.*

THE MODERN OFFICE BUILDING is a monument to energy efficiency and high technology — with ultrathick insulation, airtight windows, reduced-wattage lighting, industrial-grade carpeting, modular furnishings, extensive electrical wiring networks, temperature-controlled, recycled air, and advanced computer systems, copiers, fax machines, and other state-of-the-art office equipment. But many of the very architectural and engineering features that win awards for energy efficiency and office design also lock in toxic fumes and radiation, reduce oxygen levels, spread airborne infections, and create an alarming number of workplace "techno-stresses."

The percentage of people who spend their working days in an office is enormous — and growing faster than the rate for all other occupational workplaces worldwide. As of 1991, more than 40 million people — the majority of working men and the vast majority of working women — will be on the job in offices in the United States. Employment trends in Canada, Europe, and Asia's Pacific rim are similar. Stressful, unhealthy surroundings undercut human performance, dulling innovative thinking, eroding work quality and productivity, and leaving you more vulnerable to other sources of stress.

Alan D. Swain, senior scientist at Argonne National Laboratory in Albuquerque, New Mexico, claims that one mistaken assumption about on-the-job errors is that they are necessarily the fault of employees. He contends that the most critical errors often result from faulty workplace design.[1] Swain categorizes workplace errors as either "situation-caused" or "human-caused."

Analysis suggests that situation-caused errors — those related to the design of the work environment, including noise, lighting, posture, indoor air pollution, and related factors — account for up to half of workplace errors, and the rest are human-caused mistakes. A safe, healthful working environment is an achievable goal for all of us, and there is a growing trend among businesses to "redesign entire environments to stimulate creative productivity."[2]

"Sick-Building Syndrome"

By some estimates, up to half of the work force in Europe and North America may be affected by "sick-building syndrome."[3] The problem not only occurs in buildings constructed in recent years but also plagues stately old buildings that have been renovated. The World Health Organization estimates that at least one-third of all new and remodeled buildings worldwide are "sick."

Energy-tight, sealed windows lock in stale air. Then tobacco smoke and dangerous radon gas can accumulate. New furniture, wall paneling, draperies, and carpeting emit toxic pollutants such as formaldehyde and hydrocarbon gases. Unshielded electrical wiring increases electromagnetic radiation within the work area. Volatile organic compounds in building materials, photocopier toners, cleaning solvents, new paint, varnishes, and carpet adhesives emit toxic fumes that build up over time. Frequent exterminator visits keep baseboards and carpets doused with pest-killing chemicals, many of questionable safety to humans. Particulate matter from cleaning sprays and aerosols irritate the eyes and lungs, and poorly maintained air filters, humidifiers, and cooling towers promote the growth of biological contaminants (including viruses, bacteria, and molds) and increase the spread of airborne infections. All of these factors combine to form an onslaught of known and suspected health and performance problems.

One reason that indoor workplace environments have received scant attention by management is that most of us assume that the biggest pollution threats come from heavily industrialized *outdoor* areas and that it's up to politicians and government agencies to solve the problem.

But new studies by the Environmental Protection Agency show that *indoor* pollution levels in some commercial buildings are up to *100 times greater* than outdoor pollution levels — even in smog-filled industrial areas — and this poses a "serious risk to health."[4] In fact, adds Robert Axelrad, director of the EPA's indoor air division, during periods of peak exposure to chemicals, such as when offices are painted, indoor levels can be as much as 1,000 times higher. A growing number of studies in Europe and America have compared indoor and outdoor pollution and have reached similar conclusions to those of the EPA.[5]

Although Americans spend an estimated 90 percent of their lives indoors, no specific federal regulations have been adopted for control of air in offices. The National Academy of Sciences recently estimated that indoor air pollution may add as much as $100 billion to national health care costs every year.[6] The related costs from absenteeism and diminished productivity run into the hundreds of millions of dollars annually, and potentially damaging lawsuits are on the rise.[7]

The worst workplace pollutants include tobacco smoke, radon gas, ozone, cleaning products, formaldehyde, carbon monoxide, asbestos, pesticides, paints, and solvents. And in most cases the "tighter," more energy-efficient the building, the greater the pollution problem.

Determining the exact extent of health damage from indoor

contaminants will require many years of further study. But the levels of indoor air pollutants recently measured already "suggest significant risks" to health, warns Paul J. Lioy of Rutgers University Medical School. It appears that people who expose themselves even to low-level repeated exposure to common office chemicals may gradually develop subtle brain and nerve impairments.

With some smart, simple steps, it's possible to create a work space that is more healthful, comfortable, quiet, and inviting.

First, adopt a Performance Edge work style: Reduce your exposure to indoor pollution sources and increase available oxygen by opening some windows and taking frequent short breaks to relieve eyestrain, increase circulation, and get some fresh air; improve your nutritional health (and thereby increase your body's protection against pollutants) by eating regular small meals and light snacks; help reduce your risk of fatigue and respiratory infections by preventing dehydration; and begin planning action steps to correct specific pollution problems in your own work area.

Second, if you work for a large organization and have limited decision-making power, link up with co-workers to share information on environmental issues and to promote sensible, progressive changes toward a pollution-free work environment.

The following sections discuss some key issues involved in making workplaces healthy and safe.

Office Ventilation Systems

For many years, scientists and engineers were skeptical about worker complaints regarding the indoor air environment. But not anymore. The poor quality of indoor air in the workplace has finally been recognized as a serious public health threat.

A recent study published in the *Journal of the American Medical Association*, for example, found that people who work in modern buildings come down with respiratory infections 45 percent more often than people in older, nonrenovated structures. Other studies by the National Institute of Occupational Safety and Health (NIOSH) and the Environmental Protection Agency (EPA) confirm that there's a major problem. Research at the Walter Reed Institute of Medical Research in Washington, D.C., recently concluded that in poorly ventilated work environments absenteeism increased nearly 50 percent and productivity levels dropped sharply.

A recent NIOSH study blames about half the cases of unhealthy indoor air on poor ventilation and the other half on a combination of bad air coming in from outside, specific inside pollution sources such as tobacco smoke; microbes such as viruses, bacteria, mold, and fungi; radioactive radon gas; and irritating fumes from copying machines, carbonless paper, pesticides, paint, carpets, draperies, wall paneling, and cleaning solvents.

In poorly ventilated spaces, carbon dioxide becomes concentrated and cuts down on available oxygen. If by midafternoon, after taking Performance Edge Workbreaks as recommended in Chapter 8, you feel yourself becoming drowsy and inattentive, there is a good chance that there's not enough oxygen in your office environment. To increase your productivity and creativity, you may need more fresh air.

The ventilation system is the major determinant of indoor air quality, controlling the amount and cleanliness of outside air that is added to the building's atmosphere and the rate at which the inside air and its pollutants are either recirculated throughout the building or exhausted to the outside air. Opening some windows and increasing other air exchanges, establishing a smoke-free workplace, cleaning air filters, and removing obstacles blocking vents is often enough to make a major difference in cleaning the air.

Other ventilation problems may call for some of the following steps.

- Upgrading indoor climate control, providing a better-ventilated environment that is free from drafts and odors and in which the air is neither noticeably hot nor cold, humid nor dry (by controlling office air humidity, you can also reduce mold and mildew problems)
- Eliminating mold-harboring, virus/bacteria-breeding water in air-cooling, humidifying, and heating systems (where such organisms find fertile breeding grounds when the equipment is turned off at night and on weekends to save energy)
- Moving air-intake ducts away from loading docks (where exhaust fumes from idling trucks are drawn in and circulated through work areas)
- Installing additional windows to provide employees with in-

creased control over air exchange and an important psychological means for "visual escape" during work breaks

Minimizing Sources of Indoor Pollution

You can perform a quick investigation of the air quality in your personal office or work station area with inexpensive universal tester pumps (which have tubes filled with reagents that react with specific chemicals), vapor-monitoring badges, and a variety of detection units that measure carbon monoxide, radon, ozone, formaldehyde, and other contaminants. (For a complete list of sources, see Resources at the end of the chapter.)

Some initial action steps may include the following:

- Regularly cleaning carpets with nontoxic cleaning fluids and then ensuring that they are kept dry. Many illness-causing molds, spores, and fungi prefer moist, dark environments where there is little exposure to sunlight, and office carpets provide the perfect haven.
- Using strategically placed dust-control devices such as electrostatic preciptators and ionizers (filters should be replaced or cleaned regularly in accordance with the manufacturer's instructions).
- Keeping chemicals and cleaning fluids in tightly closed containers in a well-sealed storage closet.
- Choosing low-toxicity paints and other building materials when constructing new facilities, remodeling, or redecorating a work space.

Other principal concerns include the following:

Tobacco smoke. Nearly everyone now realizes that cigarette smoking is a major contributor to the poor quality of indoor air. The gases and particulates emitted by burning cigarettes contain some of the most toxic air pollutants known.

"The right of a smoker to smoke stops at the point where his or her smoking increases the disease risk in those occupying the same environment," concludes a recent report from the U.S. surgeon general.[8] In addition, most of us pay higher taxes and wrestle with exorbitant insurance premiums resulting in part from accidents, diseases, and early deaths attributable to the smoking habits of some policyholders.

From a health perspective, data on the harms of cigarette smoke continue to mount. The National Research Council and National Academy of Sciences have published research reports documenting many of the ways that "passive smoking" (also called "slipstream smoking," "environmental tobacco smoke," and "involuntary smoking") is linked to health risks among nonsmokers.

According to the American Cancer Society:[9]

- Workers who smoke have an absentee rate 30 to 40 percent higher and a 5 percent greater chance of hospitalization than their non-smoking colleagues.
- Thousands of nonsmokers die each year from lung cancer caused by secondhand or passive smoking.
- The cost to the economy each year from smoking is estimated at $38–95 billion by the U.S. Congress Office of Technology Assessment.
- Each smoker costs his or her employer more than $4,000 a year, according to figures compiled by William L. Weis, assistant professor at the Albers Graduate School of Business, Seattle. In addition, a recent study of nearly 4,000 Massachusetts drivers indicated that smokers had 50 percent more car accidents and got 46 percent more traffic tickets than nonsmokers.[10]

See Resources at the end of the chapter for a list of books and other information about smoking in the workplace.

Carbon monoxide. Improperly adjusted, poorly sealed, or inadequately vented heaters using carbon-containing fuels — natural gas, oil, propane, kerosene, and so on — can produce clouds of invisible carbon monoxide (CO) gas that quickly reach levels that are hazardous to health.[11] Stoves and heaters that burn charcoal and wood can also give off CO. Overall, an estimated 2 to 5 percent of workers in America, Europe, and Japan are regularly exposed to indoor CO levels that exceed the government standard.

Smokers and people in the immediate vicinity of smokers are at even greater risk, since burning tobacco can produce blood CO levels equal to or higher than EPA levels, where harm to the nervous system can set in. Carbon monoxide detectors — some as small as a key chain — are now available in pharmacies. They use small ceramic disks that change color when exposed to 50 parts per million or more, the highest CO concentration allowed by law. Although the new units are valuable because they can warn of dangerously high levels of CO exposure, they do not detect chronic low-level concentration, which may be a long-term health risk.

Formaldehyde. This preservative chemical, used in embalming fluids, is found in small amounts in hundreds of consumer and office products in America, ranging from cosmetics, perfumes, and soaps to permanent-press fabrics, upholsteries, resin-treated drapes, carpets, dry-cleaning fluids, and paper towels.[12] Building materials such as laminated wood paneling, plywood, particle board, and urethane foam insulation give off — "out-gas" — formaldehyde.

Formaldehyde is a strong irritant to the respiratory, sensory, and nervous systems and may cause brain damage and cancer. Therefore it's important for all of us to limit our workplace exposure. Improved office ventilation is the first step to take in reducing formaldehyde concentrations. Studies by the National Space Technology Laboratory reveal the surprising fact that certain common plants — notably spider plants (*Chlorophytum comosum*) — may help reduce formaldehyde levels inside closed office spaces.[13] Other common house plants — including dieffenbachia, philodendron, English ivy, and golden pothos — have reportedly been shown by NASA to help filter office air of harmful chemicals, including formaldehyde, benzene, and trichloroethylene (TCE), a solvent.[14]

Chemicals from office equipment and supplies. Many of the business machines and office supplies that we've come to depend on in recent years can be persistent sources of low-level indoor pollution.

Ozone, a sweet-smelling gas, is given off by office equipment that uses a high voltage, including photocopiers. This chemical can impair lung function and decrease the body's resistance to infection.[15] Ozone decomposes to oxygen in a relatively brief time, usually between 3 and 15 minutes. The principal solution to ozone exposure (and related photocopier problems, including heat) is limiting copy machine usage and ensuring adequate ventilation as well as making certain that no one is required to sit near the exhaust of a photocopier.

Carbonless paper, a popular office paper, has been responsible for a large number of health complaints and skin reactions,[16] and a recent report in the *Journal of the American Medical Association* indicates that in some people the allergic lung reaction can be so severe that it is life-threatening.[17]

Other office chemicals. Although the risks appear to be relatively minor during routine usage, potentially toxic chemicals — such as chloroethylene, formaldehyde, and epoxies — are found in a wide range of office products, including glues, cements, cement thinners, solid air fresheners, and liquid correction fluids. If you have suspicions that any of these chemicals may be presenting a problem where you work, contact the appropriate government agency listed at the end of this chapter.

New Light on Workplace Lighting

There is a direct relation between lighting and work productivity. More than a dozen studies confirm that, in general, the brighter the room light, the better the workers' performance.[18] The optimal level of light depends on the visual preferences and capabilities of the individual or work team and the type of work being performed.

To accommodate such variations, a good lighting system will allow individuals to control how much light they get for particular tasks. Overhead lighting fixtures should constitute only part of the light source and that the balance of the light should come from individual lamps or lighting fixtures, a design referred to as *non-uniform lighting.*[19]

"There seem to be increases in activity and productivity right until you reach the level of glare," says Jean Wineman, professor of architecture at Georgia Institute of Technology.[20] There is "a great preference for natural lighting, far beyond the contribution made by that light." The presence of windows generally helps people feel and perform better.

Eyes work best for distant seeing and must exert extra effort to focus on close work, which, without frequent breaks to rest and change eye focus to more distant objects, strains the eyes. "Some architects use the phrase 'designed for visual release,'" says Calvin W. Taylor of the University of Utah. "Physiologically, our eye muscles relax if we are looking at a far-distant view, and this effect can lead to a more generally relaxed state of the person. The physiological release or relaxation of the eye muscles often has a concomitant mental release, which can free the mind to think."[21]

Priorities for best work lighting include the following:

- An ideal lighting system will combine natural and artificial light, avoid glare (using diffusion shields and nonreflective work station surfaces), reduce shadows, and allow the individual to control at least half of his or her lighting using direct sources such as swing-arm lamps.
- To make best work use of available lighting and to reduce fatigue, maintain good posture — with relaxed muscles in the shoulders, neck, and face (which helps assure best blood flow to the brain and eyes).
- Make it convenient to select the brightest comfortable level of lighting when reading and working — in many cases, incandescent lighting is superior to unshielded fluorescent lighting in which visible flicker can be "extremely annoying and cause visual discomfort."[22] When working at a VDT, use a tiltable screen with an antiglare hood and filter that rid the monitor of "visual noise," annoying reflections of indoor and outdoor light. And choose bright, shielded direct lighting to illuminate source material next to your computer.
- Hold reading material at the proper focal length and on an angle, not horizontal. Use a clipboard, copy stand, lap desk, or adjustable book holder to make reading easiest.
- Avoid glare — high-gloss paper increases eyestrain.
- If you are nearsighted, don't wear your distance glasses for reading unless advised to do so by your ophthalmologist or optometrist; if you wear contact lenses, realize that you blink less often when you concentrate, so blink often to prevent dry eyes.
- Take frequent breaks (for a minute or more at least once every half hour) to look at distant objects and to change your visual focus and relax the eyes (see Chapter 8).

The Noise-Health-Performance Link

Loud noise is the most prevalent workplace pollution in America, and it's a primary contributor to on-the-job errors.[23] It not only damages hearing but is a psychological stressor, interfering with speech and the ability to think clearly, altering moods, reducing learning abilities, and increasing blood pressure.[24]

Columbia University researchers have repeatedly found that of all environmental factors, noise in the office has the strongest correlation with job dissatisfaction and with certain stress effects, such as irritation and anxiety.[25] More than 25 percent of complaints with the work stations studied by the researchers could be attributed to noise.

Loud noise (above 80 decibels, which includes the roar of traffic or factory machinery) and noise that may be less loud but still irritating can produce harmful physical and mental effects.[26] The sustained low-level din of urban life — moderately loud rush hour traffic, for example — can gradually destroy your hearing. This "hidden noise" has an insidious cumulative effect. The American Speech and Hearing Association estimates that 40 million Americans live or work every day around noise that is dangerously loud.

Here are some simple suggestions for reducing noise in your work environment:

- Become sound conscious, reducing or eliminating noise whenever and wherever it's reasonable to do so. Begin by noticing foot traffic routes that pass near your work area. If they are disturbing to you, take action — if possible by rerouting them. If this isn't feasible, move your work station or install carpeting, rugs, extra wall insulation, or noise-absorbing acoustical barriers to reduce sound intensity in and around your work area.
- Before buying new office equipment, compare noise levels and select a quieter model with a "sound reduction option."
- Put sound-absorbing foam pads under office machines such as typewriters, postage machines, addressing machines, and computer printers.
- Wear hearing protection whenever you must be near loud or even moderately loud noises.

Reducing Job-Related Radiation Risks

One of the most serious workplace pollution problems is radiation, which can be divided into two basic categories:

High-frequency *ionizing (atomic) radiation,* including radon gas,
x-rays, gamma rays, alpha and beta particles, and neutrons
Low-frequency *nonionizing radiation,* emitted from visible light,
electric power line emissions, televisions, computer terminals
(VDTs), ultrasound devices, microwave equipment, radio waves,
and radar

Ionizing radiation. The effects of ionizing radiation are cumulative — they keep adding up throughout a person's lifetime — and they can cause cancer and genetic mutation. Government standards for maximum levels of annual exposure have been repeatedly lowered as experts have learned more about the harmful effects of even small levels of this kind of radiation.

In general, the most serious area of concern for identifying and minimizing workplace exposure to ionizing radiation is *radon.* Over half of a typical American's exposure to ionizing radiation may come from radon.

According to government studies, this naturally occurring radioactive gas causes up to 10 percent of all lung cancer deaths and a total of 20,000 to 30,000 cancer deaths each year.[27] A colorless, odorless gas, radon is emitted from natural underground uranium deposits in soil and bedrock into at least 10 percent of all American businesses — more than 1 million — at a rate considered too high for safety, according to the National Council on Radiation Protection and Measurements, a nonprofit scientific group in Bethesda, Maryland.

Measurements in some buildings have reportedly been as high as 300 times the allowable limit in uranium mines. Excessive levels have also been found in public and private drinking water supplies in various areas of the country. The EPA estimates that about one-fourth of all U.S. homes and businesses have water that is radon-contaminated.[28]

Radon gas concentrations can be reduced by fans and heat exchangers, which vent it into the outside air where it rises and disperses into the atmosphere. In some extreme cases, buildings require more elaborate measures such as installation of a perforated pipe system beneath the building to vent radon away.

Nonionizing radiation. A number of authorities are warning about workplace health dangers from exposure to another type of radiation: nonionizing. There are two basic types — microwave and electromagnetic. These invisible forms of energy are emitted by VDTs, microwave communication equipment, microwave ovens, television and radio transmitters, radar, and electric wiring and power lines.

Microwaves are absorbed by the body and start molecules vibrating, in contrast to ionizing radiation, which knocks particles off atoms. Scientists have discovered that microwave radiation can cause significant unhealthy alterations to cell structures and functions.[29]

Researchers at New York University School of Medicine report an increase in cataracts among people working in industries in which microwaves are used.[30] That report prompted government regulatory agencies to cut acceptable exposure levels in half. Now preliminary research at Johns Hopkins Wilmer Eye Institute suggests that microwaves may cause another kind of visual damage at low levels — they destroy cells that line the cornea of the eye, blurring vision.[31] (*Note:* The danger zone for this visual damage is at higher doses than the current emission levels of household microwave ovens and cellular telephones, however.)

Over the past decade, computers and VDTs have changed the nature of work, and, according to the Arthur D. Little Corporation, by 1992 nearly 50 percent of the work force in America, Europe, and Japan will be making daily use of terminals.[32] There is some serious concern about nonionizing radiation — in particular from VDTs — causing or contributing to miscarriages, birth defects, or cancer.[33]

Electromagnetic radiation is produced by high-tension, high-voltage electric power lines; computer VDTs; electric railways, subways, and buses; and electric wires and telephone lines in businesses (wires shielded in metal conduit have significantly lower electromagnetic emissions).[34]

Evidence suggests that electromagnetic radiation may cause subtle damage by interfering with delicate electromagnetic force fields that are involved with brain and nervous system functions in the body[35] and may also stimulate human colon cancer cells to grow faster, proliferate, and survive longer.[36] Other studies show that electromagnetic fields may reduce immune system white cell activity and lower resistance to disease.[37]

If you work in or around concentrated electromagnetic fields, explore methods for shielding electrical wiring and other sources of radiation or limiting the duration of your exposure. Furthermore, some experts are even advising that children and pregnant women avoid the use of electric blankets or heating pads.[38]

If your job requires frequent VDT time at work or if you use a home computer regularly, the following practices are recommended:

- Test your computer and other devices for radiation emission levels.
- Position VDT monitors at arm's length in front of you and at least twice that far from the side or rear of your nearest neighbor's machine.[39]
- Whenever possible, turn off your computer terminal when it's not in use and, when convenient, proofread from a printout rather than the screen.
- Have an eye examination before starting to use a VDT and have annual exams thereafter.
- During VDT work periods, take at least one 15-minute rest break every hour (following the guidelines in Chapter 8), and whenever possible restrict VDT use to not more than 50 percent of the workday — up to a maximum of four hours.
- If you are pregnant, follow the preceding guidelines, and either strictly limit VDT time to less than 20 hours a week or request assignment to a non-VDT job.
- Increase your VDT productivity and decrease stress by reducing screen glare using a tiltable screen and antiglare hood and by keeping general room lighting soft. Illuminate source material with a small separate swing-arm lamp, and use window blinds when necessary to reduce glare.
- Follow the guidelines in Chapter 9 for adjusting your seat postion and work station design in ways that promote balanced posture and help prevent the tension, aches, and strains that are so common for workers who use VDTs.

Convenient Access to Pure Water

Until recently, most of us have taken water quality for granted. But new studies report that an alarming percentage of water supplies are laden with toxic chemicals, poisons capable of causing cancer, heart disease, birth defects, neurological disorders, organ damage, and other illnesses. Every business has a responsibility to ensure that safe drinking water is readily available to its employees at all times.

Drinking-water supplies in the United States, Europe, and Japan have been shown to contain toxic heavy metals (lead, cadmium, mercury, cobalt, copper, and others), cancer-causing organic chemicals, sodium, nitrates, asbestos, arsenic, radioactive substances (such as radon), and a wide range of toxic industrial chemicals. Everything that we inject into our environment — chemical, biological, or physical — ultimately finds its way into the earth's water.

Despite the publicity surrounding chemical pollution, the most serious water quality problems are usually radon and lead. Government experts warn that waterborne radon may cause more cancer deaths than all other drinking-water contaminants combined.[40]

Even if it were possible to have 100 percent pure water as it leaves the reservoir, there would still remain the serious question of whether it is fit to drink by the time it reaches the faucet. Many of us work in office buildings with an extensive network of underground pipes made from materials such as copper and lead, which can poison body tissues. Other plumbing materials, such as plastic polyvinyl chloride (PVC), have unknown health effects.

Before you decide to drink bottled water or invest in a water purifier, it's a good idea to have your office tap water tested. Pollution danger signs include brown, cloudy, or murky-looking water; smelly or bad-tasting water; foam; and sudden changes in appearance or taste. However, many toxic chemicals are invisible, odorless, and tasteless. Laboratory analysis is the only certain means of identifying safe drinking water. (If you cannot find a reputable analysis lab locally by checking with your community health department, see Resources at the end of the chapter for a list of testing kits.)

Once you have tested your workplace water supply to determine which contaminants need to be removed, you can choose a water treatment method accordingly.*

* For help in making a reliable choice, the EPA recommends contacting the National Sanitation Foundation (P.O. Box 1468, Ann Arbor, MI 48106). This organization establishes

Workplace Efforts to Reduce
Outdoor Pollution

> The challenge is . . . to mobilize, to start rebuilding a world
> that is in ecological and human equilibrium.
>
> — *Jerome B. Wiesner, president emeritus,*
> *Massachusetts Institute of Technology*

Science is uncovering hazards in our environment at a staggering pace. And the evidence is clear: Toxic pollutants do more than just damage our health; they threaten the stability — and future — of our natural world. This environmental crisis is fast becoming a major global concern. Our creative power to solve it is unlimited. Our time is not.

Until last year, it was all environmentalists seemed able to do to convince the public that the planet needs our help. But recent events — rain forest destruction, oil spills, widening hunger, global warming, food pesticides, clogged landfills, contaminated water, radon in our homes, schools, and offices, poisoned beaches, dirty air, and nuclear wastes — have persuaded tens of millions of people that it does.

The Earth's forests are shrinking, deserts expanding, and soils eroding, all at record rates. Thousands of plant and animal species are disappearing every year. The ozone layer is thinning, we're being buried alive in garbage, and the rising temperature of the Earth threatens climatic stability.

According to a recent special report in *Fortune* magazine, "in the next decade environmentalism will be the cutting edge of social reform and absolutely the most important issue for business."[41] Smart companies are doing far more than just facing this critical issue — they're joining and actively supporting the movement toward "eco-responsibility." The cost of not doing so may be fatal: The new environmental movement is a massive, mainstream, global force with tremendous consumer power.

industry standards and conducts certification tests on water treatment devices and systems. A series of specific test results and recommendations is also provided in the January 1990 issue of *Consumer Reports*.

Start by learning all you can about individual and corporate environmental priorities. Begin action by initiating office recycling programs (beginning with paper, plastics, and packaging materials), advocating eco-packaging (which includes new options for environmentally safe, recyclable, and genuinely biodegradable packing and shipping materials), and promoting water and energy conservation measures.

Resources

Workplace Environment

For job-related safety information, contact the National Institute of Occupational Safety and Health (NIOSH) (800-356-4674), your local or regional office of the Occupational Safety and Health Act (OSHA), or the OSHA National Office (U.S. Department of Labor, 200 Constitution Ave., NW, Washington, DC 20216). For answers to business pollution problems, contact your state health department or regional office of the EPA. Some good basic resources on workplace environments include the following:

- *Ergonomics: Implementing Workplace Change* (The Center for Women in Government at the University at Albany, State University of New York, Draper Hall, Albany, NY 12222).
- *Fitting the Task to the Man: A Textbook of Occupational Ergonomics,* 4th ed., by Etienne Grandjean, Ph.D. (Taylor and Francis, 1989). A leading reference book for those responsible for design, management, and safety in the workplace.
- *Indoor Air Quality and Human Health* by Isaac Turiel (Stanford University Press, Stanford, CA 94305; 1985).
- *Office Work Can Be Hazardous to Your Health: A Handbook of Office Health and Safety Hazards and What You Can Do About Them* by Jeanne Stellman, Ph.D., and Mary Sue Henifin, M.P.H., rev. ed. (Fawcett, 1989). A well-researched book by two occupational health experts.
- *The VDT Book: A Computer User's Guide to Health and Safety* (New York Committee for Occupational Safety and Health, 272 7th Ave., New York, NY 10001).
- *Formaldehyde: Everything You Wanted to Know But Were Afraid to Ask* (Consumer Federation of America, 1424 16th St., NW, Washington, DC 20036). Free booklet; send a stamped, self-addressed envelope. Also call Consumer Product Safety Commission (800-638-2772) for more information about formaldehyde.

- *Bibliography of Noise Publications* (Environmental Protection Agency, National Technical Information Service, Department of Commerce, 5285 Port Royal Road, Springfield, VA 22161). Free booklet.
- *A Citizen's Guide to Radon* (EPA publication OPA-86-004); *Radon Reduction Methods* (EPA publication OPA-86-005). EPA booklets available at public libraries and local health offices. EPA hotline for radon information (800-334-8571, ext. 713).
- *Radon: A Guide to Detection and Control* by Bernard L. Cohen (Consumer Reports Books, 540 Barnum Ave., Bridgeport, CT 06608; 1987).
- *Radiation Safety Corporation* (140 University Ave., Palo Alto, CA 94301). Markets an inexpensive but sensitive kit to test for radiation emission levels from computers and other devices.
- *Safe Drinking Water Hotline,* EPA, Water Division (800-426-4791). Toll-free number for general and technical information about the quality of drinking water.
- *WaterTest* (33 South Commerical St., Manchester, NH 03257; 800-426-8378); *National Testing Laboratories* (6151 Wilson Mills Rd., Cleveland, OH 44143; 800-458-3330); *Suburban Water Testing Laboratories* (4600 Kutztown Rd., Temple, PA 19560; 800-433-6595). Independent labs that offer simple, accurate drinking-water test kits.

Smoking Hazards

- *The Health Consequences of Involuntary Smoking* (Office of Smoking and Health, Room 1010, 5600 Fishers Lane, Rockville, MD 20857). Surgeon general's report; free.
- *The No-Nag, No-Guilt, Do-It-Your-Own-Way Guide to Quitting Smoking* by Tom Ferguson, M.D. (Ballantine, 1989). For health-concerned smokers who wish to quit, this is the best nonjudgmental guide to date.
- *The Smoke-Free Workplace* (Prometheus Books, 700 E. Amherst St., Buffalo, NY 14125). Lists addresses of about seventy-five nonsmokers' rights groups in the United States and Canada.
- *Smoke in the Workplace: An Action Manual for Non-Smokers* (Non-Smokers' Rights Association, Suite 308, 344 Bloor St. West, Toronto, Ontario M5S 1W9). Action-oriented information on nonsmokers' rights and the movement toward smoke-free workplaces.

13

Sleep and Rest: The Impact of Sleep on Alertness and Performance on the Job

> Sleep engenders energy, clarity and optimism and can provide the physical and emotional fuel needed to cope well with the day's demands.
>
> — *Lynne Lamberg,* The American Medical Association Guide to Better Sleep[1]

> Business people don't need more time management courses, they need more *time*. . . . If you can cut back sleep just one hour a day, you'll get a 14.5 percent increase in productive time every year.
>
> — *Benjamin Plumb,* Micro/Somnia

YOUR SUCCESS AT WORK — and perhaps your very survival — depends on sustained alertness and top performance hour after hour, day after day. Even a momentary lapse in attention or competence can spell defeat or, at the very least, can cause errors or communication mix-ups that add to your stress load. Few of us realize the extent to which our personal effectiveness depends on the quality of our nightly rest. Researchers have discovered that more and more of us are suffering from various kinds of *chronic partial sleep deprivation*[2] — we don't get enough sleep or, more often, we sleep *poorly* night after night.

In recent decades, one of the most powerful trends has been the movement toward a 24-hour lifestyle in which, no matter what business or profession we're in, sophisticated electronic communication devices such as cellular phones, satellite pagers, airborne phones, electronic and voice mail, portable laptop and notebook-size computers, and fax machines keep us in touch for more and more hours of the day, blurring the lines between work and family time. This not only *permits* us to work anywhere, anytime — it promotes the work ethic that we ought to.

These pressures can confuse our natural biological sleep/wake cycles, and our physiology gets pushed to the breaking point or beyond — into burnout. A recent article in the *Wall Street Journal* estimates the workplace cost to U.S. industry from reduced alertness alone at about $70 billion a year.

Even a single below-par night of sleep can cut your physical and mental performance the next day by as much as 30 percent,[3] and one recent study even links sleep loss to the human errors that contributed to catastrophes at Three Mile Island and the Chernobyl nuclear power plant and to the explosion of the space shuttle *Challenger*.[4] The sleep researchers concluded that "inadequate sleep, even as little as one or two hours less than usual, can greatly exaggerate the tendency for error."

Research confirms that poor sleep causes loss of motivation and decreased productivity; a reduced ability to learn and remember; feelings of irritability, anger, and unhappiness; increased job errors (both of commission and omission); slower healing; and lowered resistance to disease.[5] Even the effect of heavy food at lunch seems to be most pronounced when combined with sleep deprivation.[6]

Sleep loss or poor rest can also obstruct creative innovation. *Convergent* thinking — the ability to use well-established mental skills — is not nearly as dependent on optimal sleep as is *divergent* thinking, which involves spontaneity, flexibility, and originality. According to researchers, even mild sleep deprivation sabotages your ability to try different approaches to a problem or to generate new or unusual ideas.[7]

How Much Sleep Do You Really Need?

It has been estimated that most adults need between five and nine hours of sleep each night — averaging between seven and eight hours — to be optimally alert and perform well the next day. Researchers suggest that five hours a night seems to be the typical minimum for young adults. For those past age thirty, however, that falls to four hours.

The best way to know your optimum personal sleep requirement is to experiment. Can you rest completely in fewer hours than you sleep now? Probably.

First, improve your ability to handle job stress and make other changes toward a healthier lifestyle. Then, very gradually, reduce your sleep time. If you now sleep seven hours a night, try six hours and fifty minutes each night for one week, then take off another ten minutes the next week, and so on.

Most of us can gradually reduce nightly sleep by one to two hours, says James A. Horne, a sleep researcher and psychophysiologist at Great Britain's Loughborough University.[8] He contends that normal, healthy sleepers who get 7 to 8 hours of sleep a night can quite readily decrease their sleep to about 5 to 6 hours a night. But he advises that if your waking hours are a real struggle and you can't find an effective way to neutralize — or at least reduce — the negative stress you must face on and off the job, then, for now, maintain your regular sleep schedule.

Implement the sleep improvement suggestions that follow and, if you're ready to begin gradually cutting back on the hours you sleep, be certain to stop reducing your sleep time whenever you notice any prolonged sense of weariness after awakening.

Priorities for Deeper, More Revitalizing Rest

Here is a quick summary of some of the most important considerations for best sleep.

Establish a regular sleep pattern. The body's biological cycles thrive on a consistent sleep schedule — so do your best to maintain one.

Some studies suggest that the most vital hours of "anchor sleep" are from 1:00 A.M. to 5:00 A.M.

Get up at the same time every day. No matter how many hours you sleep or the actual time you fall asleep, set a regular schedule and get up at the same time every day. Even if your night's sleep has been poor or cut shorter than usual, by getting up at the same time every morning your body's biological circadian rhythm is reset and all other sleep and wake cycles are synchronized.[9]

Oversleeping or "sleeping in" on the weekends is a sure way to confuse your body clock. You'll not only become "worn out" and less alert after too much sleep, but you reduce the number of waking hours, making it more difficult to fall asleep the next night.[10] And the luxury of sleeping late on Sunday morning leads to "Sunday night insomnia" and "Monday morning blahs," says Lynne Lamberg, author of *The American Medical Association Guide to Better Sleep*.[11] If you must sleep in, limit your extra sleep to not more than an hour or so and do it as infrequently as possible.

Have a strategy for dealing with sleep loss resulting from irregular or prolonged work. If on occasion you're forced to skip most or all of a night's sleep because of prolonged, demanding work, avoid the tendency to keep at your work until you drop. Also don't try to take longer than normal sleep periods ahead of time in anticipation of the lost sleep (since evidence shows that this contributes to extra grogginess and diminished performance).[12] Instead, you may be able to dramatically extend your staying power and help prevent the buildup of sleepiness and deterioration of performance by planning ahead and taking one or two short naps (each at least 10 minutes long) *away from major sleep periods.*[13]

Exercise regularly. Studies link physical fitness with improved sleep quality.[14] Furthermore, physical and mental inactivity rank among the prime causes of insomnia.

Eat wisely. Beyond an optimal diet, discussed in Chapter 11, avoid alcohol and caffeine near bedtime; and don't go to bed hungry. A drop in blood sugar in the middle of the night can interfere with sleep. A carefully planned, moderate-size evening meal is important, and a very small midevening snack that is low in fat and protein and high in carbohydrates also helps many people have a smoother transition into deep, restful sleep.

Keep business out of the bedroom. If you want the best sleep, and especially if you suffer from insomnia, reserve your bed for sleeping and for a warm, positive sexual relationship. Nothing else. Keep heated discussions and intense brainstorming sessions out of your bedroom. Schedule a time each evening to write down concerns and challenges, planning how you will take steps to solve them *tomorrow,* and then let go of your personal and business concerns before bedtime.

Relax before falling asleep. The most common causes of sleep difficulties are related to stress.[15] If you don't release accumulated tension each evening, you prevent yourself from getting the best possible sleep and will awaken groggy or fatigued in the morning. Choose a favorite quick-relaxation technique and use it regularly before falling asleep. For example, take several minutes to consciously tighten and then relax muscles in the face, scalp, jaw, neck, and tongue down to your back and abdomen and out to your fingertips and toes.

In addition, let go of any emotional baggage you notice yourself carrying from the day's events. Relaxation and guided mental imagery tapes may help. Positive music makes it easier for some people to unwind; for others, sleep researchers at Northwestern University have found that the static "white noise" at the end of the FM radio dial is even more calming than music.[16] Finally, don't forget to bring your spiritual beliefs to light each evening — bedtime prayers and positive affirmations can help create a state of mind conducive to deep, revitalizing rest.

Design an optimal sleeping environment. Considerations include the following:

Fresh air, cool temperatures. Fresh, circulating air boosts sleep quality. Temperature is important, too. Many people find the range between 65 and 70 degrees Fahrenheit to be ideal.[17] If you're too cold, you must fumble for covers; if you're too hot, you become restless in sleep.

A *supportive bed.* Good beds can be expensive, but they're worth the investment. Firm beds are preferable to soft ones, but some extra-hard mattresses actually *contribute* to back pain rather than relieving it. Experts recommend a bed that is level, with no sags, and just firm enough to fully support the lower back. Top-quality waterbeds are also worth considering. With a thermostatically controlled heater and natural-fiber bed linens, "flotation sleep systems" can provide excellent back support and great rest all year round.

Woolen mattress cover. According to medical studies, a fleecy woolen pad placed between the mattress and bottom sheet improves sleep quality.[18] People sleeping on the wool pad tossed and turned less and felt better each morning than those who slept on a conventional mattress pad. This is apparently due to wool's ability to cushion the body and let the skin "breathe" — helping to keep you comfortably cool in summer and warm in winter.

A *dark, quiet sleeping room.* We sleep most deeply when the bedroom is dark. New curtains or window blinds may be in order if outside light filters into your room from a street lamp or the moon. Even dim light causes unnecessary eye movements that can sabotage your rest.

Noise control is also important for deep sleep. Selecting a quiet hotel room when traveling and soundproofing your bedroom at home (as well as educating family members and neighbors about nighttime peace and quiet) are good steps to take. You might also consider earplugs or, as a last alternative, a "white noise" generating device that produces ocean-like sounds to mask outside clamor.

The most comfortable sleeping position. While there are many sleep postures, the one most frequently recommended by experts is the semifetal position,[19] in which you lie on your side with the knees drawn partway up.

For best sleep, your head and neck should be well supported in a variety of sleep postures since most of us change positions during the night. Special neck-support pillows may be fine when you are sleeping on your back or side, but when you change positions they may add more pressure to your shoulders, neck, or back than traditional pillows. To help keep your head in a neutral, relaxed position when on your side, pull the side or corner of your pillow down between the top of your lowermost shoulder (the one resting directly on the bed) and the side of your chin.

A *gentle awakening.* How you wake up has a surprisingly strong influence on how you feel during the morning work hours. Awakening forces your body to go through a dramatic shifting of gears. Leaping up to shut off an alarm clock is an abrupt jolt to your entire being — triggering racing heartbeat, muscle tension, and other stress "emergency" symptoms. In fact, as you merely *step* out of bed, two pints of blood go into your legs, your blood pressure shoots up by 30 points, and a cascade of hormones enters your system.[20]

Positive music — set to come on with a timer and with the volume just loud enough that you'll notice it and awaken — is a better choice than a traditional alarm clock. If possible, wake up at least a minute or two early to lie in bed and allow your body to slowly shift into being wide awake.

Chronobiologists — medical researchers who study the body's biological cycles — continue to make new discoveries that are important to business productivity. For example, between 2:00 P.M. and 4:00 P.M. most of us are affected by a sense of sleepiness brought on by what is called the *midafternoon circadian trough*. The effects of this natural cycle can be reduced with optimal work breaks (Chapter 8) and other Performance Edge guidelines. Nonetheless, whenever possible it makes strategic sense to schedule active rather than passive tasks during this time — and important meetings should be placed at other times on the daily calendar if you want the participants to be alert and attentive.

Understanding human sleep/wake cycles is an essential part of the Performance Edge. We can no longer afford to underestimate the impact of sleep and rest on job performance. Our high-stress, high-speed technological age has dramatically increased the need for alertness and vigilance — to prevent serious accidents and errors *and* to increase innovation, quality control, and productivity. There's a direct link here to the competitive advantage. It's time for businesses to pay attention.

"If you must assume people are adaptable and they'll manage somehow," says Harvard University sleep researcher Martin Moore-Ede, "then you end up asking them to do things which are really — even given unlimited willpower — still beyond their present capabilities."[21]

14

Self-Renewal and Social Support: Dealing More Successfully with the Competing Demands of Work and Family

Making yourself a better person — more diverse in your interests, more reflective, perhaps even more loving — may well make you a better manager.

— Fortune *magazine*[1]

CHANCES ARE that there are times when you feel trapped or tormented by the competing demands you face at work and at home, times when your personal and family priorities seem to be totally at odds with your work responsibilities. Finding effective ways to deal with this perplexing issue is one of today's top corporate and personal challenges.

Research is showing that your productivity and satisfaction *on* the job are determined to a great extent by three concerns that require your attention *off* the job: self-renewal, social support, and balancing the opposing needs of work and family.

Self-Renewal

With so many of us working harder and longer than ever, putting such enormous energy into our jobs, one of the great risks is that the work can end up controlling our lives. Parents already dizzied by work demands feel additional pressure as they struggle to find some spare minutes for themselves and to spend more time with their loved ones while climbing the career ladder.

One of the most serious consequences of this contest is *burnout*, with symptoms that include mental and physical exhaustion, anxiety, and feelings of being overwhelmed by stress.[2] It often begins like this: You feel as if you're not getting enough accomplished, so you put in more work hours, which makes you more tired and ineffective, so you feel as if you're *really* not getting anything done, so you put in more work hours. . . .

Burnout is an insidious problem, says a report in *Fortune* magazine, "because it is most likely to affect a company's best people. Managers who care deeply about their jobs, who put in long hours, who sincerely want to make things better, are the ones most likely to wipe out."[3] Burnout often stems from a lack of awareness and respect for your needs and personal priorities.

"The process of preventing and overcoming burnout and performing up to our capacities involves not only external management of difficult situations and working together with others, but also some inner reflection on such questions as who we are, what we need, and what we want from our lives," say organizational psychologists Dennis T. Jaffe and Cynthia D. Scott. "We also need to take proper care of ourselves — physically, emotionally, and spiritually — and replenish the energy we expend every day."[4]

Self-renewal consists of the conscious, regular steps you take to rejuvenate and revitalize yourself. It's the primary way to prevent burnout and rekindle your spark of excitement about your work — keeping it flourishing, even in tough, trying work settings.

To managers and professionals who think they're rocketing toward the top, blocking out regular time slots to slow down may appear foolhardy. It isn't. Says Dan Stamp, chairman of Priority Management: "I think the people who reject long hours will be the real leaders in the years to come — they're the brightest, the innovators. The guys logging really long hours aren't seen as heroes anymore. They're seen as turkeys."[5]

As discussed in Chapter 5, setting both work and personal priorities and then learning to say no to nonimportant intrusions on your time is absolutely crucial to the delicate juggling act of excelling on the job while you concurrently take care of your personal and family needs.

Besides, self-discovery and self-renewal are integral aspects of leadership, says Warren Bennis, professor of business administration at the University of Southern California. Implicit in his findings, based on more than a decade of research, is the realization that becoming a leader depends on becoming yourself — getting in touch with yourself, becoming keenly aware of your personal work strengths and your specific needs for support and assistance from others. In fact, being in sync with yourself, notes Bennis, is prerequisite to — and sometimes even more crucial than — being in sync with the organization, department, or work team you lead.

We've already looked at the value of stress management, communication skills, regular exercise, balanced posture, good food, deep sleep, mental development, frequent work breaks, less-polluted indoor environments, and other factors as integral ways to improve your health and provide a buffer against the pressures of work. But these factors alone aren't enough.

You may be startled to learn that new research suggests the uppermost priority for self-renewal may, in fact, be *healthful pleasures* — finding ways to do more of what you love to do and taking greater advantage of life's unvarnished golden moments to lift your spirits and put a little more fun back into your life. Yes, *fun*, pure and simple.

Healthful Pleasures

> Strength through joy.
>
> — *Robert Ley (1890–1945)*

Many of us bet our lives on getting ahead, getting to the top, and getting rich. But does the time, training, and effort pay off in terms of our health and happiness? Not very often. We need to modify our thinking.

Feeling good is good for you.* In the past decade, a wave of research data has been published in support of that simple sentence. Yet for the most part, the message continues to fall on a society with deaf ears. The dominion of work has become so complete that it often dampens even the most innocent, joyful pursuits.

For example, how would your co-workers, boss, or family react if you told them you were going to a movie over the lunch hour or were headed out to race a model boat in a nearby pond or into the park to kick off your shoes and listen to Mozart while you stretch out under a tree? In truth, stolen moments and simple pleasures like these are genuinely health-promoting[6] — *and* they contribute to work productivity.

Positive moods and pleasurable expectations are the inner threads of *joie de vivre*. Yet rarely do we consciously invest in our mental and emotional life in the same way we invest our money or our time. "Why not devote your free time to something better than merely resting up so you'll be ready to go back to work?" asks Walter Kiechel III in *Fortune* magazine. By better managing your time and leaving the office earlier "you will have the energy to cultivate other interests — playing a musical instrument, making furniture, going on nature walks with your kids — that should help make you a more diverse, competent, interesting person."[7]

We need to shift our judgments toward increased optimism and "stop searching for happiness in the extreme highs of emotion, money, and status," say health researchers Robert E. Ornstein, a psychologist at the University of California, San Francisco Medical School, and Dr. David S. Sobel, a regional director of patient education and health promotion at the Kaiser Permanente Medical Care Program.

"Your company can go out of business," they warn. "Your division can get merged into another and you be let go. Many people work from dawn to dusk and find little room for sensual enjoy-

---

* In case you opened the book to this chapter first, let me point out that I recognize well that wearing seat belts, exercising regularly, eating a low-fat diet, not smoking, not taking drugs, not drinking alcohol to excess, managing stress, actively developing your mind, and a variety of other factors all contribute to a long, healthy, and productive life. Even so, a missing ingredient for lifelong vitality and meaningful work is healthful pleasure — and the strength of the research data makes it warrant our attention.

ment or mental pleasure. For many their entire business can rise and fall on international economic tides over which they have little control. So, we need to surround ourselves with little rewards that mean something, that we can keep separate." [8]

Scientists are proving that healthful pleasures are an essential complement to productive work. Studies show that a life filled with a variety of simple happinesses can better absorb the difficult times and contribute to ongoing well-being and productivity. If you stop to think about it, you'll recognize how many chances there are to capture — or begin *re*capturing — these small healthful pleasures:

Playing hide and seek with your children or grandchildren
Roller skating, hitting some golf balls, or shooting baskets
Writing poetry, painting a landscape, savoring a novel, or tackling a crossword puzzle
Puttering in the garden or going on a bicycle ride
Swinging in a hammock or stretching out on the sofa
Sitting on the lawn watching the stars or seeing the sun come up or go down
Sipping lemonade in the shade or hot cider in front of the fireplace
Listening to your favorite music or composing a song
Watching old movies
Playing a musical instrument (even badly)
Taking a walk through your favorite park
Holding hands with your spouse, cuddling with your pet, or smelling the flowers
Knitting a sweater, building a model, or flying a kite
Baking an exotic loaf of bread or testing a new recipe
Playing a board game or dancing old dances
Whatever gives your heart — and psyche — a boost

It also pays to laugh more, not just for your own benefit but also for your company's. It's time to revive our natural sense of humor. Very few things so instantly form a bond between people as laughter. People who know how to have fun are generally healthier and better able to bounce back from stressful situations. [9] And research suggests that laughter can enhance workplace productivity. When we're in a good mood we are more helpful and generous toward others and experience improved cognitive processes such as judgment, problem solving, and decision making.[10]

Humor can improve group as well as individual performance. When it's related to the task at hand, laughter tends to increase productivity, says organizational psychologist Howard Pollio of the University of Tennessee, Knoxville.[11] He speculates that laughter rallies spirits and provides a brief break without being too diverting. If the work task is tedious, humor relieves boredom, which promotes increased alertness and problem solving. Even during intensive cognitive tasks, says Pollio, when laughing may not facilitate the group's output, it doesn't interfere with it either.

Humor helps keep things in perspective and works as an antidote to drudgery, depression, and conflict in the workplace. One way to defuse anger with co-workers, for example, is to momentarily shift the conversation to a time when you laughed together. But avoid telling jokes based on ridicule — they inflict pain (and, as a form of cynicism, can backfire and increase your own risk of heart attack and early death).[12] And skip hurtful sarcasm. A good pun that gives you a twist of expectancy can be wonderful. And cosmic humor — an appreciation of work's (and life's) paradoxes and absurdities — is the most fun of all.

In short, loosen up. Self-renewal means putting your own inner happiness on a level with your highest work priorities. Schedule regular appointments with yourself for letting go of work concerns long enough to revitalize your body and mind through simple, healthful pleasures. And take advantage of unexpected schedule openings, such as airplane delays, to do the same.

It comes down to some pure and simple advice: *It's not so important to be serious as it is to be serious about important things.* What aspects of life on the job and at home can you take with a little more humor and a little less intensity? Your health and personal effectiveness depend on it.

Social Support

Human connectedness — a positive and supportive social network — helps us work more productively, resist disease, enjoy life, and live longer.[13] Studies confirm that personal relationships make a significant difference in how we feel at work and how effective we are on the job.[14] People who value power over friendship appear to have a harder time fighting off disease and get sick more often.[15]

"Researchers have repeatedly demonstrated a vital link between the strength of our social support systems and our emotional and physical resilience under severe stress," says psychologist Julius Segal. In reviewing the evidence to date, Hebrew University psychiatrist Gerald Caplan adds that "when the stress level is high, people without psychological support suffer as much as ten times the incidence of physical and emotional illness experienced by those who enjoy such support."[16]

Positive Support of — and Then from — Others

There are four principal types of support networks:

- Your intimate loved ones and extended family
- Your friendship and community networks
- Your co-workers and job mentors
- Service and professional contacts

In each of these categories, good relationships are those that can deal well with differences in values, perceptions, and interests. In contrast, bad relationships are filled with conflict, selfishness, disruption, frustration, and emotional trauma.

Support from others adds many important dimensions to our lives and work, including love, nurturance, and friendship; role models; motivation and encouragement; help in meeting everyday demands as well as those that arise in times of crisis; mentoring; and referrals for finding assistance outside our usual circle of contacts.

In their book *Getting Together: Building a Relationship That Gets to Yes,* Roger Fisher and Scott Brown, leaders of the Harvard Negotiation Project, advise strengthening qualities essential to coping successfully with the inevitable differences found in all personal and work relationships.[17]

First, although it takes two or more people to have a relationship, it's important to realize it takes only one to change the quality of that relationship. Second, try to separate people from problems. Don't entangle substantive issues (money, dates, time, property, terms, conditions) with human aspects (how we deal with each other).

Third, learn to be unconditionally constructive, which means checking partisan perceptions; don't forget how differently we each see things. In a relationship with another person, do whatever is good for the relationship and you — whether or not the other person reciprocates.

The extensive research by Fisher and Brown suggests that the following actions will help strengthen a relationship: Even if the other person is acting emotionally, try to balance emotions with reason. Even if you feel you are being misunderstood, keep trying to understand the other person. Even if you think the other person isn't listening, consult him or her before making decisions on matters that affect you both. Be reliable, whether or not you trust or feel deceived by the other person. Operate beyond coercion; try to persuade the other person and be open to persuasion yourself. Even if you feel that you and your concerns are being rejected, care about others, accept them and their ideas as worthy of your consideration, and be open to learning from them.

Expanding and Strengthening Your Support Networks

According to Dr. Tom Ferguson, an award-winning medical writer, there are some quick, simple ways to nurture and enlarge your support network. He offers these suggestions: Take three pieces of paper. Draw a circle in the center of one and, inside this circle, write your name. In circles near yours, write the names of the people with whom you have the strongest, closest bonds. Include those who have been sources of warmth and approval during earlier periods of your life as well as those who actively support you now — at work, in your family, and among your broad circle of friends.

"List the people you have warm feelings for," advises Dr. Ferguson. "People you are comfortable with. Nurturing people. People you would like to be able to talk with if you were having a hard time. All the people you have enjoyed working with. All the people you'd enjoy receiving a letter from. Don't worry about being 'fair' or reasonable or logical — this exercise is for you alone." [18]

As you list the names, you may find yourself wishing you were closer in touch with some of them. If so, list these people on the second sheet of paper. Entries may include former co-workers or friends you haven't seen in a long time or new friends or co-workers you'd like to get to know better.

There may be some people for whom you would like to do something special — a note of appreciation, a hug, a phone call, a letter, or a gift to let them know how much you value their friendship and support. If such feelings come to mind, list them with the names of these people on the third sheet of paper.

When you've finished your social support system diagram, take several minutes to review each name, remembering the kinds of support you've received from and given to that person. Is there anyone you'd like to be in touch with right now? What ongoing use can you make of your lists?

Resources

- *Do I Have to Give Up Me to Be Loved by You?* by Jordan Paul, Ph.D., and Margaret Paul, Ph.D. (CompCare, 2415 Annapolis Lane, Minneapolis, MN 55441; 1983). One of the best books on self-discovery and building intimate relationships.
- *Getting Together: Building a Relationship That Gets to Yes* by Roger Fisher and Scott Brown (Houghton Mifflin, 1988). Offers proven guidelines for solving disputes at home and at work, avoiding cycles of hard feelings, keeping emotions from getting in the way of agreement, and learning how to accept and be accepted.
- *How to Talk So Your Kids Will Listen and Listen So Your Kids Will Talk* by Adel Faber and Elaine Mazlish (Avon, 1980). Based on their parenting workshops, the authors give guidelines for family communication, including helping children deal with their feelings, giving praise, encouraging cooperation and autonomy, and alternatives to punishment.
- *LifeMates: The Love Fitness Program for a Lasting Relationship* by Harold H. Bloomfield, M.D., and Sirah Vettese, Ph.D. (New American Library, 1989). A valuable book on intimate relationships.
- *Making Peace with Your Parents* by Harold H. Bloomfield, M.D., and Leonard Felder, Ph.D. (Ballantine, 1983). Deals with the most funda-

mental relationship in your life — coming to terms with your parents, no matter how old you are and whether or not they are alive.

• *Managing the Equity Factor . . . Or "After All I've Done for You . . ."* by Richard C. Huseman, Ph.D., and John D. Hatfield, Ph.D. (Houghton Mifflin, 1989). A readable and helpful guide to improving workplace relationships, written by two professors at the University of Georgia Business School.

Self-Help Groups in the Computer Age

The computer age has ushered in the era of high-speed networking. Self-help groups are being formed for special needs of all kinds. In fact, there's a support group for virtually every problem and interest these days — workplace concerns, job burnout prevention, physical and psychological health issues of all descriptions, sports and fitness interests, adult learning, communication skills, family needs, education, politics, hobbies, travel, and spiritual growth.

Computer databases* can put you in instant contact with groups in your community who share your interests or needs. To link up with these groups, talk to co-workers, relatives, friends, psychologists, physicians, and community service offices.

---

* *The Self-Help Sourcebook* lists 500 national groups, 50 call-in clearinghouses, and more than 80 toll-free help lines (the book is available from the Self-Help Clearinghouse, St. Clares-Riverside Medical Center, Pocomo Road, Denville, NJ 07834; 201-625-9565 or 800-367-6274).

To volunteer to help lead a group or contribute your support, check the white pages of your phone book under "Volunteer Bureau" or "Volunteer Center." Or send a stamped, self-addressed envelope to VOLUNTEER — The National Center (1111 N. 19th St., Suite 500, Arlington, VA 22209). VOLUNTEER provides groups with information sharing, training, and promotion.

Dealing Successfully with the Competing Needs of Work and Family

> To make a living is no longer enough. Work also has to make a life.
>
> — *Peter F. Drucker*, Management

> Conflicts between work and family may be one of the primary ways through which traditional organizations limit their effectiveness. By fostering such conflict, they distract and disempower their members — often to a far greater degree than they realize.
>
> — *Peter M. Senge, Ph.D., Director of the Systems Thinking and Organizational Learning Program at MIT's Sloan School of Management*

On the job, you're expected to be on time and on top — meeting your responsibilities to the letter and working productively. The company is counting on you. Your work performance is the number one priority, and you're supposed to arrange the rest of your life so that you can be effective on the job.

At the same time, you have very pressing family responsibilities. Your children and other family members need your time and attention to meet *their* physical and emotional needs. And what about time for yourself? There never seems to be enough time or energy to achieve a satisfying balance among work, family, and personal life.

National surveys indicate that 72 percent of men and 83 percent of women experience "significant conflict between work and family." [19] However, most organizations have been slow to acknowledge this growing concern.

That's because the myth about separate and nonoverlapping work and home worlds has a long history in the corporate mind. [20] It's time for that to change. Convincing new research shows that stress at home interferes with work performance and, conversely, that work stress creates or magnifies problems at home. [21] The intensity and single-mindedness that make for corporate achievement are often the opposite of the qualities needed to be an effective husband, wife, or parent.[22]

Let's admit it, today's working parents and family caregivers have to perform like triathletes. We've got to be in exceptional shape just to handle the stress. More than ever, we need the Performance Edge to consistently stay on top of the demands we face — at work and at home — and to meet our responsibilities in the best possible way.

Personal Actions to Help Balance Work and Family Life

Nearly every study on family stress puts time pressures near the top of the list. "When a couple suffers from lack of time together," writes Dolores Curran in *Stress and the Healthy Family*, "communication suffers. When communication suffers, couples are less able to deal with their own concerns or with issues like children's behavior and financial worries. When your personal time gets squeezed out by work and excessive community activities, predictable feelings like fatigue, tension, and futility give rise to sharp retorts, temperamental outbursts, and an atmosphere of walking-on-eggs at home."[23]

Successful families, like successful organizations, require careful thought and planning and persistent attention, explains Barrie S. Greiff, who teaches courses at Harvard University on work-family concerns. "When a man or woman asks the other to defer life until they make it in the work world — to hang on, things will get better — it assumes that the rewards of work will justify the neglect of self and family. Pure fantasy. And it assumes that after a number of years in which the family accepts second-best because it has no other choice, the professional can then pick up where he or she left off. Equal fantasy."[24]

According to researchers, those people who most effectively balance work and nonwork demands develop creative techniques for allocating time for personal, couple, and family activities. Here are several strategies for creating your own balance.*

* One of the most thorough professional presentations on this subject is "Business and the Facts of Family Life" by Fran Sussner Rodgers and Charles Rodgers (*Harvard Business*

Determine your commitment to work-family balance. "The first task," says Peter M. Senge from MIT's Sloan School of Management, "is asking yourself if, given your ambitions, it is really your *vision* to have a balance between work and family. How serious are you? This is not a trivial question. If it were simple to achieve this balance, more people would do it. Many people lament the problem, but few have made a conscious choice to achieve the balance they espouse."

Become an advocate for performance-based pay and flexible work hours. There is a growing corporate trend toward performance-centered compensation, whereby managers, professionals, and employees are rewarded at least in part based on contribution rather than status. There is a strongly held belief that this not only is fairer than other pay plans but actually encourages higher levels of quality control, productivity, and customer responsiveness — as people learn that they will actually get back more if they put more in.[25]

Flexible scheduling is another way to better enable workers to handle nonwork pressures and, in turn, be more focused and productive on the job. *Flextime* can be tightly structured to allow a daily schedule shift of a half hour or hour or more broadly designed to allow extensive variations from day to day. Introduced in this country by Hewlett-Packard, flextime is now offered by about two-thirds of all large American corporations and used by nearly one-fifth of all workers. The effects on lateness, absenteeism, and employee morale have generally been very positive.[26]

Bosses give high marks to employees working flexible schedules and predict that more and more managers, professionals, and workers will break out of 9-to-5 routines in the next few years — and that this will become critical if companies want to keep their top workers.

In a recent national survey of 521 firms by the Conference Board of New York,[27] 93 percent said they now offered at least one flextime option and that more than 8 out of 10 personnel chiefs say

Review [Nov.-Dec. 1989]: 121–29). See also *The Worth Ethic* by Kate Ludeman, Ph.D. (Dutton, 1989). For general reading, two other good publications are *Stress and the Healthy Family* by Dolores Curran (Winston Press, 1985) and *Achieving Balance: How to Handle the Stress of Work and Family Life* (Work/Family Directions, Inc., c/o Great Performance Inc., 14964 N.W. Greenbrier Parkway, Portland, OR 97006; 503-690-9181; 1990).

that flextimers are high performers. According to Kathleen Christensen, a City University of New York psychologist and director of the study, "Corporate culture is going to have to change from the assumption that visibility and long hours are the criteria for commitment. Instead, commitment will have to be judged by tasks, meeting deadlines, and how much you can trust someone."

In another recent study of 50 major companies, 47 offered part-time work, job sharing (in which two workers share all responsibilities of one full-time job), and telecommuting (working at home via computer hookup). Two out of three personnel chiefs said that part-time schedules actually boost productivity. "They say people are working harder and smarter, being more focused. They can't stay until 7, so they don't fool around," says Julie Harris of New York–based Catalyst, a research and business advisory group that directed the study.[28]

Demonstrate your commitment to personal and family priorities. The same skills that contribute to your effectiveness at work — setting priority objectives, communicating clearly, saying no to nonessential demands on your time — can help you stay in control of your personal and family life.

First, take some strategic actions to establish increased workplace respect for your life *off* the job. When the opportunity presents itself, you may appropriately point out the value to your company of a balanced life. You might begin by scheduling exercise on your lunch hour. "Unless your boss is prepared to confess that he doesn't care if you drop dead at your desk," explains one recent report, "he can hardly argue with your pursuit of fitness. Heading off to the gym (or for a walk around the block) sends a message that you're putting your own needs ahead of the company, at least for an hour or so, and helps you establish some personal time in your day. Once it's clear that you are not available to hop every moment the boss gets a brainstorm, you could use the time for other needs — seeing your spouse or kids at lunch, for instance."[29]

Second, establish an "emotional bank account," a metaphor used by Stephen R. Covey to describe the amount of trust that can be built up in a relationship. According to Covey, chairman of the Institute for Principle-Centered Leadership and author of *The Seven Habits of Highly Effective People,* "If I make deposits into an

Emotional Bank Account with you (or my coworkers or family members) through courtesy, kindness, honesty, and keeping my commitments to you, I build up a reserve. Your trust toward me becomes higher, and I can call upon that trust many times if I need to . . . and communication is more effective.

"But if I have a habit of showing discourtesy, disrespect, cutting you off, overreacting, ignoring you, becoming arbitrary, or betraying your trust . . . eventually my Emotional Bank Account is overdrawn. The trust level gets very low. Then what flexibility do I have?"[30]

Covey suggests six major deposits that build the emotional bank account: understanding the individual, attending to the little things, keeping commitments, clarifying expectations, showing personal integrity, and apologizing sincerely when you make a withdrawal. *Make family time a higher priority on your schedule.* One widespread delusion is that home life takes care of itself naturally and that the best way to deal with it is to let it take its own course. Effective couples recognize that family time is a controllable resource that can quickly get out of control. The time that we spend with our family deserves — but rarely receives — a priority ranking right up there with predominant business responsibilities.

Schedule nonwork time in advance — and say no to requests that take away from family time. In the home, time needs to be recognized by one and all as a resource that requires the same attention as money — and this includes talking about it in regularly scheduled family meetings (in which every family member has a chance to speak, and may share, without fear of judgment, whatever he or she thinks about an issue); airing feelings and needs that arise from insufficient nonwork time; budgeting time; allocating time for specific family activities (some decisions are reserved as the parents' right to decide, but others are made by the whole group); and even instituting a savings plan where you reserve time on your schedules for unanticipated family needs. Post a large family calendar in the kitchen where everyone can see and use it. List all of the family members' activities for each week.

To streamline traditional family cooperative functions and take advantage of everyone pitching in to help free up some extra time, establish daily and weekly routines for shopping, cooking, cleaning, lawn care, babysitting, taking out the garbage, and doing laundry. Don't make these routines rigid, but design them with the goal of providing a comfortable pattern for getting things done each week. This reduces organizational tension and enables each family member to anticipate and prepare for family priorities.

To review a variety of practical time management strategies, see Chapter 5.

When you're away from work, let go of work concerns. Few things hurt our loved ones more than when, at the end of the day, our bodies come home from work but our minds remain locked on job concerns. Don't imagine for a second that you can hide it. None of us can. Our eyes glaze over, we listen poorly, if at all, and our family members must wonder which is worse — our being away so many hours at work or the fact that, even when we're home, we often can't seem to give them the attention they deserve.

"There's just no way around it," says Walter Kiechel. "Your undistracted presence is required if you are to get together with friends and laugh, talk the day over with your spouse or significant other — and what is a good marriage if not an extended conversation? — attend to the needs of your parents, or listen to the discoveries of your children. In thinking about you, your kids in particular will remember not the excuses you offered, but the time you spent with them. Or didn't spend." [31]

If in order to leave your job at a decent hour you're forced to bring home work projects, schedule a specific work time later in the evening — after the kids are in bed, for example — to wrap things up for the day. But between the time you arrive home and the beginning of this work period, shift *all* your attention to family and personal nonwork matters.

First, as discussed in Chapter 6, listen carefully to the messages you hear at home and learn to show your affection and concern by tuning in to the unique conversational style of each loved one. Some of your family members may indeed perceive the world differently than you do, and even if at work you insist that co-workers and employees get to the point whenever they talk with you, individuals in your family may need — or at least genuinely prefer — to take a different communication approach. If you are patient enough not to interrupt, tune out, or shut down the conversation in some other hurtful way, you'll be rewarded with a stronger, warmer sense of connection and clearer two-way communication with your loved ones.

Another way to help this process along is through an increased skill in *present-moment awareness*. This calm, attentive skill is the opposite of distraction, and it can be a sterling attribute in the workplace as well as the home. Your mind is alert, your body relaxed and efficient. You can unknot tension patterns and quickly catch — and correct — negative thoughts because you're aware enough to notice them. When you feel yourself becoming distracted from something important, you can clear your mind to focus on the subject at hand without concern about what's coming up later or what happened before.

Practical suggestions for increasing your ability to let go of workplace stress and become more present-moment aware are provided in Chapters 3 and 16.

Corporate Actions to Address Work-Family Concerns

At the same time that you are taking personal steps to deal more effectively with the competing demands of work and family, it's a priority to initiate or increase company support for your efforts. There are four principal reasons for the growing corporate interest in work-family issues:

First, *work force demographics are changing*. In some parts of the United States, Europe, and Japan, labor is already so scarce that companies are using innovative family policies as a means of attracting and keeping qualified employees. With the baby boom over, businesses are being forced to address the needs of talented people who are trying to act responsibly at home as well as at work.

Second, *employee perceptions are changing*. "Unless we rethink our traditional career paths," write Fran Sussner Rodgers and Charles Rodgers in the *Harvard Business Review*, "the raised aspirations of many women are now clearly on a collision course with their desire to be parents. . . . [A] shift in women's perceptions greatly changes the climate for employers. Women and men in two-career and single-parent families are much better able to identify policies that will let them act responsibly toward their families and still satisfy their professional ambitions. Companies that don't act as partners in this process may lose talent to companies that do rise to the challenge." [32]

Third, there is increasing evidence that *inflexibility about work-family issues has an adverse effect on productivity and health.* According to a recent study at Merck and Company, employees who perceived their managers or supervisors as unsupportive about family issues reported higher levels of stress, lower job satisfaction, and greater absenteeism.[33] Other studies report that supportive companies attract new employees more easily, have them return more quickly to the job after maternity leave, and generally benefit from higher work force morale.[34]

Fourth, there is *rising concern about children.* The number of single-parent families is growing, childhood poverty is up, scholastic aptitude test scores are falling, suicide rates are rising, and childhood obesity, physical fitness, and literacy levels are all moving in the wrong direction.

To date, businesses have expressed their concern primarily through efforts to assist schools or offer community education programs. But a number of studies, including those by Work/Family Directions, Inc., a leading research and consulting firm on dependent care and the changing workplace, show that up to one-half of parents complain that they don't have the workplace flexibility to attend important school events and parent-teacher conferences. "It is certainly possible," conclude the researchers, "that adapting work rules to allow this parent-school connection — and trying to influence schools to schedule events with working parents in mind — might have as great a positive effect on education as some direct interventions."[35]

"For companies that want to use and fully develop the talents of working parents and others looking for flexibility," say the Rodgerses, "the agenda is well defined."[36] There are three broad areas that require attention (few companies are active in all of them — many are active in none):

Dependent care, including infants, children, adolescents, and the elderly. A number of studies show that many working parents have difficulty arranging child care and that those with the most trouble also experience the most frequent work disruptions and the greatest absenteeism.

Companies can help provide, or support, effective child care programs in many ways. These include help in finding existing child care services and efforts to increase the availability of top-quality care (including care for sick children) in the community at large and especially in locations convenient to company employees; financial assistance for child care, particularly for entry-level employees; involvement with schools and other community programs to increase the number and quality of programs available for school-age children whose parents work; and support for government initiatives that provide greater investment in children.

Studies at IBM and Traveler's Insurance Company indicate that 20 to 30 percent of employees have some responsibility for the care of an adult dependent. And, as in the case of pressures caused by child care responsibilities, studies show that productivity suffers when people try to balance work and the care of parents.[37]

To make matters worse, elder care is often complicated by distance: Many elderly dependents live more than 100 miles away from the person concerned about them. Companies can help by connecting with agencies in the dependent's city that can provide referrals and arrangements in case of questions or emergencies. This helps spare employees time, expense, and distress — and, correspondingly, increases productivity and job satisfaction.

Greater flexibility in work design and career path options. A recent study at two high-technology companies showed that employed parents work the equivalent of two full-time jobs.[38] The average working mother puts in a total work week (combining work at home and on the job) of 84 hours, compared with 72 hours for male parents and about 50 hours for married men and women with no children.

A Swedish research team at a Volvo plant[39] recently found significant signs of stress in both men and women during the day. When the men went home, however, their blood pressure and stress hormone levels usually returned to normal, while the women's levels more often remained elevated, possibly because of added responsibilities and stresses at home. And because stress has been linked to silent heart disease and heart attack — and nearly half of those killed by heart attack in the United States each year are women (six times as many as will die from breast cancer) — it's especially important for working mothers to learn how to effectively manage stress and, whenever possible, to reduce their at-home workload by delegating responsibilities and arranging for brief, regular periods of quiet time and self-renewal.

These and other findings have ignited new corporate interest in flexible schedules, part-time employment options, and new career path alternatives. In addition to time away from work to care for newborn or newly adopted children, employees with dependent-care responsibilities have several primary needs for flexibility.

First, it's important to have a schedule that can accommodate the normal and special requirements of children, such as school conferences, medical and dental appointments, and artistic and sporting events. Second, it's essential to be able to respond to unexpected emergencies and requests that are an integral part of family life — glitches in child care arrangements, illnesses, and early school closings in bad weather.

The most common and successful corporate response to both needs has been flextime, discussed earlier in this chapter. In terms of career path alternatives, it's important for companies to find new ways to integrate flexible work schedule options into long-term career tracks. This includes abolishing the antiquated notion of judging productivity by time spent at work. "Nothing is more frustrating to parents," write Rodgers and Rodgers in the *Harvard Business Review*, "than working intensely all day in order to pick up a child on time, only to be judged inferior to a co-worker who has to stay late to produce as much."[40]

Confirmation of family issues as an organizational concern. The message that upper management sends to employees is extremely important. Every company needs to develop a corporate work-family policy and communicate it to all employees; and it must then hold every manager and supervisor accountable for the implementation and responsiveness to this policy in departments and work teams.

In today's business world, narrow approaches to personal effectiveness and performance enhancement just don't work. Through research, a new view is emerging of what it takes for an individual to become an outstanding workplace performer, and it includes such long-overlooked areas of attention as self-renewal, social support, and balancing the needs of work and family. Each makes a basic but indispensable contribution to creating — and sustaining — the Performance Edge.

15

High-Stress Business Travel

In the years ahead, more and more CEOs, managers, and professionals will have to maintain tough personal travel schedules, with longer, more frequent flights and stressful performance criteria.

— Fortune *magazine*

THE DEMANDS of business travel have never been higher. Each year, 40 million Americans embark on business-related trips — by plane, train, and automobile — more than a billion times. These numbers are rising and so are the risks to our health and performance.

According to a recent national study,[1] nearly two-thirds of us feel that business travel has become so stressful that we often lose our effectiveness and feel pressured, tired, nervous, tense, or uptight. This travel stress is costing untold billions of dollars in lost productivity and errors in strategic planning, quality control, and customer service. Worst of all, we're paying this price at a time when we can least afford it.

Going Global, Competing Against Time

Some are calling this the Era of Possibilities. Across the planet, authoritarian governments and centralized economies are on the run while democracies and free markets are on the rise. As battles for world markets replace wars over territory, economic competition — and opportunities — are unprecedented.

Going global has become the only way for many companies to survive. Those that lag behind will find doors slamming shut. Therefore, many corporations are now investing more heavily overseas than at home. As a result, more and more people — from CEOs and managers to engineers and sales representatives — are hitting the road, being expected to handle frequent, long-distance travel.

Adding to the challenges of business travel is the fact that it's turning into an all-out race: Those who get there faster, perform better, and get back sooner are "running circles around their slower competition, enabling them to use this time advantage to upset the traditional leaders of their industries and to claim the number one competitive and profitability positions," says one recent business report.[2]

Travel Pressures Keep Growing

The business traveler must excel in some of the toughest work environments, performing in unfamiliar surroundings where the assignments are often dictated by someone else's schedule. Even worse, frequent travel attacks the heart of a healthy lifestyle — exercise and sleep routines get interrupted, healthful diets are difficult to maintain, dehydration and air pollution are constant threats, there's an increased risk of sudden death from stress-related heart attack, and the nonstop pressures drain energy and can quickly dull the mind.

In spite of these factors, corporate travelers are expected to

- meet tighter travel deadlines
- remain highly alert and productive under adverse conditions
- have the mental and physical stamina to cope with unexpected delays and upper management's rising expectations of accomplishment
- handle personal relationship strains and feelings of worry or guilt about being away from home and family.

Adding to the pressure is the fact that there's no longer any imposed downtime during business travel — voice mail, pagers, facsimiles, and electronic messages can reach us 24 hours a day. "Technology is increasing the heartbeat of society," says Manhattan architect James Trunzo, who designs "automated environments." "We are inundated with information. The mind can't handle it all. The pace is so fast now — at work and when traveling — that I sometimes feel like I'm a gunfighter dodging bullets." [3]

With the cost of travel — and company stakes — climbing so high, there's an urgent new boardroom demand: No more performance slack on business trips. Corporate travelers are now expected to arrive at each destination on time and on top, fully capable of getting things accomplished more quickly and effectively than ever before. [4]

But it remains to be seen whether this executive manifesto will be successful. Although the rules of the corporate travel game may be changing, up to this point the travel fitness of the players has not — and job burnout is increasing at an alarming rate. Right at a time when companies most need their skills, an unprecedented number of executives, managers, sales reps, and service professionals are worn out, complaining of anxiety, mental and physical fatigue, and ennui. [5]

Practical Guidelines for Corporate Travelers

Fortunately, there are many simple, practical ways for individual business travelers to protect their health and enhance their performance.

At the time of this writing, I am in the midst of a comprehensive research project on business travel designed to draw together the newest scientific discoveries from experts in the United States, Canada, Europe, and Asia. The goal is to develop a comprehensive personal blueprint for mastering the pressures of corporate travel — in the air and on the road — including practical solutions to dozens of travel-related concerns. My associates and I have already pinpointed a variety of simple, innovative ways for business travelers to increase their energy and stamina, sharpen their mental powers, and protect their health, arriving at each destination with a fresh sense of vitality and a stronger competitive advantage. Just as important are other guidelines that can enable you to arrive back home with energy to spare.

Many of the basic priorities for effective business travel are presented throughout *The Performance Edge* — such as dealing with stressful "crisis moments"; gaining control of time pressures; stopping tension and pain; balancing your posture; improving communication exchanges; capturing decision-making and innovation opportunities; taking frequent, brief work breaks; and so on. The remainder of this chapter offers some insights into several other areas of special concern to business travelers.

Quick-Release Stress Control

Stress is a primary hazard for frequent business travelers. Many aspects of travel — schedule delays, crowds, long lines, lost baggage, noise, and so on — are to a large extent beyond your personal control as an individual traveler. Without some quick-release stress management skills, these pressures can quickly turn into *negative* stress — the most damaging kind.

Consequently, business travelers need to be especially alert to stress hot spots and early warning signals such as anger, frustration, anxiety, or fatigue, and they should rely on a practical collection of on-the-spot stress management methods. Here are three examples.

The Instant Calming Sequence (ICS). During travel, mishandled stressful crisis moments pile up, steadily breaking down your work effectiveness, blocking your ability to rest or relax, and magnifying pressure. On the road, few of us have time for traditional stress management methods, such as taking 20 to 30 minutes twice a day to go off somewhere to meditate or listen to a relaxation tape.

The Instant Calming Sequence (ICS), presented in Chapter 3, is designed to let you catch the first stimulus or signal of distress and trigger an immediate control response. Because the ICS is performed while you are fully alert, with eyes open, the technique may be used unobtrusively in a wide range of business travel circumstances.

As you'll recall, the five ICS steps are: (1) uninterrupted breathing, (2) positive face, (3) balanced posture, (4) release muscle tension, and (5) mental control. They combine to form a powerful automatic reflex that is ideal for two broad types of travel stress situations: (1) when forced to make a sudden critical decision or deal with unexpected problems — of which traveling seems to provide an endless supply, and (2) handling scheduled peak pressure situations, such as walking off the airplane and immediately making a key sales call or presentation at a business meeting.

Strategies for winning the waiting game. Benjamin Franklin's expression "Time is money" has come to symbolize the new corporate currency — and travel-related waiting costs us lots of it. In fact, billions of dollars are wasted annually because so few of us have figured out effective ways to minimize waiting and turn what seems to be "down wait time" into highly productive breaks. During business travel, waiting occurs frequently and it's a learned aggravation. Fortunately, there are some simple things all of us can do to take better advantage of unavoidable travel delays.

First, take a lesson from Albert Einstein. A friend once needed his advice and arranged for the two of them to meet one evening. But the friend told Einstein that he wanted to make certain that the esteemed professor wasn't forced to waste any time waiting. Einstein replied: "Don't worry, the kind of work I do can be done anywhere." Grasping this simple perception can help you master wait time and minimize impatience.

If you often find yourself in circumstances where unexpected waits occur, prepare in advance. Take along work or leisure projects that can be pursued anywhere — a book or memos to read, a Dictaphone for organizing your thoughts on a new project or catching up on correspondence, a music or learning tape with pocket-size cassette player and headphones, or a notebook to do quick business work or jot out a letter to someone special. Even without these materials, you can capitalize on wait time to shift mental gears and use your imagination to boost your creative powers and expand your "time horizons" (Chapter 7) or simply take a brief, invigorating "mental vacation" like a trip to the beach. With some awareness and planning, wait time can be used to bring out the best, instead of the worst, in you.

When you find yourself unexpectedly faced with a delay, consider one final tactic recommended by researchers in this field.[6] Turn your mind from *clock time* — counting minutes — to *event time,* where you begin and end activities when circumstances warrant. "Remind yourself why you are waiting," advises psychologist Perry W. Buffington, "focus on the positive things that have come to you while waiting, and plan what you want to happen as you wait. By focusing on the positive event, time moves faster and is easier to justify."[7]

Turn off techno-stress. The shift to an electronically assisted lifestyle is gathering momentum. Communication breakthroughs keep us on call everywhere we go on business trips. Airport business centers, mobile cellular phones, pagers, dictation machines, laptop and notebook-size computers, remote phone answering machines, voice mail, electronic mail, computer bulletin boards, facsimiles, and vehicle navigation systems are guaranteeing that even when we're out of sight, we're never out of touch.

Beyond the obvious advantages of the new "portable office" is a serious pitfall — burnout from traveler's techno-stress. Compelling evidence suggests the need to break the cycle of working on the move by taking regular self-renewal breaks.[8]

"I suspect that the key personality variable is self-discipline," says James Campbell Quick, professor of organizational behavior at the University of Texas at Arlington.[9] Quick theorizes that the executive, manager, or professional who can say no as well as yes is likely to get more positive results from the new electronic gadgetry. "We need to turn off often enough to rejuvenate ourselves," he says. "The risk in being able to work around the clock anywhere in the world is that you'll do just that. You may get a lot done, but you may also be dead sooner." So be certain to schedule private daily downtime (when you close off communication with everyone except your immediate family), shifting your posture and mind away from work, and take a 60-second work break routine, as discussed in Chapter 8, at least once every half hour.

Exercise — Keeping on Track When You're Traveling

Frequent business travel makes it difficult to maintain a consistent fitness program. But exercising on the road pays solid dividends.

Beyond the health and performance benefits noted in Chapter 10, new evidence suggests that regular exercise contributes to physiological adaptability and "toughness" — and that means an increased ability to cope more effectively with the stresses of business life, including travel.[10]

But let's face it, away-from-home exercise sessions need to be made as convenient as possible. Even when you have time for a workout, finding a gym or fitness area in an unfamiliar city can be frustrating. Fortunately, more and more hotels are putting greater emphasis on meeting customers' fitness needs, and a host of travel-related fitness services are appearing in major cities throughout North America, Europe, and Asia.

Most of us who travel on business emerge from airplanes, cars, and trains ready to relieve cramped muscles and move stiff joints. But often all we can do during layover or transfer times is walk in circles around the terminal building, dragging our briefcases and carry-on luggage, fighting the crowds as we go.

When this seems to be your only option, consider renting a locker, storing your bags, loosening your collar, and taking a brisk but comfortable fitness walk for 20 minutes or so. Try to avoid wrestling with your luggage or carrying a heavy purse or briefcase since this is one of the surest ways to strain your neck and shoulder muscles.

When you're waiting to board your plane or train, you can go through a 60-second Performance Edge Workbreak (Chapter 8) and include a few quick abdominal exercises, neck ovals, or other joint range of motion exercises.

Travelers passing through many major airports and train stations these days are finding another option — full-service fitness centers that for a nominal fee offer a complete circuit of weight training equipment and aerobic options (treadmills, climbers, rowers, stationary cycles, cross-country ski machines, racquetball courts, and more) along with a locker room, steam room, sauna, showers, towels, and toiletries. Some clubs also provide a free baggage check (or staff members will keep an eye on your luggage while you exercise), workout clothes (shirts, shorts, and socks), and professional massage therapy services.

When you're booking a hotel, be sure to ask about nearby walking and jogging trails, and inquire about the hotel's fitness facilities. Ask for details such as the size of the pool and the specific type, brand, and number of fitness machines. You may also want to inquire about whether there are waiting lines to use equipment during peak time periods such as early morning and the noon hour.

If you enjoy heading into the urban outdoors for a short bicycle ride or brisk walk, first check with your hotel staff on the safest and most scenic fitness routes in the area. Second, minimize smog-related health stress by avoiding rush hour and choosing to exercise outdoors on summer mornings and winter evenings since these are the best times to avoid air that's thick with car exhaust, carbon monoxide, ozone, and other toxic fumes.[11]

Even if you don't have time to leave your hotel room, there's still no excuse for not exercising. You can do push-ups, abdominal exercises, flexibility stretches, and aerobic activities such as jumping rope, chair stepping, or spending a few minutes walking in place.

Resources

- *Birnbaum's Guides for Business Travelers* (Houghton Mifflin, published annually). Offer concise but limited information on fitness centers and jogging/walking routes in dozens of cities. Separate editions for the United States, Europe, and Asia.
- *FastTracks* (DWH, 528 Hennepin Ave., Suite 506, Minneapolis, MN 55403; 612-341-9843). A newsletter devoted to reviewing and rating fitness facilities and walking/running/cycling routes in major cities worldwide.
- *Fodor's* recently announced plans to begin publishing a new guide for travelers on exercise opportunities in thirty-five U.S. cities.

Travel Nutrition

During business travel, your food and beverage choices strongly influence your mental and physical stamina. Previous chapters of *The Performance Edge* have included practical advice on eating frequent small meals and light snacks; controlling fat and cholesterol levels; drinking plenty of extra water to prevent dehydration; and other nutritional considerations.

An area of special concern for corporate travelers is the mind-mood-food connection[12] — how specific meals and snacks affect the production of brain chemical messengers called neurotransmitters and how this influences your state of mind and emotions. As discussed in Chapter 11, compelling evidence suggests that you can gain greater control of your alertness and performance by choosing certain foods and beverages at specific travel times.

- *Foods for increased alertness* are the best choice right before that important midafternoon business meeting or crucial 2:00 A.M. conference call from Asia or Europe. Meals and snacks that are low in fat and include a small amount of protein-rich food can reportedly promote faster thinking, greater energy, increased attention to detail, and quicker reaction speed.
- *Foods for increased calmness* are a good preparation for entering rush hour traffic or for right after takeoff on a flight when you're ready to relax and unwind. Here, meals or snacks that are low in fat and low in protein while being high in complex carbohydrates can often help produce a calm, focused state of mind and relaxed emotions (although in late afternoon these snacks make some people drowsy, so be certain to experiment to find which snacks are best for you).

Choose your best meals and snacks for traveling. When dining out on a business trip, follow the suggestions given in Chapter 11. During travel on commercial airlines, see what your options are for advance-request special meals, such as low-fat, seafood, kosher, or vegetarian. Recognize that there's often no way to control the fat content or ensure the freshness of the food in these in-flight meals (medical authorities warn that many cases of traveler's "24-hour stomach flu" are actually the result of food poisoning, so freshness really *does* matter when you need to perform at your best on a business trip).

Like a growing number of savvy corporate travelers, you might begin packing some of your own meals and snacks, particularly when pressures are high and deadlines tight. When it's inconvenient to prepare your own favorite meals and snacks at home prior to departure, you may be able to locate a nearby "gourmet-to-go" take-out restaurant where you can choose from a variety of delicious low-fat options. For a full range of ideas and recipes, see *America's New Low-Fat Cuisine* by Leslie L. Cooper (Houghton Mifflin, 1991).

Replenish fluids. In Chapter 8, dehydration was discussed as a serious cause of mental and physical fatigue and poor work performance.[13] This is especially true for corporate travelers. The steady loss of water during airline flights is more than double that which occurs in an average office building. In fact, if you're a frequent business flyer, the rapid circulation of dry airplane air may cause your body to lose as much as two pounds of water in a three-to-four-hour flight.[14]

Get into the habit of drinking six to eight glasses of water every day. Add an extra glass of water for each caffeinated or alcoholic beverage you consume. Keep a glass of spring water next to you throughout each airline flight. Sip it regularly and have the flight attendant refill your glass several times during the flight. As a general guideline, avoid drinking tap water on any commercial airline and, in addition, skip ice cubes in beverages on most foreign and international flights since there is a potentially serious risk of contamination.

Flying the Frenzied — and Often Unfriendly — Skies

The government agencies that regulate air travel conditions maintain that the controlled environment of airplane cabins at 38,000 feet is no less "healthy" than that of the average business office. However, in our age of "sick building syndrome" — where, as noted in Chapter 12, researchers say that up to half of the work force in America and Europe suffers from pollution-related ailments in the workplace — this is hardly reassuring.

Physicians, radiation experts, environmental medicine researchers, and others insist that there's a serious problem — and it's getting worse. Despite recent improvements in some air cabin conditions, including smoking bans on many flights, passengers are still exposed to dozens of substances that cause mental and physical fatigue and adversely affect health. These irritants include high-altitude radiation, carbon monoxide, ozone, carbon dioxide, bacteria, fungi, viruses, and other contaminants.*

For the moment, the best we can do as individuals is to keep our personal resistance high. The following are several further guidelines:

Increase your protection against toxic air and high-altitude oxygen deprivation. Fresh air is sucked into commercial airliners through two airpacks, compressors that run off the jet engines, and circulated throughout the cabin. A recent study by the National Academy of Sciences reports that, on average, pilots in the cockpit receive 150 cubic feet of fresh air a minute, first-class passengers get 50, and those in coach as little as 7. And this limited air flow gets cut in half when, as often happens, pilots turn off one of the plane's two airpacks to save fuel.

To make matters worse, Federal Aviation Administration regulations on cabin oxygen content and on carbon dioxide and other air pollutants often fail to meet even the modest standards set by the federal Occupational Safety and Health Administration. And many of the newest planes are designed to conserve fuel by recirculating at least 50 percent of the cabin air.

This poses a number of potentially serious health risks. Hypoxia (reduced availability of oxygen) causes symptoms ranging from dizziness and drowsiness to agitation and impaired reasoning.[15] Factors such as fatigue, vibration, noise, and dehydration tend to make the symptoms worse.

In addition, a new study by the National Academy of Sciences shows that air travelers face significantly increased risk of respiratory infections from the extremely dry air and the germs from other passengers and crew members circulating through the aircraft's ventilation system.[16]

The most practical advice to date is to make advance reservations to select a seat near the front of the plane (either in first class, business class, or the most forward rows of coach), and upon boarding the plane to let the head flight attendant know that for your health you need plenty of fresh air and oxygen during the flight, requesting that he or she ask the pilot not restrict the flow of fresh air by turning off any of the airpacks.

* The Department of Transportation has just completed a major new study that involved secretly measuring the in-flight cabin environment on seventy-five different domestic and international flights. The evidence confirms some of our worst suspicions.

In addition, if you wear contact lenses, consider removing them during long flights. This will help prevent the low-humidity cabin air, which approximates the moisture content of the Gobi Desert, from drying out your contact lenses and causing corneal abrasions that can make your eyes bloodshot, tired, and sore.

Reduce noise and vibration stress. Studies show that aircraft noise and vibration cause significant discomfort and stress reactions.[17] It's common to experience short-term interference with hearing during flight, and frequent travelers run the risk of some permanent hearing loss. To minimize these problems, select comfortable earplugs to wear during takeoff and landing — and consider keeping them in throughout the flight. (Commercially available "sonic ear valves" feature a unique membrane that screens out loud noise but enables you to hear loudspeaker messages or to talk with someone next to you.) To dampen vibrational stress during takeoff and while aloft, place a small pillow or foam pad between any body areas and hard surfaces of the seat or armrests.

Prevent cramped posture problems, including "leg travel lag." During airline flights, pay special attention to your seating position. Follow the guidelines on balanced posture provided in Chapter 9. Wear loose, comfortable clothing. And if you're dressed in business attire, unbutton your shirt and loosen your tie to avoid restricting blood flow to your eyes.[18] Adjust your seating position and reduce vibrational stress points using several small pillows or a padded back support.

If you're planning to rest during the flight, once the plane levels off tilt your seat back about 20 degrees and position small pillows against your lower back and at the base of your neck. This helps unload the force of your body weight from your spine and put it on the seat.[19]

Recent British medical studies report a rare but alarming health risk for those who travel long distances in cramped airline seats.[20] For a number of corporate travelers, "including those who are relatively young and without a past history of cardiovascular disease," there is an increased risk of heart attack and sudden death due to blood clots resulting from restricted circulation in the lower legs (caused by the downward pull of gravity, lack of movement, poor seat design, alcohol, dehydration, and other factors).

"The hazards of long airline trips, often under such cramped conditions (especially in economy class seats), are not appreciated by most travelers," say Drs. John M. Cruickshank, Richard Gorlin, and Bryan Jennett, who headed a recent British study. Flights as short as three hours may be potentially dangerous.

Whenever possible when flying economy class, try to select flights with roomier, more comfortable seats, such as the Boeing 767 and McDonnell-Douglas MD-80, advises Ed Perkins, editor of *Consumer Reports Travel Letter*.[21] Make an advance reservation for an aisle seat or other "preferred" seat as far forward as possible. If these are unavailable, choose an aisle seat over the wing, where the ride is generally more stable than in the rear of the aircraft.

Make it a special point to be physically active during the hour preceding your airline departure. Walk through the airport for 15 to 20 minutes before your flight. Few of us think of walking around the gate area in the final minutes before boarding, but it's a convenient way to use these downtime minutes to invigorate your body and help make the travel miles easier.

Once on board, loosen any restrictive clothing and periodically release tension and increase flexibility by going through some gentle, fairly inconspicuous exercises in your seat — neck ovals, shoulder shrugs, torso turns, wrist and ankle rotations, knee lifts, and so on. Then, every half hour or so during the flight, get up to move around the cabin and further stretch your legs, shoulders, and back.

Airborne time management. With more and more corporate managers and professionals spending time in plane seats than ever before, being effective during those in-flight hours requires careful planning. Few of us can afford the luxury of reading a novel, watching the movie, or chitchatting with the traveler next to us. Instead, travel time has become, of necessity, work time — a chance to catch up on paperwork, prepare for an upcoming meeting, or do some deep strategic thinking.

If you don't want your neighbor bothering you, as soon as you're settled into your seat and have said a friendly word or two, pull out your work and put your pen or pencil in hand. If the person in the adjoining seat misses the hint, respond warmly but clearly by saying that you have to meet some work deadlines during the flight time. If necessary, put on the earphones with the volume off and then go ahead with your work.

Insights on Winning the Time Zone War

When you travel on business, some of your most valuable competitive assets — such as alertness and stamina — come under serious attack. This is particularly true whenever you fly long distances east to west or west to east. Flying across multiple time zones creates physiological disturbances that adversely affect the human body and brain.

Internal "biological clocks," synchronized to your home time zone, govern the cycles of millions of hormonal and biochemical processes in your body and mind. On a long-distance easterly or westerly flight, the "hands" of literally billions of body clocks get thrown out of balance, causing a period of adjustment that scientists call a *transient state of dyschronism*, commonly known as *jet lag*.

Symptoms include physical and mental fatigue (a kind of all-over, all-consuming weariness), headaches, poor concentration, thwarted creativity, memory loss, dulled vision, irritability, slowed physical reflexes, and sharply reduced productivity. One recent study[22] showed that 94 percent of all travelers who cross three or more time zones suffer jet lag; and 45 percent said it was severe.

In intercontinental travel between Europe, Asia, and North America, jet lag is the major stress factor, and this performance threat will grow if, as predicted, aviation technology steps up to faster and faster aircraft. Supersonic planes can already cut transatlantic flight times almost in half. If commercial hypersonic aircraft (which are closely related to spacecraft) are developed, a transatlantic crossing might take only 15 minutes.

This will certainly be convenient for attending a brief afternoon meeting on another continent and then returning home in time for the evening family meal. But for those of us who need to remain overnight or longer in a new time zone, these lightning-quick flights through multiple time frames will produce even more of a shock to the body's internal clocks than present-day flights do.

Beating jet lag — preventing or minimizing its symptoms and dramatically reducing adjustment time for your internal biological clocks — depends on some newly discovered guidelines, a collection of simple strategies to arrive at your destination fresh and ready to perform at your best.

Here are some basic guidelines that chronobiologists (scientists who study the body's biological cycles) and other professionals researching jet lag refer to as *zeitgebers* (pronounced "tsight-gay-bers," from the German for "time givers").

1. *Preset your watch — and mind — to your destination time zone.* This is a simple, effective way to help your body clock adjust to a new time frame. During the days preceding a trip involving a change of three to eight time zones, gradually adjust your schedule while you're still at home to the time frame of your destination. For example, when you have advance notice of a business trip, modify your sleep/wake cycle. If you're headed east, you can help prepare your biological clocks for the trip by going to bed and waking up earlier each day, gradually moving your internal body rhythms toward your destination time zone. For westbound trips, the opposite pattern is appropriate.

2. *Take advantage of light/dark cycles.* "Changes in the light/dark cycle have profound effects on circadian rhythms," says Dr. F. S. Preston, director of medical services for British Airways, "particularly when you're required to work or perform well in a new time environment. These changes include effects on sleep, mental performance, including judgment and decision making, and physical performance."[23]

"The body has hundreds of biochemical and hormonal rhythms, all keyed to light and dark," explains Dr. Michael Irwin, medical director of the United Nations. A Harvard medical team recently discovered that the human body clocks can be adjusted by exposure to bright light[24] (the researchers used light with an intensity between 7,000 and 12,000 lux, which is comparable to daylight just after dawn).

What this means, according to Professor Richard Kronauer and Dr. Charles Czeisler, the two scientists who headed the three-year Harvard study, is that travelers' body clocks can be reset by as much as 12 hours by means of a series of "bright-light treatments" using either daylight or commercially available light boxes. The findings confirm the conclusion that there is a neurological link between the retina of the eye and a small area of the brain known as the suprachiasmatic nuclei, which are thought to play a key role in the timing of body clocks. Therefore, say researchers, you can use natural or artificial light to help move your body clocks forward or backward by up to two full hours a day in order to resynchronize your wake/sleep schedule to the new time frame.

Scientists offer some preliminary advice: First, on the day of your flight, avoid exposure to morning daylight and if possible avoid exposure to all bright light until the first afternoon or early evening at your destination time zone. Wearing dark sunglasses — indoors and out — is helpful, although some of the researchers prefer welder's goggles, which, rather obviously, are inappropriate attire for most business settings. (One of Dr. Czeisler's Harvard Medical School colleagues was taken in for questioning by security personnel at London's Heathrow Airport when he arrived on a recent flight wearing welder's goggles to ward off the morning sunlight.)

Second, maximize your exposure to bright light in the afternoon at your destination time, especially during the critical period between 1:00 P.M. and 5:00 P.M. In many cases, the simplest suggestion is to go for a brisk walk outdoors where you can flood your eyes with daylight — without sunglasses but shielding exposed skin by using a broad-spectrum sunscreen with a skin protection factor of at least 15 — or to keep the window shades open during this time period on your flight.

On an eastbound evening flight, such as from New York to Zurich, for example, arrange to avoid bright light on the morning of your departure. On arrival in Zurich, stay out of bright indoor light or daylight until at least 10:00 A.M. local time. Then arrange to spend some time in bright light during the afternoon and early evening hours. If it's nighttime in Zurich when you arrive, immediately assume the destination schedule and get to your room, terminate all social or business conversations, turn off the lights, and shut your eyes until dawn.

On a westbound flight, such as from Los Angeles to Tokyo, follow the same basic light/dark rules: Avoid daylight in the morning on the day of departure. That afternoon and early evening, maximize your light exposure — walking outside in bright light, choosing a window seat on the plane, keeping the shade open, and not watching the in-flight movie during this period. If you're flying during nighttime in your destination time zone, then pull down the window shade, stop conversing with anyone near you on the flight, turn out the reading light, and close your eyes to rest (some business travelers use a special foam sleep mask to block out light). Even if you don't sleep, your body clock will continue adjusting to your destination time frame.

Dr. Czeisler strongly recommends repeating this light-exposure procedure for several days after arriving at your destination. Professor Kronauer predicts that there will soon be light and darkness facilities in airports and hotels "and even headsets that will administer light directly to the eye while the user is traveling." A number of companies are already manufacturing portable light screens for the home or office (you can use this method while working, reading, or watching television), but the current size makes them impractical for in-flight use.

If your flight is scheduled during the afternoon or early evening, you may want to request a window seat in the south-facing aisle (for the Northern Hemisphere) for greater access to bright light; the opposite, darker aisle if you're on an early morning flight.

3. *Select healthful meals and snacks according to mind-mood-food principles.* Follow the nutritional guidelines discussed earlier in this chapter and in Chapter 11. Choose a jet-lag-beating strategy of knowing which foods may safely influence changes in your brain chemistry and state of alertness or drowsiness.[25]

▪ Basic advice for *both* eastbound and westbound flights:

The day before your flight
1. Eat a hearty breakfast, a light midmorning snack, a hearty lunch, and a light midafternoon snack that are all *low in fat and high in protein.* Researchers have found that these foods help promote increased energy and alertness. For examples of specific meal and snack choices, see Chapter 11.
2. Eat supper (and, if you wish, a light evening snack) that is low in fat, low in protein, and high in carbohydrates. A variety of suggestions are given in Chapter 11. Scientists report that these foods help promote a calm, relaxed state of mind and emotions and, on a biochemical level, they can help prepare you for restful sleep.

The morning of your flight

Arise an hour or so earlier than usual and repeat your routine from the previous day, *but make the meals and snacks smaller in quantity — about half the normal size.* Researchers have found that this helps prime your biochemistry so that you are more highly sensitive to influences such as light/dark cycles, activity patterns, and certain foods in order to promote the most rapid adjustment to your destination time zone.

The first breakfast at your destination

Resume the meal and snack schedule of your day before departure — a hearty breakfast, light midmorning snack, hearty lunch, and midafternoon snack that are all low in fat and high in protein. Then eat a hearty evening meal that is low in fat, low in protein, and high in carbohydrates.

4. *Drink extra water — and use coffee and tea strategically.* Dehydration is a typical problem on all airline flights. Therefore, on the days preceding, during, and following your flight, drink extra water (choose bottled or spring water since contamination risks warrant avoiding tap water on all airline flights and even skipping ice cubes in your beverages on some international flights).

Methylated xanthines — chemicals such as theophylline, theobromine, and caffeine, which are found naturally in coffeee and tea and can be obtained in nonprescription caffeine tablets — have a powerful ability to reset the body's internal clock timers. Researchers have found that, for those who tolerate methylated xanthines, these naturally occurring chemicals can be used to help rapidly resynchronize your body clock from home time to destination time, sharply reducing symptoms of jet lag.

However, to make this strategy most effective, you must give up or cut back on methylated xanthines for several days prior to your departure to encourage your biochemistry to become more sensitive to mind-mood-food influences. Cutting back also helps your evening meal prompt deeper, more restful sleep and helps ensure that, at the right moments, the methylated xanthines are maximally effective to push your internal biological clocks forward or backward to destination time.

- For *both* eastbound and westbound flights: Two to three days before the flight, stop consuming beverages, foods, or drugs containing methylated xanthines. If you want to have coffee or tea between 3:00 P.M. and 4:30–5:00 P.M., feel free to do so, since research indicates that "for reasons not yet fully understood, methylated xanthines taken during 'British tea time' in the afternoon seem to have little or no effect on the timing of body clocks."[26]

Then:

- *For eastbound flights:* Chronobiologist Charles F. Ehret, former senior scientist at the Argonne National Laboratory in Illinois, advises that on the day of your flight between 6:00 P.M. and 7:00 P.M., "no matter where you are or what you are doing, whether you are still in the airplane or not, drink two to three cups of black coffee or strong, plain tea."[27] Then, during the arrival day at your destination do not have any methylated xanthines all day — except, if you wish, during British tea time in the afternoon.

- *For westbound flights:* On the day of the flight, between 10:30 A.M. and 11:30 A.M. home time, drink two to three cups of black coffee or strong, plain tea. Then do not consume any more methylated xanthines for the rest of this travel day.

5. Schedule activity/rest cycles to match destination time zone. Physical and mental activity has a strong influence on your body's internal clocks. If you find yourself on the airplane during the active, "stay awake" phase of your program to beat jet lag, keep your brain producing alertness chemicals by choosing the corresponding meals and snacks, keeping the lights on and the window shade up, by increasing your physical and mental activity level — read, write, talk to your neighbors, and frequently get up to stretch and move around the plane. Recent studies suggest that physical activity may be one of the most important single factors in resetting your internal body clocks.[28]

This is also why it's so critical that when you arrive at your destination, you immediately merge with the activity phase *matching that time of day in your new location* — even if you feel the urge to slow down and rest, keep walking and talking and stay awake until it's time in this new locale to fall asleep.

- *For eastbound flights:* On the morning of the flight, arise 30 to 60 minutes earlier than usual. Get up and exercise. Then, during the travel day when your watch tells you it's bedtime in your destination time zone — at 11:00 P.M., for example — try to darken your area of the plane, stop moving around, close your eyes, and try to sleep (using a sleep mask if necessary). Even if you don't feel tired, if you rest quietly until morning destination time, your internal body clocks will work to reduce jet lag.
- *For westbound flights:* Do not arise earlier than usual on the morning of your flight (although you may wish to sleep an extra hour or more to encourage your body to adjust to your destination time zone).
- *For both eastbound and westbound flights:* The first morning at your destination, get up at the same hour on the local time clock that you would normally arise back at home. Do *not* oversleep. Get up, go to the restroom and splash some cold water on your face, and get moving — for 15 to 30 minutes before breakfast. Plunge into some stimulating mental activities as well — animated conversation, an important work project, a fast-paced card game, a tough crossword puzzle, or an exciting book — any mental activity that requires your full concentration. Without stopping to take a nap, keep active all day. Then, by the time you fall asleep in the evening, your body clocks will be on track in adjusting to your new time frame.

Increasingly in the 1990s, American managers and business professionals will be expected to maintain tough personal travel schedules, with long flights, meetings, and phone conferences at inconvenient hours. They must be able to perform at their best at all times.

— *"Going Global,"* Business Week

16

The Further Reaches of the Mind: More New Ways to Awaken Your Sleeping Mental Giant

The greatest unexplored territory in the world is the space between our ears.

— *Bill O'Brien, president, Hanover Insurance*

Creativity is not a luxury. Ideas are as important as genes. . . . Wisdom is becoming the new criterion of fitness.

— *Jonas Salk*[1]

NO MAGIC PILL unlocks the further reaches of your brain power. Only a wide array of challenging mental exercises and experiences will enable you to break down the barriers to your mind's optimal function. This chapter expands on the guidelines presented in Chapter 7 on innovative thinking and decision making and shares some practical new ideas for developing and sharpening your mental powers.

Developing Your Brain/Mind at Any Age

Most of us have been led to believe that once we reach maturity, brain growth ceases, signaling the beginning of a steady, unavoidable loss of nerve cells as we grow older. Finally, or so the assumption goes, we end up elderly and trapped in some inevitable web of senility, confusion, fatigue, and boredom. But scientists are discovering that, in most cases, there is absolutely no need for this mental collapse.

Here's why. Without the specific, necessary types of stimulation, the brain will steadily deteriorate, becoming "flabby" in certain vital areas like underused muscles do. But scientists at Yale University School of Medicine, the National Institute on Aging, and other research centers have discovered that with the right mental exercises, active intellectual interests, and a challenging environment, your mind can keep developing toward its full potential and be as sharp — or *sharper* — at age ninety as at age twenty.[2]

In long-term human studies, researchers have found that people who are healthy and mentally active can improve on intelligence tests at age sixty and beyond.[3] "A brain cell needs to be stimulated," explains Marian Cleeves Diamond, professor of neuroanatomy at the University of California, Berkeley. "If you cut off that stimulation, you lose the dimensions of that cell. . . . You lift weights to get more efficient muscles, and you challenge the brain to get more efficient brain cells."[4] Lifelong learning actually changes the qualities of nerve cell endings and increases the strength of nerve impulse transmission.[5]

Aging business executives whose work required sharp concentration and diversified intellectual focus showed little or no weakening of their brain and nervous system when compared in a study with production workers of the same age.[6] Even in our later years, from the time we reach sixty into our nineties, brain cells can keep creating new growth connections, reports Paul Coleman of the University of Rochester.[7]

Drawing Together the Pieces of the Puzzle

Maximizing your mental powers depends on cultivating the habit of welcoming change; acquiring the flexibility to appreciate challenges, ambiguity, and unpredictable experiences; and continuing to seek out and assimilate new information and skills. The whole idea is to turn typical business thinking inside out and shake it — to be able to regard difficult circumstances and other viewpoints with acute curiosity and an open mind.

When you reach that point, conflicts diminish and you'll find it far easier to "go beyond the information given" to make innovative breakthroughs.

In addition to the insights and suggestions offered in previous chapters, the following focus areas warrant consideration:

1. A creative attitude
2. Brain-building physical exercises
3. Mindfulness and concentration
4. Mental imagery skills

---

1. A Creative Attitude: Some Additional Insights

You never know where your next great idea will come from or how far it will take you. For most of us, being consistently creative depends on a work style characterized by concentration and persistence as well as a thinking style conducive to generating new possibilities.

Creativity is related to variety, which researchers say is the spice of memory. In fact, much age-related memory loss can reportedly be prevented if people seek a great diversity of enjoyable, challenging activities.[8]

In Chapter 7, we discussed ten innovation-enhancing heuristics:

- Establish and maintain an open mind and spirit of inquiry.
- Remove hidden obstacles to creative thinking.
- Laugh more: humor can increase creativity.

- Look for anomalies and reject old explanations.
- Ask creative questions.
- Listen carefully — and pay attention.
- Continually expand and develop your work expertise.
- Be willing to be uncertain.
- Gather data.
- Be goal-guided, not goal-governed.

To further develop a more creative attitude, experts in this field set forth some additional heuristics.

- *Let your mind wander.* On every work break and at opportune moments throughout the day, let your mind shift gears and wander, looking at difficult challenges and routine procedures from odd angles and fresh, unusual vantage points.
- *Take time to play.* It may sound a bit odd to suggest that to boost creativity and productivity you might work less and play more. But it's true — the wondrous human spirit is full of surprises. "Rest and reflection are crucial to productivity," says Stephen Colarelli, a psychologist at Central Michigan University. "We are obsessed with busyness, but some of the most productive corporate and public figures took time to rest."[9] Mixing in laughter, humor, and play with your work can be a powerful stimulus to enhancing the creative process.[10]
- *Stretch your mind in as many directions as possible.* Studies[11] confirm that in the modern world we've come to neglect many time-honored habits of lifelong learning, such as creative writing and poetry. For the most part, this is because it's far more convenient to rely on telephones, tape recorders, fax machines, videocameras, computers, and television. We've failed to recognize that the power of communication is not simply to transmit information or pass it along but also to *create* it.

    Writing stimulates innovative thinking because it expands the mind through a disciplined means of expression, explains Mihaly Csikszentmihalyi, professor and former chairman of the Department of Psychology at the University of Chicago. After more than twenty years of research on what is known as the *flow* of optimal experience, he strongly recommends developing intellectual interests that can broaden and deepen your perspectives on work and life. Among his suggested areas of focus are history, philosophy, science, and creative writing, both poetry and prose.

In addition, says Csikszentmihalyi, even such simple endeavors as working crossword puzzles — which in their best form resemble ancient riddle contests — can increase your "flow of thought." Beyond the fact that this game is inexpensive and portable, its challenges can be precisely adjusted so that novices and experts alike can enjoy it. But the key is to move past the confines of simply *solving* crosswords and begin to create your own. This enables you to break free of patterns imposed from the outside and to enjoy a more profound and mentally stimulating experience.

- *Take more risks and be willing to fail early and often.* Being creative is risky — and essential. Cultivate the habit of taking mental chances, of choosing an idea and allowing the possibility that it may be a bad idea. "Anyone who is willing to propose a new theory," says Roger C. Schank, professor of computer science and psychology at Yale University, "to suggest a different way of doing things, to mention that the current wisdom might be wrong, also has to be willing to fall flat on his face." [12]

    AT&T and other corporations have even begun issuing "amnesty certificates" to managers and employees, openly empowering them to take risks without repercussion if they fail. "To encourage mindfulness at work," suggests Ellen J. Langer, professor of psychology at Harvard University, "we should make the office a place where ideas may be played with, where questions are encouraged, and where an 'unlucky throw of the dice' does not mean getting fired." [13]

- *In your own mind, test out a variety of rash generalizations — not to be right, but to be thinking.* In most circumstances, it's a costly mistake to jump to conclusions, but in terms of brainstorming and creativity you can elicit the sparks of innovation when you pose a quick hypothesis in your mind and then are forced to find data to support it, especially if you have to change your hypothesis to account for the new data. "The idea," says Schank, "is not to come up with new creative ideas at first try, but during the process of elaboration, defense, conjecture, refutation, and re-categorization, one might be reminded and begin a totally new process of creative adaptation of an old pattern. The idea is to keep thinking . . . to keep the creative process running."[14]

• *Use brainstorming.* "The ability to analyze and judge the products of our intuition is of crucial importance," writes Philip Goldberg in *The Intuitive Edge.* "But we tend to do it too quickly and peremptorily, forcing premature closure and killing fragile intuitive ideas before they have a chance to develop and reproduce. . . . To counteract this critical urge, it is a good idea to set aside a judgment-free period for generating solutions to specific problems."[15]

Brainstorming, a technique developed in 1948 by Alex Osborn for business settings, is a formal method whereby the collective interaction yields extra power because each person's thoughts can ignite the others'. The rules are easily enforced, and the principles can be adapted to individual use. There are essentially four rules:

1. There is to be no judgment or criticism of any ideas presented. Evaluation is done in a subsequent session — otherwise you interfere with the creative flow.
2. Quantity is desirable; the more ideas the better. As the Chinese proverb aptly states, The best way to catch a fish is to have many lines.
3. No idea is too bizarre, too wild, or too irrelevant. The purpose is not to be correct but to fuel the process of generating imaginative alternatives.
4. Combinations, modifications, and improvements on previously mentioned ideas are encouraged.

• *Get away from it all.* Historically, for the artist, writer, composer, philosopher, inventor, and business entrepreneur, the spark of creativity has burned most brightly in a mind working in solitude.[16] Scheduling time to break away from others and be alone, even just for a few quiet minutes, can open the mind to new perspectives and enable you to reflect more clearly on the challenges and possibilities at hand.
• *Sidestep creativity-stifling criticism.* When you come up with new ideas, you invite criticism. This criticism ultimately causes many

of us to forgo even our fondest dreams and projects. One way to head off critical remarks or deal with them more effectively is to anticipate such responses, says Vincent R. Ruggiero, professor at the State University of New York. This can help us prevent discouragement when we hear it and enable us to improve certain aspects of our ideas before making them public. In his book *The Art of Thinking*, Ruggiero suggests knowing — and perhaps changing — your ideas in advance if they are impractical; too expensive; illegal; immoral; inefficient; unworkable; disruptive of existing procedures; unesthetic; too radical; unappealing to others; or prejudiced against one side of a dispute.[17]

- *Know when to choose individual or group efforts.* When it comes to innovative thinking, whether groups are more effective than individuals depends on the criteria you use for defining success. If decision effectiveness is defined in terms of speed, individuals are superior. If effectiveness means the degree of acceptance the final solution achieves, groups tend to be better. The evidence also indicates that, on average, groups make better quality-oriented decisions than individuals.[18] This doesn't mean, of course, that groups will outperform *every* individual — no matter what the situation, group decisions are seldom better than the performance of the best individual.[19]

2. Brain-Building Physical Exercises

When most people think of building mental power, they think of mental exercises. But you can also strengthen your mind by developing your body. The more sensitively aware the surface of your body is, for example, and the more toned your muscles, the larger the "map" in your brain. Recent discoveries suggest that this map can be expanded in many directions and at virtually any age. For example, you can augment the area of the brain assigned to your fingers simply by increasing and varying the use of your fingers.[20]

One recent study showed that regular bouts of aerobic exercise can trigger brainstorms of innovative thinking, concluding that exercise is "not frills, but should be central to our learning and work processes."[21] Regular exercise increases mental creativity in the workplace, says Thomas E. Backer of the UCLA School of Medicine. "In working with thousands of creative people, I now recommend a regular exercise program as the single best way both to increase resistance to stress and to facilitate personal creativity."[22]

To increase your overall physical and mental coordination, schedule a regular exercise program (Chapter 10) that includes a variety of aerobics and strengthening activities. Beyond that, neuroscientists recommend other enjoyable ways to improve your dexterity and hand-eye coordination,[23] including playing the piano, hand-eye coordination drills, stacking coins, using tweezers to pick up small objects, playing jacks, or completing dot-to-dot or connect-the-numbers puzzles or mazes.

Activities such as these help develop *fluid intelligence*,[24] discussed in Chapter 7. To a great extent, fluid intelligence depends on your degree of physical fitness and the proficiency of your nervous system. At both young and older ages, more fit individuals consistently display higher levels of fluid intelligence.[25]

3. Mindfulness and Concentration

> If there is any one "secret" of effectiveness, it's concentration.
>
> — *Peter F. Drucker*, The Effective Executive

Mindfulness is the ability to focus your complete attention on the world around you and within you exactly as it is this moment — slowing your pace and releasing tensions while increasing your energy, objective intelligence, and productivity. This mental performance attribute is revered in Asia — and it's something that we sorely need in the helter-skelter Western workplace. "The most sophisticated marketing plan, the most complex strategic analysis, the most up-to-the-minute personnel policies are moot in comparison with the power of a manager's attitudes and *visible attention*," says Robert H. Waterman, Jr., in *The Renewal Factor*.[26]

"Mindfulness means being open to an awareness of the moment as it is and to what the moment could hold," explains Joan Borysenko, business consultant and director of the Mind/Body Clinic at Harvard Medical School. "It is a relaxed state of attentiveness to both the inner world of thoughts and feelings and the outer world of actions and perceptions. The joy is not in finishing an activity — the joy is in doing it. You can train yourself to be mindful by cultivating awareness of where your mind is and then making a choice about where you want it to be."[27]

Concentration is defined as bringing one's faculties and efforts into focus on a single task or thought. Many of us assume that it's possible to pay attention to several events simultaneously — for example, studying a business report while listening to news on the radio or writing detailed notes while attending a corporate lecture or workshop. But what actually happens is that your mind must shift back and forth between the two stimuli, causing your attention to oscillate, creating fatigue. When you add other distractions — sights, sounds, scents, uncomfortable seating, and so forth — the stress is even higher. By strengthening your concentration, you can cut down on random, energy-wasting shifts in attention. "*Learn to control your attention*," says a top Soviet sports psychologist, "*and you learn to control your destiny.* Concentration is all-important to achievement because it adds power to any effort, mental or physical."[28]

With heightened concentration, you increase your control over *where* and *when* you focus your mind on the job — on what, precisely, you wish to see, hear, think, feel, and do.

The following sensory-enhancement exercises are examples of those suggested by neuroscientists. While for most of us there's no need to begin any kind of rigorous regimen of these activities, it's certainly worthwhile to consider devoting 5 minutes or so every week to stimulating your powers of sensory alertness.

Vision-Sharpening Exercises

Nerve cells in some of the cortical areas of the brain can be activated only by specific features of what the eyes see, according to Nobel laureates David Hubel and Torsten Wiesel.[29] Here are several simple exercises to help sharpen your vision.

Seeing hidden details. Place a single object on a table. Study it meticulously for about one minute and then close your eyes. Visualize it in your mind for about 15 seconds and then open your eyes and compare your exact image with reality. Over a period of weeks, expand the exercise: increase the number of objects visualized at one time, varying the colors, lighting, positioning, and distance from you as you reduce the allotted time.

You can train your eyes and brain to take in greater detail each time you look quickly and closely at a person, place, or object — and this can enhance your skills as a leader and innovator. This exercise takes less than a minute. Pick up a small object — a pen, pencil, key, watch, small book, or anything else you have nearby. Look at it from all angles, really concentrating on every detail. As you look describe its features — colors, textures, size, shape, usefulness, imprinting, and so on. After 10 to 20 seconds, put this object down and pick up another. Repeat the exercise.

Shifting focus. The eyes register the most information in the first several seconds of looking at an object, scene, or person. When your gaze remains fixed, your eyes become strained and good vision diminishes. In most business situations, it's best to keep fluidly shifting your gaze to help your eyes stay relaxed and take in more information from the scenes around you. Perform a simple focus-shifting exercise by looking at a person or object and moving your gaze every second or two, blinking your eyes often to lessen fatigue, smoothly guiding your vision from one feature to another.

Visual scanning exercises. Crossword and jigsaw puzzles are excellent for stimulating your scanning ability. Another enjoyable mental exercise is to take a newspaper or magazine article and cross out all of any single letter of the alphabet you find on the page. For example, find and cross out the letter *a* wherever you find it. Time yourself so that you go as rapidly as possible.

Auditory-Sharpening Exercises

The acuity of your hearing — and ability to concentrate on what you hear — can often be improved through training.[30] Here are several simple exercises.

Attention-focusing exercises. By listening to two radios, each on a different news channel with the volumes set equally, you can practice "tuning in" one station and "tuning out" the other. Alternate your focus from one station to the other every 20 seconds or so for up to two minutes once or twice a week. Progressively reduce the volume as your hearing sharpness improves.

Extend your hearing exercise. First, relax in a comfortable position. Sit quietly with your eyes closed, listening to the sounds all around you for several minutes. Extend your hearing radius outward from your body (where you can hear your breathing) to as far away as you can stretch it — perhaps to a car horn honking or a dog barking several blocks away.

Selective awareness exercise. This activity helps you develop selective awareness, zeroing in on a certain sound while diminishing your attention to others. Put on your favorite music — ensembles first, working up to full orchestra. Focus your attention for 30 seconds or so on the music line of only one instrument or voice rather than the total sound. Then switch to another performer. Then another. Once this becomes reasonably comfortable, you might try tracking two voices or instruments at the same time while blocking out the rest. Then switch to other voices or instruments. And so on.

4. Mental Imagery Skills

Creative thinking often begins when you remove yourself mentally from the day-to-day business routine. "A brilliant idea, a pivotal decision, a simple solution . . . in a few key minutes you can often accomplish more than shuffling papers for sixty hours," say Dr. Harold H. Bloomfield and Leonard Felder, authors of *The Achilles Syndrome.*[31]

We each have the natural ability to stimulate our creative innovation and problem-solving skills through the power of mental imagery. Beginning in the 1950s, researchers in Europe, the United States, Asia, and the Soviet Union began systematically exploring the role of mental imagery in health, education, and workplace innovation and productivity. Neuroscience literature is filled with evidence that the mind's internal gaze can be harnessed to change human thoughts, feelings, and performance.[32]

"*Thoughts* are basically short-lived electrical events in the brain; like electric sparks, they *come* quickly and they *go* quickly — dozens in each moment," says Dr. Emmett E. Miller, author of *Power Vision: Mastering Life Through Mental Image Rehearsal.* "Look back at the thousands of thoughts you've already had today. They can easily distract you. But if you guide and hold your thoughts to a single *focus* for a while, something quite interesting and important occurs . . . a *mental image* begins to form. This image is represented in the brain by a pattern of chemicals . . . hormone-like substances secreted by the nervous system. The quality of this chemical state influences how we *feel.* Thus, each image stimulates the creation of a particular chemical state, which in turn produces emotions and behaviors consistent with that image. Our emotions, in turn, have a direct effect on our muscular system . . . on how we stand, speak, and approach our work." [33]

"Imaging abilities are vastly underdeveloped in most of us," says Harvard University psychologist Stephen Kosslyn, who has directed several recent studies. "With training and a bit of practice, people can improve immensely in their capacity to use images." [34] Kosslyn recommends finding the separate parts of a mental picture, fitting them together properly, then scanning the image, moving it around, zooming in on one aspect of the image, moving it farther away, panning it to capture a better view of the whole picture, and so on.

For innovative business thinking, it has become extremely important to be able to create detailed mental images — richly woven sensory tapestries filled with sounds, lights, colors, touches, textures, temperatures, movements, and emotions. The ability to quickly and vividly envision a future product, process, system, or service is the first step to solving the business challenges of the future.

Four Steps to Successful Positive Imagery

Mental imagery skills are expanded through practice. In the beginning, mental training often works best using audiotapes. Without a tape, you need to give yourself specific suggestions as well as carry them out. Sometimes this slows results.

You can either create your own written scripts and listen to a friend's voice or your own voice reading them on a recorded tape or memorize the instructions "in a loose fashion, then close your eyes and let yourself drift through the message."[35] As an alternative, consider purchasing previously recorded tapes. In every case, the voice (including your own internal voice) should be calm, interested, and pleasing.

Powerful, positive mental images can be formed using four key steps.

1. *Establish a relaxed, receptive state.* The most effective guided imagery training is preceded by deep relaxation, which helps free the brain from unnecessary chatter and distraction. Breathing helps you relax quickly and deeply, changing the body's center of gravity, increasing the feeling of inner calm, and enhancing your ability to focus your senses.

2. *Recall a successful past experience.* "To take charge of your life and create your own positive future, it is absolutely essential that your images generally be based on a foundation of high-quality, successful experiences from your past," says Dr. Miller.[36] To tackle something new or a task you have never been able to do, you can invent a positive image by watching or reading about others performing the feat successfully, or relating some similar experience from your past. For example, athletic confidence in one sport can often be transferred to another. Images of speaking eloquently to a close friend can be used to help prepare for a major public speaking appearance. And so on.

"We all have within us the key to feeling stronger, more confident, more resourceful, and more successful," explain organizational psychologists Bernie Zilbergeld and Arnold A. Lazarus. "By recalling and focusing on times when you were successful, you recreate the feelings of confidence, power, and accomplishment that are associated with these successes, and that helps to ensure good feelings and positive results in the present and future. Recollection of past achievements is one of the most powerful kinds of imagery available to anyone. All of us have been successful and effective at something, but it's amazing how quickly we forget or minimize these experiences."[37]

Assemble a collection of past success images to call on whenever you need a boost of confidence or strength. This sets a positive emotional tone for the next step in the mental training sequence.

3. Imagine a positive outcome. Imagining a desired outcome — also called *goal imagery* or *result imagery* — helps you focus on what you really want. This unlocks your creative energy, aligns your precise direction, and aids you in organizing the steps necessary to achieve that result. If you regularly, vividly imagine achieving your goal — your vision of the future — you will begin to think about yourself in a brighter light, improving your self-image or perception.

For best results, you must believe the image is an achievable one, something you truly think could happen, something motivating, satisfying, fulfilling that serves your higher values and purposes. Use all of your senses and describe the image as if it were happening right now (using the future perfect tense as recommended in "Your Time Horizon" in Chapter 7).

If you are recording your own audiotape, be certain to give enough detail to get yourself deeply involved with this step and be certain to include positive reinforcements: "You're doing fine," "That's great," "Very good," and so on.

There are three little-known but essential principles for creating genuinely constructive, forward-moving mental images:

(a) *Avoid negative-on-negative imagery and thinking.* Bleak negative-on-negative statements and images are easy to spot. They usually surface when we're in a down mood, and they tend to be a judgmental put-down of yourself, someone else, current circumstances, or the world in general, followed by an image of failure or suffering.

The problem, of course, is that negative suggestion works. It's a self-fulfilling prophecy, bringing about in reality the inadequacy, worthlessness, and other victimizing traits that are imagined.

The way to turn this around is to choose to champion constructive attributions and images and to use negative thoughts as a trigger for positive responses — acting immediately to do something productive instead of destructive; and then identify the source of negative thoughts and whenever possible remove the origins. For example, negative thoughts caused by tension or anxiety tend to get bigger if you use mental warfare, but they can often be controlled through stress management techniques or relieved by physical exercise.

(b) *Notice negative-on-positives,* the saboteurs of imagery and self-talk. It is important to catch and correct the mixed-up statements and mental pictures that slip by most of us in everyday self-talk and work conversations. Here, one part of the image or comment is positive, another negative. The net result is often negative.

For example, even if you mentally picture yourself in a positive way, how do you describe your choices and actions? Are you preventing or avoiding a problem (negative focus) or building a specific, constructive outcome (positive focus)? This common problem was discussed in Chapter 7.

(c) *Choose positive-on-positive thinking patterns.* Pictures in the mind generally have two predominant emphases: the subject and the event. Both must be positive to avoid self-sabotage:

1. Is the subject of your attention (the specific person, group, place, feeling, action, or circumstance) constructive and positive?
2. Does something good happen (the actual statement about the subject of your thought) once your concentration is focused there?

The first part of your mental picture. How do you envision yourself and others throughout the day? Take a minute right now to relax and examine some of your statements and images in slow motion. When you think of yourself or say the pronoun *I*, do you automatically sense your best self? Or do you tend to see a composite self-image that you don't like very much?

Slow down your mind so you can look at your mental pictures more closely. As you review them, do you notice any patterns in your thoughts and images of yourself, other people, places, and circumstances? Is there a predominant negative or positive slant? Many of us have an unconscious tendency to amplify — and hold on to — the distrustful, anxious, angry, hurtful parts of our experiences.

Sit quietly, relaxing, and roll your mental videotape in slow motion. Here comes the subject of your thought. Imagine: yourself, your boss, a co-worker, a loved one, or other subject. What is the view of this person in your mind? Your imagery choice will quickly affect your mood.

With some practice, you can teach your mind to choose the most vivid, constructive, competent view of yourself (and most other subjects) every time you think or say the name or pronoun. Whenever possible, choose meaningful, useful images and give them a little extra magnitude. Remember, you're not required to permanently banish bad memories — you're just choosing to stop dragging up the negative again and again. The same principles apply to events and situations.

All right, you may be thinking, but what about those people and circumstances for which you have no positive memories at all? In these cases, imagery experts frequently suggest "rewriting the script" of the past to create a more positive mental picture or feeling. You can imagine the past mistake or situation as if the outcome had been positive. This can help you let go of emotional baggage and find some growing room right now. The bottom line is that images are a choice.

The second part of the picture. Now look at the predicate — what's happening to the subject in each image or sentence. Apply the same imagery principles here, choosing accurate, empowering descriptions. Start a mental campaign to cut out chronic pessimism and cynicism — not just the obvious negative-on-negative complaining but also the more subtle, distorted thinking that locks us in stress closets. Choose honest, specific statements that prompt the best feelings, perceptions, and actions — in yourself and those around you.

4. Imagine the process to achieve your positive outcome. This part of the guided imagery experience, called *outcome imagery,* clearly identifies the challenges you face in achieving your goal and creates a specific action plan of thoughts, behaviors, and resources that will help it become a reality. Precisely what skills, feelings, attitudes, words, performance adjustments, shifts in awareness, and so on are essential to the results you desire? Be clear and supportive. Seek out precise ways to solve each challenge or problem rather than getting tangled up dwelling on the problem itself.

A sad refrain of think tank seminars and op-ed pages today is that, by and large, we've lost much of our creativity and instinct for innovation. But, if it's true, there's no reason for this situation to persist. According to the experts, each of us possesses a vast, untapped inner creative resource. To draw it forth in our work requires personal exploration, a keen sense of awareness, and a commitment to break old habits and broaden our horizons. But few business efforts pay greater dividends — because it's the personal spark of creativity that lights the way to the future.

Resources

In addition to the mental development and performance psychology resources recommended in Chapter 7, the following publications (listed alphabetically) offer guidance in increasing your brain power and creativity.

- *American Imagery Institute* (P.O. Box 13453, Milwaukee, WI 53213). This institute, directed by Dr. Anees Sheikh, chairman of the department of psychology at Marquette University, offers publications in a variety of mental imagery areas.
- *Brain Power: A Neurosurgeon's Complete Program to Maintain and Enhance Brain Fitness Throughout Your Life* by Vernon H. Mark, M.D., with Jeffrey P. Mark, M.Sc. (Houghton Mifflin, 1989). A highly readable and useful book.
- *Mind Power: Getting What You Want Through Mental Training* by Bernie Zilbergeld, Ph.D., and Arnold A. Lazarus, Ph.D. (Little, Brown, 1987). A practical, step-by-step guide. Accompanying audiotapes are available from MindPower Distribution Services (2847 Shattuck Ave., Berkeley, CA 94705).
- *Mindfulness* by Ellen J. Langer, Ph.D. (Addison-Wesley, 1989). Langer, a professor of psychology at Harvard University, presents highlights of her years of research on the dangers and detriments of mindlessness and ways to create more mindful, optimal work.
- *Power Vision: Mastering Life Through Mental Image Rehearsal* by Emmett E. Miller, M.D. (Nightingale-Conant, 1988). Audiotape album and manual by a leading stress management authority. A complete series of Dr. Miller's audiotape and videotape programs is available from Source Cassette Learning Systems (P.O. Box W, Stanford, CA 94309; 415-328-7171).

17

Welcome to the Future

We are what we repeatedly think and do.

— *Artistotle*

I know of no more encouraging fact than the unquestionable
ability of man to elevate his life by conscious endeavor.

— *Henry David Thoreau*

"THE FUTURE never just happened," observe Will and Ariel Durant in *The Lessons of History*. "It was created." That is true not only for societies and organizations but also for individuals. Through our work, we each create the future.

Above the din of the global business battles rising up around us on all fronts, an urgent edict is being heard:

Do absolutely everything possible — and do it smarter and faster and better than ever before — to gain, and keep, the Edge — in leadership, innovation, strategic thinking, speed, productivity, quality control, and customer service.

The corporate landscape has never been so competitive and unpredictable. Yet new possibilities are emerging with unprecedented frequency, and the barriers to innovation and accomplishment are being knocked down one by one.

Chief Justice Oliver Wendell Homes once said, "I don't care at all about the simplicity on this side of complexity; but I would give everything for the simplicity on the other side of complexity." In this book, I have sought to present some of the latest thinking about that simplicity on the *other* side of complexity, and to share a number of the most accessible and powerful tools to create your own Performance Edge. You can begin using these principles and guidelines right away, without waiting for your company to implement changes.

I hope that *The Performance Edge* has helped guide you on a journey resulting in a new, energized sense of what's truly possible in your work — no matter what your industry or profession. In the turbulent business times ahead, your own personal performance *capabilities* — your effectiveness under pressure — will mean much more than your job title or position.

Graham Greene once wrote that "there always comes a moment in time when a door opens and lets the future in." We have arrived at one of those critical turning points, moving into a world with far fewer boundaries. This fact will provide special rewards for those who think, plan, and act in ways unrestricted by yesterday's limitations. The brightest possible future depends not nearly as much on organizational resources as on your untapped *human* resources — your own Performance Edge.

Notes

Chapter 1/ Introduction

1. The professional practices of management, sales, and service are growing more challenging and complex every day, and there's no doubt that a wide range of factors — many requiring years of education and experience — contribute to corporate leadership, quality control, productivity, and customer service.

   It's also clear that to build a foundation for consistent breakthrough achievement on a company-wide scale, most organizations need to make fundamental changes in corporate organization and culture, including such areas as market-driven strategic planning and product/service development; improved operations management (technology, capacity, quality standards, scheduling, inventory, distribution, and control); purpose-oriented objectives and missions that motivate; and greater empowerment, recognition, and performance-based compensation.

   But, as important as these underlying organizational changes are, they're not enough.

   When managers who believe they are already pushing the limits of what can be achieved are asked to produce improvements, most think immediately of adding costly resources — new systems, new equipment, better measurements, new people, additional training, or increased support from other departments or suppliers. But worldwide scientific research shows that there are some simple, practical new strategies that you can use immediately — *with the resources you have in place right now* — to meet the urgent demands you face for greater innovation, zero-defect quality control, productivity breakthroughs, and total customer responsiveness.

   But to do this requires a bold new emphasis on developing *human capital* — what a number of experts are calling the greatest untapped organizational resource.

   In traditional management science, an organization's *capacity* — the ability to yield output — depends on the right combination of work elements:

(1) financial and information resources; (2) access to raw materials and finished products; (3) physical technology (equipment, buildings, and related assets); and (4) human performance technology (the performance capabilities of the organization's people — in all positions and at all levels).

Whichever one of these four basic elements is in shortest supply determines the productive capacity of the organization.

In today's relentlessly competitive, high-velocity global marketplace, company-to-company differences in the first three areas are rapidly narrowing. Again and again, new players from near and far are successfully attacking long-established companies deep in their prized markets — and beating them in the race for new ones. Turbulence and uncertainty have reached every boardroom in America. Even the most dramatic advances in physical technology have become difficult to protect and sustain — competitive advantages are now measured in weeks or months instead of years.

In short, in most cases *the weakest link in corporate capacity is human performance.* And improving human performance is the focus of this book.

2. Stewart, C. A. "New Ways to Exercise Power." *Fortune* (Nov. 6, 1989): 52–64.
3. Schlesinger, L. A. "The Art of Managing for the Long Run." In Collins, E. G. C., and Devanna, M. A. (Eds.). *The Portable MBA* (New York: Wiley, 1990): 1–16.
4. Schaffer, R. H. *The Breakthrough Strategy* (New York: Ballinger, 1988): 11–12.
5. Walton, R. E. Quoted in "The Payoff from Teamwork." *Business Week* (Jul. 10, 1989): 62.
6. Schaffer. *Breakthrough*: 2.
7. Hillkirk, J. "Firms Learn That Quick Development Means Big Profits." *USA Today* (Nov. 22, 1989): 103.
8. Dumaine, B. "What the Leaders of Tomorrow See." *Fortune* (Jul. 3, 1989): 58.
9. Parker, M., and Slaughter, J. "Management by Stress." *Technology Review* 91(7) (Oct. 1988): 36–44.
10. Parker and Slaughter. "Management by Stress": 40–41.
11. Gill, M. S. "Stalking Six Sigma." *Business Month* (Jan. 1990): 42–46.
12. Bolger, N., et al. "The Contagion of Stress Across Multiple Roles." *Journal of Marriage and the Family* (Feb. 1989): 175–83; Robbins, S. P. *Organizational Behavior*, 4th ed. (Englewood Cliffs, NJ: Prentice Hall, 1989): 267; Thomas, K. W., and Schmidt, W. H. "A Survey of Managerial Interests with Respect to Conflict." *Academy of Management Journal* (Jun. 1976): 317.
13. Kanter, R. M. *When Giants Learn to Dance: Mastering the Challenges of Strategy, Management, and Careers in the 1990s* (New York: Simon and Schuster, 1989): 267–68.
14. "Special Report: Where Did the Gung-Ho Go?" *Time* (Sep. 11, 1989): 52–56; Farnham, A. "The Trust Gap." *Fortune* (Dec. 4, 1989): 56–78; Kanter, D. L., and Mirvis, P. H. *The Cynical Americans: Living and Working in an Age of Discontent and Disillusion* (San Francisco: Josey-Bass, 1989).
15. Yankelovich, D. Quoted in *Psychology Today* (Sep. 1988): 34.
16. Marks, M. L. Quoted in *Psychology Today* (Sep. 1988): 34–39.
17. Kanter. *Giants*: 232.
18. "The Payoff from Teamwork." *Business Week* (Jul. 10, 1989): 56–62; Dumaine, B. "Who Needs a Boss?" *Fortune* (May 7, 1990): 52–60; "Work Design: The Quiet Revolution." *Enterprise* (Spring 1990): 33–37.

19. Zemke, R., with Schaaf, D. *The Service Edge: 100 Companies That Profit from Customer Care* (New York: New American Library, 1989): 31.
20. "King Customer: At Companies That Listen Hard and Respond Fast, Bottom Lines Thrive." *Business Week* (Mar. 12, 1990): 88–94.
21. "Stop Whining and Get Back to Work." CEO Poll. *Fortune* (Mar. 12, 1990): 49–50.
22. Eliot, R. S., and Breo, D. L. *Is It Worth Dying For?* Rev. ed. (New York: Bantam, 1989); "Stress on the Job." *Newsweek* (Apr. 25, 1988): 40–45; "Stress: The Test Americans Are Failing." *Business Week* (Apr. 18, 1988): 74–78.
23. "Stress: The Test Americans Are Failing." *Business Week* (Apr. 18, 1988): 74–77; "Stress: Can We Cope?" *Time* (Jun. 6, 1983): 48; Weiss, J. "Stress: The Invisible Killer." *Gallery* (Feb. 1985): 44; "Stress on the Job." *Newsweek* (Apr. 25, 1988): 40–45.
24. Silent heart disease includes silent myocardial ischemia (SMI) and other conditions. For general reading, see Eliot and Breo. *Is It Worth Dying For?* and Karpman, H. L. *Preventing Silent Heart Disease: Detecting and Preventing America's Number One Killer* (New York: Crown, 1989).
25. Eliot, R. S. Report from the Institute of Stress Medicine (8055 East Tufts Ave., Suite 1400, Denver, Co 80237; 1989): 2.
26. Eliot and Breo. *Is It Worth Dying For?*: 14.
27. Horowitz, J. M. "A Puzzling Toll at the Top." *Time* (Aug. 3, 1987): 46.
28. Pelletier, K. R., and Lutz, R. "Healthy People — Healthy Business: A Critical Review of Stress Management Programs in the Workplace." *American Journal of Health Promotion* 2(3) (Winter 1988): 5–12; "Stress: The Test": 74–76; "Stress on the Job": 40–45.
29. Kanter, R. M. *Work and Family in the United States* (New York: Russell Sage Foundation, 1977).
30. Bolger, N., et al. "The Contagion of Stress Across Multiple Roles." *Journal of Marriage and the Family* 51(Feb. 1989): 175–83; and "Marital Problems Affect Job." American Psychological Study reported in *USA Today* (Nov. 8, 1989).
31. Yankelovich, D., and Harman, S. *Starting with the People* (Boston: Houghton Mifflin, 1988); Ludeman, K. *The Worth Ethic* (New York: Dutton, 1989); Covey, S. R. *The Seven Habits of Highly Effective People* (New York: Simon and Schuster, 1989); Kiechel, W. III "The Workaholic Generation." *Fortune* (Apr. 10, 1989): 50–62; O'Reilly, B. "Why Grade 'A' Executives Get an 'F' as Parents." *Fortune* (Jan. 1, 1990): 36–46; O'Reilly, B. "Is Your Company Asking Too Much?" *Fortune* (Mar. 12, 1990): 38–46.

Chapter 3/ Performance Turning Point #1: Stressful "Crisis Moments"

1. Tipgos, M. A. "The Things That Stress Us." *Management World* (Jun.–Aug. 1987): 17–18.
2. DeCarlo, D. "Don't Let Stress Claims Broadside You." *Business and Health* (Jan. 1989): 43–44; McCarthy, M. J. "Stressed Employees Look for Relief in Worker's Compensation Claims." *Wall Street Journal* (Apr. 7, 1988).
3. *Advances* (Journal of the Institute for the Advancement of Health) 6(1) (Spring 1989): 9.

4. Kemery, E. R., et al. "Outcomes of Role Stress." *Academy of Management Journal* (Jun. 1985): 363–75.

5. Wang, P., et al. "A Cure for Stress?" *Newsweek* (Oct. 12, 1987): 64–65.

6. Pelletier, K. R. *Healthy People in Unhealthy Places: Stress and Fitness at Work* (New York: Delacorte, 1984); Windom, R., et al. "Examining Worksite Health Promotion Programs." U.S. Office of Disease Prevention and Health Promotion. *Business and Health* 4(9) (1987): 26–37.

7. Lazarus, R. S. *American Psychologist* 30 (1975): 553–61; DeLongis, A., et al. "Relationship of Daily Hassles, Uplifts, and Major Life Events to Health Status." *Health Psychology* 1 (1982): 119–36; Kanner, A. D., et al. "Comparison of Two Modes of Stress Measurement: Daily Hassles and Uplifts Versus Major Life Events." *Journal of Behavioral Medicine* 4 (1981): 1–39; Pelletier. *Healthy People*: 42–44; Sheehan, D. W. *Science News* 11(2) (Aug. 1981): 119; London, P., and Spielberger, C. "Job Stress, Hassles, and Medical Risk." *American Health* (Mar.–Apr. 1983): 58–63.

8. Brodish, A., et al. *Brain Research* 426 (1987): 37–46.

9. Nathan, R. G., Staats, T. E., and Rosch, P. J. *The Doctors' Guide to Instant Stress Relief* (New York: Ballantine, 1987): 6.

10. Eliot, R. S., and Breo, D. L. *Is It Worth Dying For?* Rev. ed. (New York: Bantam, 1989); Eliot, R. S. "The Dynamics of Hypertension — An Overview: Present Practices, New Possibilities, and New Approaches." *American Heart Journal* 116(2) (Aug. 1988): 583–89; Morales-Ballejo, H. M., et al. "Psychophysiologic Stress Testing as a Predictor of Mean Daily Blood Pressure." *American Heart Journal* 116(2) (Aug. 1988): 673–81; Eliot, R. S. "Lessons Learned and Future Directions." *American Heart Journal* 116(2) (Aug. 1988): 682–86. Dr. Eliot and his staff at the Institute of Stress Medicine have launched a corporate screening and treatment program for businesses in the United States and abroad. For details, contact the ISM (8055 East Tufts Ave., Suite 1400, Denver, CO 80237; 303-770-1414).

11. "A Killer of Women, Too: Half of All Americans Who Die of Heart Attack Are Women." *U.S. News & World Report* (Dec. 18, 1989): 75–76.

12. Stone, A. A. *Journal of Personality and Social Psychology* 52 (1987): 988–93; "Mood Immunity." *Psychology Today* (Nov. 1987): 14.

13. Brodish, A., et al. *Brain Research* 426 (1987): 37–46.

14. Carlzon, J. *Moments of Truth* (New York: Ballinger, 1987).

15. Bandura, A., and Mahoney, M. J. "Maintenance and Transfer of Self-Reinforcement Functions." *Behaviour Research and Therapy* 12 (1974): 89–98; Denney, D. R. "Self-Control Approaches to the Treatment of Test Anxiety," in Sarason, I. G. (Ed.). *Test Anxiety: Theory, Research and Applications* (Hillsdale, NJ: Erlbaum, 1980): 209–43; Goldiamond, I. "Self Reinforcement." *Journal of Applied Behavior* 9 (1976):509–14; Stroebel, C. F., Luce, G., and Glueck, B. C. "Optimizing Compliance with Behavioral Medicine Therapies." *Current Psychiatric Therapies* (1983/1984); Stroebel, C. F. *QR: The Quieting Reflex* (New York: Berkley, 1983).

16. Backer, T. E. "Creativity and Stress." Cited in "Workplace Creativity," in Klarreich, S. H. (Ed.). *Health & Fitness in the Workplace* (New York: Praeger, 1987): 328.

17. Heide, F. J. "Relaxation: The Storm Before the Calm." *Psychology Today* 19 (1985): 18–19; Heide, F. J., and Borkovec, T. D. "Relaxation-Induced Anxiety." *Journal of Counseling and Clinical Psychology* 51(2) (1983): 171–82; Heide, F. J., and Borkovec, T. D. "Relaxation-Induced Anxiety: Mechanisms

and Theoretical Implications." *Behavior Research Therapy* 22(1) (1984): 1–12.

18. Labich, K. "The Seven Keys to Business Leadership." *Fortune* (Oct. 24, 1988): 58–66.

19. Ford, M. R., et al. "Quieting Response Training: Predictors of Long-Term Outcome." *Biofeedback and Self-Regulation* 8(3) (1983): 393–408; Ford, M. R., et al. "Quieting Response Training: Long-Term Evaluation of a Clinical Biofeedback Practice." *Biofeedback and Self-Regulation* 8(2) (1983): 265–78; Stroebel, C. F., Ford, M. R., Strong, P., and Szarek, B. L. "Quieting Response Training: Five-Year Evaluation of a Clinical Biofeedback Practice." (Institute for Living, Hartford, CT 06106; 1981); Stroebel et al., "Optimizing Compliance"; Pribram, K. H. *Holonomic Brain Theory* (Hillsdale, NJ: Erlbaum, 1988); Pribram, K. H. Lecture at the Center for Health & Fitness Excellence, Bemidji, MN (Jun. 13–14, 1987).

20. *The Behavioral and Brain Sciences* 8 (1986): 529–66; "Brain Shows Activation Before Conscious Choice." *Brain/Mind Bulletin* (May 5, 1986): 1; Cattell, R. B. *Abilities: Their Structure, Growth and Action* (Boston: Houghton Mifflin, 1971); Pribram. Lecture (Jun. 1987).

21. Winter, A., and Winter, R. *Build Your Brain Power* (New York: St. Martin's, 1986): 90.

22. Jaret, P. "Mind: Why Practice Makes Perfect." *Hippocrates* (Nov.–Dec. 1987): 90–91; Salthouse, T. *Scientific American* (Feb. 1984).

23. Jaret. "Mind."

24. Csikszentmihalyi, M., and Csikszentmihalyi, I. S. (Eds.). *Optimal Experience: Psychological Studies of Flow in Consciousness* (New York: Cambridge University Press, 1988); Csikszentmihalyi, M. *Flow: The Psychology of Optimal Experience* (New York: Harper and Row, 1989); Jaret. "Mind"; Teich, M., and Dodeles, G. "Mind Control: How to Get It, How to Use It, How to Keep It." *Omni* (Oct. 1987): 53–60.

25. Pribram. *Holonomic Brain Theory*; Pribram. Lecture (Jun. 1987).

26. "Breathing Linked to Personality." *Psychology Today* (Jul. 1983): 109; Teich and Dodeles. "Mind Control."

27. Ekman, P., Levenson, R. W., and Friesen, W. V. "Autonomic Nervous System Activity Distinguishes Among Emotions." *Science* (Sep. 16, 1983): 1208–10; Greden, J., et al. *Archives of General Psychiatry* 43 (1987): 269–74; Teich and Dodeles. "Mind Control"; Zajonc, R. B. "Emotion and Facial Efference: A Theory Reclaimed." *Science* 228(4695) (Apr. 5, 1985): 15–21; Duclos, S. E., et al. "Emotion-Specific Effects of Facial Expressions and Postures of Emotional Experience." *Journal of Personality and Social Psychology* 57(1) (1989): 100–108.

28. Hingsburger, D. "Learning How to Face That Stressful Situation." *Management Solutions* 33(2) (1988): 41–45.

29. Duclos et al. "Emotion-Specific Effects"; Riskind, J. H., and Gotay, C. C. "Physical Posture: Could It Have Regulatory or Biofeedback Effects on Motivation and Emotion?" *Motivation and Emotion* 6(3) (1982): 273–98; Weisfeld, G. E., and Beresford, J. M. "Erectness of Posture as an Indicator of Dominance or Success in Humans." *Motivation and Emotion* 6(2) (1982): 113–31; Bhatnager, V., et al. "Posture, Postural Discomfort, and Performance." *Human Factors* 27(2) (Apr. 1985): 189–99.

30. Rippe, J. M. *Fit for Success* (New York: Prentice Hall, 1989): 114.

31. Garfield, C. *Peak Performance* (New York: Warner, 1984): 95; Csikszent-

mihalyi. *Flow*; Csikszentmihalyi and Csikszentmihalyi. *Optimal Experience*.

32. Logan, R. "The Flow Experience." *Journal of Humanistic Psychology* 25(4) (1985): 79–89; Logan, R. "Flow in Solitary Ordeals," in Csikszentmihalyi and Csikszentmihalyi. *Optimal Experience*.

33. Nadler, G., and Hibino, S. *Breakthrough Thinking* (Rocklin, CA: Prima, 1990): 93.

34. Fischman, M. G. *Journal of Motor Behavior* 16 (1984): 405–23; Fitts, P. M., and Peterson, J. R. *Journal of Experimental Psychology* 67 (1964): 103–12; Greenwald, A. G., and Schulman, H. G. *Journal of Experimental Psychology* 101 (1973): 70–76; Keele, S. W. "Motor Control," in L. Kaufman, J. Thomas, and K. Boff (Eds.). *Handbook of Perception and Performance* (New York: Wiley, 1986); Newell, K. M., et al. *Journal of Motor Behavior* 12 (1980): 47–56; Quinn, J. T., and Sherwood, D. E. *Journal of Motor Behavior* 15 (1983): 163–78; Rosenbaum, D. A. *Journal of Experimental Psychology* 109 (1980): 444–74; Schmidt, R. A. *Psychological Bulletin* 70 (1968): 631–46; Schmidt, R. A. *Motor Control and Learning: A Behavioral Analysis* (Champaign, IL: Human Kinetics, 1988).

35. Csikszentmihalyi. *Flow*: 204.

36. Basmajian, J. V. "Control of Individual Motor Units." *American Journal of Physical Medicine* 46 (1967): 1427–40; Basmajian, J. V. "Electromyography Comes of Age: The Conscious Control of Individual Motor Units in Man May Be Used to Improve His Physical Performance." *Science* 176 (1972): 603–9; Lynch, J. J. *Language of the Heart: The Body's Response to Human Dialogue* (New York: Basic Books, 1985); Sheikh, A. A. (Ed.). *Imagery: Current Theory, Research, and Application* (New York: Wiley Interscience, 1984); Marks, D. F. (Ed.). *Theories of Image Formation* (New York: Brandon House, 1986); Sheikh, A. A. (Ed.). *Imagination and Healing* (Farmingdale, NY: Baywood, 1984); Sheikh, A. A., and Sheikh, K. S. (Eds.). *Imagery in Education* (Farmingdale, NY: Baywood, 1985); Sheikh, A. A. (Ed.). *Imagery in Sports* (Farmingdale, NY: Baywood, 1988); Suinn, R. M. *Seven Steps to Peak Performance* (Lewiston, NY: Hans Huber Publishers, 1986).

37. Langer, E. J. *Mindfulness* (Reading, MA: Addison-Wesley, 1989).

38. *The Neuropsychology of Achievement* (Sybervision Systems, Inc., 6066 Civic Terrace Ave., Newark, CA 94560; 1985).

39. Csikszentmihalyi. *Flow*; Csikszentmihalyi and Csikszentmihalyi. *Optimal Experience*.

40. Csikszentmihalyi. *Flow*: 119, 211.

Chapter 4/ Performance Turning Point #2: Tension and Pain

1. Matteson, M. T., and Ivancevich, J. M. *Controlling Work Stress: Effective Human Resource and Management Strategies* (San Francisco: Josey-Bass, 1987): 6; Linet, M. S., et al. "An Epidemiological Study of Headache." *Journal of the American Medical Association* (Apr. 21, 1989): 2211–16.

2. Monmaney, T. "Bouncing Back from Bad Backs." *Newsweek* (Oct. 24, 1988): 69; Zamula, E. "Back Talk: Advice for Suffering Spines." *FDA Consumer* (Apr. 1989): 28–35.

3. Zamula. "Back Talk": 28.
4. Nicholson, N., and Johns, G. "The Absence Culture and the Psychological Contract: Who's in Control of Absence?" *Academic Management Review* 10(3) (1985): 79–84.
5. Raymond, C. "Mental Stress: 'Occupational Injury' of the 80s That Even Pilots Can't Rise Above." *Journal of the American Medical Association* 259(21) (1988): 3097–98.
6. Nikiforow, R., and Hokkanen, E. "Effects of Headache on Working Ability." *Headache* 19(4) (1979): 214–18; Croog, S., et al. "Work Performance, Absenteeism, and Antihypertensive Medications." *Journal of Hypertension* 5(1) (1987): 547–54.
7. Anderson, J. "Back Pain and Sickness Absence." *Annals of Rheumatic Disease* 35(3) (1976): 327–28.
8. Haynes, R., et al. "Increased Absenteeism from Work After Detection and Labeling of Hypertensive Patients." *New England Journal of Medicine* 299(14) (1978): 741–44.
9. "On-the-Job Straining: Repetitive Motion Is the Information Age's Hottest Hazard." *U.S. News & World Report* (May 21, 1990): 51–53.
10. The standard medical text in this field is *Myofascial Pain and Dysfunction: The Trigger Point Manual* by Janet G. Travell, M.D., and David G. Simons, M.D. (Baltimore: Williams and Wilkins, 1983). This highly technical manual, complete with more than 2,500 scientific and medical references, is the result of decades of research by the authors and is strongly endorsed by the author of the book's foreword, Dr. Rene Cailliet, an international leader in physical and rehabilitative medicine and chairman of the Department of Rehabilitative Medicine at the University of Southern California School of Medicine.

Other recent studies on myofascial pain and dysfunction include Simons, D. G. "Myofascial Pain Syndromes." *Archives of Physical Medicine and Rehabilitation* (Sep. 1984): 561; Simons, D. G. "Myofascial Pain Syndromes: Where Are We? Where Are We Going?" *Archives of Physical Medicine and Rehabilitation* 69(3, Pt. 1) (Mar. 1988): 207–12; Simons, D. G. "Familial Fibromyalgia and/or Myofascial Pain Syndrome?" *Archives of Physical Medicine and Rehabilitation* 71(3) (Mar. 1990): 258–59; Simons, D. G. "Trigger Point Origin of Musculoskeletal Chest Pain." *Southern Medical Journal* 83(2) (Feb. 1990): 262–63; Smythe, H. "Referred Pain and Tender Points." *American Journal of Medicine* 81(3A) (Sep. 29, 1986): 7–14; Fisher, A. A. "Documentation of Myofascial Trigger Points." *Archives of Physical Medicine and Rehabilitation* 69(4) (Apr. 1988): 286–91; Mennell, J. "Myofascial Trigger Points as a Cause of Headaches." *Journal of Manipulative and Physiological Therapeutics* 11(2) (Apr. 1989): 63–64; Friction, J. R. "Myofascial Pain Syndrome." *Neurological Clinics* 7(2) (May 1989): 413–27; Campbell, S. M. "Regional Myofascial Pain Syndromes." *Rheumatic Diseases Clinics of North America* 15(10) (Feb. 1989): 31–44.
11. Travell and Simons. *Myofascial Pain*: 5.
12. Sola, A. E., et al. "Incidence of Hypersensitive Areas in Posterior Shoulder Muscles." *American Journal of Physical Medicine* 34 (1955): 585–90.
13. Kraft, G. H., et al. "The Fibrositis Syndrome." *Archives of Physical Medicine and Rehabilitation* 49 (1968): 155–62.
14. Travell and Simons. *Myofascial Pain*: 13.
15. Travell and Simons. *Myofascial Pain*: 31.
16. Travell and Simons. *Myofascial Pain*: 87.

17. Travell and Simons. *Myofascial Pain*: 18.
18. Sola. "Incidence"; Travell and Simons. *Myofascial Pain*: 13.
19. Nachemson, A. Quoted in *Newsweek* (Oct. 24, 1988): 69.
20. Travell and Simons. *Myofascial Pain*: 114–43.
21. Travell and Simons. *Myofascial Pain*: 149.

Chapter 5/ Performance Turning Point #3: Time Pressures

1. "The Rat Race: How America Has Run Out of Time." *Time* (Apr. 24, 1989): 58–67.
2. Stalk, G., and Hout, T. M. *Competing Against Time: How Time-Based Competition Is Reshaping Global Markets* (New York: Free Press, 1990).
3. Dumaine, B. "How Managers Can Succeed Through Speed." *Fortune* (Feb. 13, 1989): 54–59.
4. Cooper, C. Quoted in Worthy, F. "You're Probably Working Too Hard." *Fortune* (Apr. 27, 1987): 133–40.
5. Kanter, R. M. *When Giants Learn to Dance* (New York: Simon and Schuster, 1989): 232.
6. Oncken, W., Jr. *Managing Management Time* (Englewood Cliffs, NJ: Prentice Hall, 1983).
7. Covey, S. R. *The Seven Habits of Highly Effective People* (New York: Simon and Schuster, 1989): 149.
8. "No They Can't Stop Time, But They Can Help You Manage It." *Business Week* (May 22, 1989): 178–79.
9. Zaleznik, A. Quoted in *Fortune* (Apr. 27, 1987): 140.
10. Kanter, R. M. *Work and Family in the United States* (New York: Russell Sage Foundation, 1977).
11. Bolger, N., et al. "The Contagion of Stress Across Multiple Roles." *Journal of Marriage and the Family* 51 (Feb. 1989): 175–83; and "Marital Problems Affect Job." American Psychological Study reported in *USA Today* (Nov. 8, 1989).
12. Kanter. *Giants*; Ludeman, K. *The Worth Ethic* (New York: Dutton, 1989).
13. Covey. *Seven Habits*: 174.
14. Douglass, M., and Baker, L. *The New Time Management* (Chicago: Nightingale-Conant, 1983): 25.
15. "Don't Let Time Management Be a Waste of Time." *Business Week* (May 4, 1987): 144.
16. Dotto, L. *Asleep in the Fast Lane* (New York: Morrow, 1990): 179.
17. Horne, J. A. *Why We Sleep* (Oxford: Oxford University Press, 1988).
18. Wurman, R. S. *Information Anxiety* (Garden City, NY: Doubleday, 1989).
19. Cole, D. "Meetings That Make Sense." *Psychology Today* (May 1989): 14–15; Tropman, J. *Meetings: How to Make Them Work for You* (New York: Van Nostrand Reinhold, 1988); Calonius, E. "How Top Managers Manage Their Time." *Fortune* (Jun. 4, 1990): 250–62; Worthy, F. S. "How CEOs Manage Their Time." *Fortune* (Jan. 18, 1988): 88–97; Frank, M. O. *How to Run Successful Meetings in Half the Time* (New York: Simon and Schuster, 1989).
20. Oppenheim, L. Quoted in Cole. "Meetings."
21. Frank. *Successful Meetings*: 23.
22. "Information Management: At These Shouting Matches, No One Says a Word." *Business Week* (Jun. 11, 1990): 78.

Chapter 6/ Performance Turning Point #4: Communication Exchanges

1. Smeltzer, L. R. "The Relationship of Communication to Work Stress." *Journal of Business Communication* 24(2) (Spring 1987): 47–58.
2. Kanter, D. L., and Mirvis, P. H. *The Cynical Americans: Living and Working in an Age of Discontent and Disillusion* (San Francisco: Josey-Bass, 1989); Spector, P. E., et al. "Relation of Job Stressors to Affective, Health, and Performance Outcomes: A Comparison of Multiple Data Sources." *Journal of Applied Psychology* 73(1) (1988): 11–19.
3. Eliot, R. S., and Breo, D. *Is It Worth Dying For?* Rev. ed. (New York: Bantam, 1990).
4. Hellweg, S. A., and Phillips, S. L. "Communication and Productivity in Organizations: A State-of-the-Art Review." In *Proceedings of the 40th Annual Academy of Management Conference,* Detroit (1980): 188–92.
5. Kanter, R. M. *When Giants Learn to Dance* (New York: Simon and Schuster, 1989): 206.
6. Kanter. *Giants:* 275.
7. Stewart, T. A. "CEOs See Clout Shifting." *Fortune* (Nov. 6, 1989): 66.
8. Mintzberg, H. *The Nature of Managerial Work* (New York: Harper and Row, 1973).
9. Farnham, A. "The Trust Gap." *Fortune* (Dec. 4, 1989): 70.
10. Bolger, N., et al. "The Contagion of Stress Across Multiple Roles." *Journal of Marriage and the Family* (Feb. 1989): 175–83.
11. Robbins, S. P. *Organizational Behavior,* 4th ed. (Englewood Cliffs, NJ: Prentice Hall, 1989): 267; Thomas, K. W., and Schmidt, W. H. "A Survey of Managerial Interests with Respect to Conflict." *Academy of Management Journal* (Jun. 1976): 317.
12. McCall, M. M., Jr., and Lombardo, M. M. "What Makes a Top Executive?" *Psychology Today* (Feb. 1983): 26, 28–31.
13. Rippe, J. M. *Fit for Success: Proven Strategies for Executive Health* (Englewood Cliffs, NJ: Prentice Hall, 1989): 163.
14. McGill, M. E. *American Business and the Quick Fix* (New York: Holt, 1988): 143.
15. McGill. *American Business:* 214.
16. Eliot and Breo. *Is It Worth Dying For?*
17. Paul, S., quoted by Gallagher, W. "The Dark Affliction of Mind and Body." *Discover* (May 1986): 76.
18. Lynch, J. J. *The Language of the Heart: The Body's Response to Human Dialogue* (New York: Basic Books, 1985).
19. Sommers-Flanagan, J., and Greenberg, R. *Journal of Nervous and Mental Disease* 177 (1989): 15–24.
20. Lynch. *Language:* 3–4.
21. Nichols, R. G., and Stevens, L. A. "Listening to People." *Harvard Business Review* (Sep.–Oct. 1957).
22. McGill. *American Business:* 214–15.
23. Clynes, M., and Nettheim, N. "Neurobiological Patterns of Communicating Feeling." In Clynes, M. (Ed.). *Music, Mind, and Brain: The Neurophysiology of Music* (New York: Plenum, 1982): 47–82.
24. Kiechel, W. III. "Learn How to Listen." *Fortune* (Aug. 17, 1987): 107–8.

25. Brown, A. Quoted in Kiechel. "Learn How to Listen": 108.
26. Bazerman, M. Quoted in Kiechel. "Learn How to Listen": 108.
27. McKay, M., Davis, M., and Fanning, P. *Messages: The Communication Book* (Richmond, CA: New Harbinger, 1983): 24–28; Brennan, E. J. *Performance Management Workbook* (Englewood Cliffs, NJ: Prentice Hall, 1989): 171–84.
28. Grove, A. S. *One-on-One with Andy Grove* (New York: Penguin, 1987): 94.
29. Blanchard, M., and Tager, M. J. *Working Well* (New York: Simon and Schuster, 1985): 140–41.
30. Elgin, S. H. *Success with the Gentle Art of Verbal Self-Defense* (Englewood Cliffs, NJ: Prentice Hall, 1989): 133.
31. Elgin. *Success*: 135.
32. Leeds, D. *Smart Questions* (New York: Berkley, 1988): 41.
33. Leeds. *Smart Questions*: 41.
34. Zemke, R., with Schaaf, D. *The Service Edge: 100 Companies That Profit from Customer Care* (New York: New American Library, 1989): 31.
35. Zemke and Schaaf. *Service Edge*: 23–24.
36. Zemke and Schaaf. *Service Edge*: 24.
37. Elgin. *Success*: 8, 28.
38. "The Art of Negotiating." *The Royal Bank Letter* (Canada) (Jul.–Aug. 1986): 3.
39. Kotkin, J., and Kishimoto, Y. *Inc.* (Apr. 1986).
40. Tannen, D. *That's Not What I Meant!* (New York: Morrow, 1986): 27.
41. Tannen. *That's Not What I Meant!*: 19.
42. Walsh, J. P., et al. "Feedback Obstruction: The Influence of the Information Environment on Employee Turnover Intentions." *Human Relations* (Jan. 1985): 23–46.
43. Krackhardt, D., and Porter, L. W. "The Snowball Effect: Turnover Embedded in Communication Networks." *Journal of Applied Psychology* (Feb. 1986): 50–55.
44. Schuler, R. S. "A Role Perception Transactional Process Model for Organizational Communication-Outcome Relationships." *Organizational Behavior and Human Performance* (Apr. 1979): 268–91.
45. Weiss, D. H. *How to Deal with Difficult People* (New York: American Management Association, 1987): 5–6.
46. Fisher, R., and Ury, W. *Getting to Yes: Negotiating Agreement Without Giving In* (New York: Penguin, 1983).
47. Cherney, M. B., and Tynan, S. A. *Communicoding* (New York: Donald Fine, 1989): 7, 17, 39.
48. Luthans, F., and Lockwood, D. L. "Toward an Observational System for Measuring Leader Behavior in Natural Settings," in Hunt, J. G., et al. (Eds.). *Managers and Leaders: An International Perspective* (New York: Pergamon, 1984); and Yukl, G. A. *Leadership in Organizations* (Englewood Cliffs, NJ: Prentice Hall, 1981).
49. Quinn, R. E. *Beyond Rational Management: Mastering the Paradoxes and Competing Demands of High Performance* (San Francisco: Josey-Bass, 1988); Quinn, R. E., and Cameron, K. S. *Paradox and Transformation: Toward a Framework of Change in Organization and Management* (Cambridge, MA: Ballinger, 1988).
50. Knapp, M. L., et al. "Compliments: A Descriptive Taxonomy." *Journal of Communication* 34 (Fall 1984): 12–31; Knapp, M. L., et al. "I Really Loved

Your Article, But You Missed Your Deadline." *Psychology Today* 19 (Aug. 1985): 24–28.

51. Crum, T. F. *The Magic of Conflict* (New York: Simon and Schuster, 1987): 120.

52. Ray, M., and Myers, R. *Creativity in Business* (New York: Doubleday, 1986): 48–49.

53. Hawkins, J. D. Quoted in Buffington, P. W. "Compliments." *Sky* (Jan. 1989): 63–66.

54. Buffington. "Compliments": 65–66.

55. Buffington. "Compliments": 66.

56. Kierchel, W. III. "Facing Up to Executive Anger." *Fortune* (Nov. 16, 1981): 208.

57. Grove. *One-on-One*: 25.

58. Tavris, C. *Anger: The Misunderstood Emotion* (New York: Simon and Schuster, 1982).

59. Williams, R. *The Trusting Heart* (New York: Times Books, 1989): xiii, 11.

60. Julius, M., et al. *American Family Physician* (May 1986).

61. Kello, J. Quoted in Kiechel. "Learn How to Listen": 108.

62. Baron, R. Quoted in Goleman, D. "Why Job Criticism Fails: Psychology's New Findings." *New York Times* (Jul. 26, 1988).

63. Grove. *One-on-One*: 100.

64. Weisinger, H. *Dr. Weisinger's How to Give Criticism and Get Results* (New York: Morrow, 1986); Blanchard, K., and Johnson, S. *The One Minute Manager* (New York: Berkley, 1983); Leeds. *Smart Questions*; Weisinger, H. *The Critical Edge* (Boston: Little, Brown, 1989).

65. Weisinger. *Critical Edge*: 36.

66. Weisinger. *Critical Edge*: 43.

67. Nickerson, P. *Nickerson's Four Star Management Workshop* (Englewood Cliffs, NJ: Prentice Hall, 1989): 77.

68. Grothe, M., and Wylie, P. *Problem Bosses: Who They Are and How to Deal with Them* (New York: Fawcett, 1987); Elgin. *Success*: 99; Branson, R. M. *Coping with Difficult People* (New York: Ballantine, 1981).

Chapter 7/ Performance Turning Point #5: Decision-Making and Innovation Opportunities

1. Winter, A., and Winter, R. *Build Your Brain Power* (New York: St. Martin's, 1986): 1.

2. Nightingale, E. "Our Changing World." Radio program. (Chicago: Nightingale-Conant, 1974).

3. *Discover* (Sep. 1987): 87.

4. Rossi, E. *The Psychobiology of Mind/Body Healing* (New York: Norton, 1987): 102; Sagan, C. *The Dragons of Eden: Speculations on the Evolution of Human Intelligence* (New York: Random House, 1977).

5. Black, I. B., et al. "Neurotransmitter Plasticity at the Molecular Level." *Science* 225(4668) (1984): 1266–70; Kandel, E. R., and Schwartz, J. H. "Molecular Biology of Learning: Modulation of Transmitter Release." *Science* 218(4571) (1982): 433–43.

6. Merzenich, M. Quoted in Hooper, J., and Teresi, D. *The Three-Pound Universe* (New York: Macmillan, 1988): 61.
7. Cattell, R. B. *Abilities: Their Structure, Growth, and Action* (Boston: Houghton Mifflin, 1971).
8. Suarez, R., Mills, R. C., and Stewart, D. *Sanity, Insanity, and Common Sense* (New York: Fawcett, 1987); Emery, G. "Rapid Cognitive Therapy of Anxiety." Research monograph. (Los Angeles Center for Cognitive Therapy, 630 S. Wilton Pl., Los Angeles, CA 90005; 1987): 39–52; Beck, A. T. *Cognitive Therapy and Emotional Disturbances* (New York: International Universities Press, 1976); Emery, G., and Campbell, J. *Rapid Relief from Emotional Distress* (New York: Fawcett, 1986); Dobson, K. S. (Ed.). *Handbook of Cognitive-Behavioral Therapies* (New York: Guilford Press, 1988); Freeman, A., and DeWolf, R. *Woulda, Coulda, Shoulda* (New York: Morrow, 1989).
9. Basmajian, J. V. "Control of Individual Motor Units." *American Journal of Physical Medicine* 46 (1967): 1427–40; Basmajian, J. V. "Electromyography Comes of Age: The Conscious Control of Individual Motor Units in Man May Be Used to Improve His Physical Performance." *Science* 176 (1972): 603–9; Lynch, J. J. *Language of the Heart: The Body's Response to Human Dialogue* (New York: Basic Books, 1985).
10. Isen, A. M. "Toward Understanding the Influence of Positive Affect on Social Behavior, Decision Making, and Problem Solving: The Role of Cognitive Organization." Paper presented at the annual meeting of the American Association for the Advancement of Science, Boston (Feb. 11–15, 1988); Carlson, M., et al. "Positive Mood and Helping Behavior: A Test of Six Hypotheses." *Journal of Personality and Social Psychology* 55(2) (1988): 211–29.
11. Davis, R. T. "Marketing Management: Becoming a Market-Driven Company." In Collins, E. G. C., and Devanna, M. A. (Eds.). *The Portable MBA* (New York: Wiley, 1990): 174–218.
12. Schank, R. C. *The Creative Attitude* (New York: Macmillan, 1988): ix–x, 348.
13. Adams, J. L. *The Care and Feeding of Ideas: A Guide to Encouraging Creativity* (Reading, MA: Addison-Wesley, 1986): 4–7.
14. These creativity enhancement heuristics are drawn from a variety of sources, including Schank. *Creative Attitude*: 349–62; Adams. *The Care and Feeding of Ideas*; Dormen, L., and Edidin, P. "Original Spin." *Psychology Today* (Jul.–Aug. 1989): 47–52; Benderly, D. L. "Everyday Intuition." *Psychology Today* (Sep. 1989): 35–40; Langer, E. J. *Mindfulness* (Reading, MA: Addison-Wesley, 1989); and Ray, M., and Myers, R. *Creativity in Business* (New York: Doubleday, 1986).
15. Ray and Myers. *Creativity in Business*: 39–66.
16. Kanter, R. M. *When Giants Learn to Dance* (New York: Simon and Schuster, 1989): 209.
17. Backer, T. E. "How Health Promotion Programs Can Enhance Workplace Creativity." In Klarreich, S. H. (Ed.). *Health and Fitness in the Workplace* (New York: Praeger, 1987): 325–37.
18. Isen, A. M., et al. "The Influence of Positive Affect on the Unusualness of Word Associations." *Journal of Personality and Social Psychology* 48 (1985): 1413–26; Isen, A. M., et al. "Positive Affect Facilitates Creative Problem Solving." *Journal of Personality and Social Psychology* 52 (1987): 1122–31; Isen, A. M. "Positive Affect, Cognitive Processes, and Social Behavior." *Advances in Experimental Social Psychology* 20 (1987): 203–53.

19. Adams. *Care and Feeding*: 52–53.
20. Richards, R. Quoted in Dormen and Edidin. "Original Spin."
21. Ray and Myers. *Creativity in Business*: 91.
22. Benderly. "Everyday Intuition."
23. Csikszentmihalyi, M. *Flow: The Psychology of Optimal Experience* (New York: Harper and Row, 1990).
24. Langer. *Mindfulness*: 143.
25. Langer. *Mindfulness*: 138.
26. Langer, E. Quoted in *Psychology Today* (Mar. 1989): 44.
27. Kahneman, D., and Tversky, A. "The Psychology of Preferences." *Scientific American* (Jan. 1982): 160–73; Kahneman, D., and Tversky, A. "The Framing of Decisions and the Psychology of Choice." *Science* 211 (1981): 453–58; Kahneman, D., and Tversky, A. "Judgment Under Uncertainty: Heuristics and Biases." *Science* 185 (1974): 1124–31.
28. A summary of Herbert Simon's wide-ranging views on decision making is presented in two volumes of invited lectures: *The Sciences of the Artificial*, 2nd ed. (Cambridge: MIT Press, 1981), and *Reason in Human Affairs* (Stanford: Stanford University Press, 1983).
29. Kahneman, D., et al. *Judgment Under Uncertainty: Heuristics and Biases* (London: Cambridge University Press, 1982); Arkes, H. R., and Hammond, K. R. (Eds.). *Judgment and Decision Making: An Interdisciplinary Reader* (London: Cambridge University Press, 1986); Bel, D., et al. (Eds.). *Decision Making: Descriptive, Normative and Prescriptive Interactions* (London: Cambridge University Press, 1988); Bazerman, M. H. *Judgment in Managerial Decision Making* (New York: Wiley, 1986); Hogarth, R. *Judgment and Choice*, 2nd ed. (New York: Wiley, 1987); Dawes, R. M. *Rational Choice in an Uncertain World* (New York: Harcourt, 1988); Russo, J. E., and Schoemaker, P. J. H. *Decision Traps* (New York: Doubleday, 1989); Quinn, R. E. *Beyond Rational Management: Mastering the Paradoxes and Competing Demands of High Performance* (San Francisco: Josey-Bass, 1988).
30. Keinan, G. "Decision Making Under Stress: Scanning of Alternatives Under Controllable and Uncontrollable Threats." *Journal of Personality and Social Psychology* 52(3) (1987): 639–44; Janis, I. L., et al. "Decision-Making Under Stress," in Goldberger, L., and Breznitz, S. (Eds.). *Handbook of Stress: Theoretical and Clinical Aspects* (New York: Free Press, 1982): 69–80; Mandler, G. "Stress and Thought Processes," in Goldberger and Breznitz. *Handbook of Stress*: 69–80.
31. Cohen, A. R. "Managing People: The R Factor." In Collins and Devanna. *Portable MBA*: 19–44.
32. Pelton, W. J., Sackman, S., and Boguslaw, R. *Tough Choices: The Decision-Making Styles of America's Top 50 CEOs* (Homewood, IL: Dow-Jones Irwin, 1990): vii, 13.
33. Kiechel, W. III. "Corporate Strategy for the 1990s." *Fortune* (Feb. 29, 1988): 34–58; "The New America." *Business Week* Special Edition (Sep. 25, 1989); Saporito, B. "Companies That Compete Best." *Fortune* (May 22, 1989): 36–44; "Innovation in America." *Business Week,* Special Edition (Fall 1989); Pelton et al. *Tough Choices*: 11.
34. Kahneman and Tversky. "Framing": 453.
35. Drucker, P. *Management: Task, Responsibilities, Practices* (New York: Harper and Row, 1974).
36. Pascarella, P., and Frohman, M. A. *The Purpose-Driven Organization* (San

Francisco: Jossey-Bass, 1989); Vaill, P. B. *Managing as a Performing Art* (San Francisco: Jossey-Bass, 1989); Nadler, G., and Hibino, S. *Breakthrough Thinking* (Rocklin, CA: Prima, 1990).

37. Quinn. *Beyond Rational Management*: xvii–xviii.

38. Quinn. *Beyond Rational Management*: 24.

39. Miller, R. C., and Berman, J. S. "The Efficacy of Cognitive Behavior Therapies: A Quantitative Review of the Research Evidence." *Psychological Bulletin* 94 (1983): 39–53; Beck, A. *Cognitive Therapy and the Emotional Disorders* (New York: International Universities Press, 1976); Beck, A., and Emery, G., with Greenberg, L. *Anxiety Disorders and Phobias* (New York: Basic Books, 1985); Burns, D. D. *Feeling Good: The New Mood Therapy* (New York: Signet, 1980); McKay, M., Davis, M., and Fanning, P. *Thoughts and Feelings: The Art of Cognitive Stress Intervention* (Richmond, CA: New Harbinger, 1981).

40. Seligman, M. E. P. Quoted in "Mind Over Illness: Do Optimists Live Longer?" *American Health* (Nov. 1986): 50–53.

41. Pelton et al. *Tough Choices*: 4.

42. Ingvar, D. "Memory of the Future: An Essay on the Temporal Organization of Conscious Awareness." *Human Neurobiology* 4 (1985).

43. Nadler and Hibino. *Breakthrough Thinking*: 136.

44. Luria, A. R. *The Human Brain and Psychological Processes* (New York: Harper and Row, 1966): 531.

45. Jaques, E. "The Development of Intellectual Capacity: A Discussion of Stratified Systems Theory." *The Journal of Applied Behavioral Science* 22(4) (1986): 364.

46. Jaques, E. (Ed.). *Levels of Abstraction in Logic and Human Action* (London: Heinemann, 1978): 258–61.

47. Melges, F. T. "Future Oriented Psychotherapy." *American Journal of Psychotherapy* 26 (1972): 22–33.

48. Quinn. *Beyond Rational Management*.

49. Peterson, P., and Seligman, M. E. P. "Causal Explanations as a Risk Factor for Depression: Theory and Evidence." *Psychological Review* 91(3) (1984): 347–74; Seligman, M. E. P. "Helplessness and Explanatory Style: Risk Factor for Depression and Disease." Paper presented at the annual meeting of the Society for Behavioral Medicine, San Francisco (Mar. 1986); Burns, M. O., and Seligman, M. E. P. "Explanatory Style Across the Lifespan: Evidence for Stability over 52 Years." *Journal of Personality and Social Psychology* 56(3) (1989): 471–77.

50. Eliot, R. S., and Breo, D. T. *Is It Worth Dying For?* Rev. ed. (New York: Bantam, 1989): 14.

51. Lichtenstein, S., et al. "Calibration of Probabilities: The State of the Art," in Kahneman et al., *Judgment*.

Chapter 8/ Performance Turning Point #6: Mental and Physical Stamina

1. Editorial Note. *Industrial Management* 30(1) (Jan.–Feb. 1988): 32.

2. Parker, M., and Slaughter, J. "Management by Stress." *Technology Review* 91(7) (Oct. 1988): 36–44; Turner, L. "Three Plants, Three Futures." *Technology Review* 92(1) (Jan. 1989): 38–45; Forbes, D. "The Lessons of NUMMI." *Business Month* 129(6) (Jun. 1987): 34–37.

3. Turner. "Three Plants": 41.

4. Parker and Slaughter. "Management by Stress": 42.

5. Backer, T. E. "Workplace Creativity," in Klarreich, S. H. (Ed.). *Health and Fitness in the Workplace* (New York: Praeger, 1987): 325–27.

6. "On-the-Job Straining." *U.S. News & World Report* (May 21, 1990): 51–53.

7. Stephens, R. Quoted in "On-the-Job Straining." *U.S. News & World Report* (May 21, 1990): 51.

8. Zinchenko, V. P., et al. *The Psychometrics of Fatigue* (London: Taylor and Francis, 1985).

9. Zinchenko et al. *Psychometrics*: 70, 73.

10. Janaro, R. E., and Bechtold, S. E. "A Study of the Reduction of Fatigue Impact on Productivity through Optimal Rest Break Scheduling." *Human Factors* 27(4) (1985): 459–66.

11. Janaro, R. E., et al. "A Technical Note on Increasing Productivity Through Effective Rest Break Scheduling." *Industrial Management* 30(1) (Jan.–Feb. 1988): 29–33; Penc, J. "Motivational Stimulation and System of Work Improvement." *Studia-Socjologiczne* 3(102) (1986): 179–97; Foegen, J. H. "Super-Breaktime." *Supervision* 49 (Oct. 1988): 9–10; Bechtold, S. E., and Sumners, D. L. "Optimal Work-Rest Scheduling with Exponential Work-Rate Decay." *Management Science* 34 (Apr. 1988): 547–52; Krueger, G. P. "Human Performance in Continuous/Sustained Operations and the Demands of Extended Work/Rest Schedules: An Annotated Bibliography." *Psychological Documents* 15(2) (Dec. 1985): 27–28; Boothe, R. S. "Optimization of Rest Breaks: A Productivity Enhancement." *Dissertation Abstracts International* 45 (9-A) (Mar. 1985): 2927; Gustafson, H. W. "Efficiency of Output in Self-Paced Work, Machine-Paced Work." *Human Factors* 24(4) (Aug. 1982): 395–410; Janaro and Bechtold. "Study of the Reduction of Fatigue Impact"; Okogbaa, O. G. "An Empirical Model for Mental Work Output and Fatigue." *Dissertation Abstracts International* 15(2) (Dec. 1985): 27–28; Thatcher, R. E. *Journal of Personality and Social Psychology* 52 (1987): 119–25; Zarakovski, G. M., et al. "Psychophysiological Analysis of Periodic Fluctuations in the Quality of Activity Within the Work Cycle." *Human Physiology* 8(3) (May 1983): 208–20; Bechtold, S. E., et al. "Maximization of Labor Productivity through Optimal Rest-Break Schedules." *Management Science* 30(12) (Dec. 1984): 1442–48.

12. Grandjean, E. *Fitting the Task to the Man,* 4th ed. (London: Taylor and Francis, 1988): 205.

13. Gill, M. S. "Stalking Six Sigma." *Business Month* (Jan. 1990): 42–46.

14. Hoffer, W. "Errors on the Job Can Be Reduced." *Nation's Business* 76(4) (Apr. 1988): 62–64.

15. Grandjean. *Fitting the Task*: 206–7.

16. Romert, W., et al. "Das Anlernen sensumotorischer Fertigkeiten." *Europaische Verlagsanstalt* (Frankfurt, 1971); Grandjean. *Fitting the Task*: 208.

17. Miller, P. M. *The Hilton Head Executive Stamina Program* (New York: Rawson, 1986): 37; Miller, P. M., director of Hilton Head Health Institute. Personal communication (Oct. 2, 1987).

18. Kramer, J. "Biomechanische Veranderungen in lumbalen Bewegungssegment." (Stuttgart: Hippokrates, 1973).

19. Thompson, D. Quoted in Roach, M. "Do You Fit In Your Office?" *Hippocrates* (Jul.–Aug. 1989): 42–46.

20. Stellman, J., and Henifin, M. S. *Office Work Can Be Dangerous to Your Health* (New York: Ballantine, 1989): 25–26.
21. Thompson: 46.
22. Stellman and Henifin. *Office Work*: 28.
23. Thompson: 46.
24. Kelly, J. R., and McGrath, E. "Effects of Time Limits of Task Types on Task Performance and Interaction of Four-Person Groups." *Journal of Personality and Social Psychology* 49(1985): 395-407.
25. Langer, E. J. *Mindfulness* (Reading, MA: Addison-Wesley, 1989): 137.
26. McArdle, W. D., Katch, F. I., and Katch, V. L. *Exercise Physiology: Energy, Nutrition, and Human Performance* (Philadelphia: Lea and Febiger, 1986): 451; Miller. *Hilton Head*: 26; Swarth, J. *Stress and Nutrition* (San Diego: Health Media of America, 1986): 23; Brooks, G. A., and Fahey, T. D. *Exercise Physiology: Human Bioenergetics and Its Applications* (New York: Macmillan, 1985): 462.
27. Mark, V. H., and Mark, J. P. *Brain Power: A Neurosurgeon's Complete Program to Maintain and Enhance Brain Fitness Throughout Your Life* (Boston: Houghton Mifflin, 1989): 152.
28. Goldman, B. *The "E" Factor* (New York: Morrow, 1988): 5.
29. Miller. *Hilton Head*: 26.
30. McArdle et al. *Exercise Physiology*: 451.
31. Sports and Cardiovascular Nutritionists, American Dietetic Association. Report in *American Health* (May 1987): 109.
32. Grandjean. *Fitting the Task*: 213.
33. Jenkins, D. A., et al. "Nibbling Versus Gorging: Metabolic Advantages of Increased Meal Frequency." *New England Journal of Medicine* (Oct. 5, 1989): 929–34.
34. Wurtman, J. J. *Managing Your Mind and Mood Through Food* (New York: Rawson, 1986); Drewnowski, A., Report to the American Heart Association Scientific Sessions (Nov. 1989), reported in *USA Today* (Nov. 11, 1989).
35. Wurtman. *Managing Your Mind and Mood*.
36. Janaro et al. "Technical Note."
37. Bechtold and Sumners. "Optimal Work-Rest Scheduling."
38. Foegen, J. H. "Super-Breaktime." *Supervision* 49 (1988): 9–10.
39. Imai, M. *Kaizen: The Key to Japan's Competitive Success* (New York: Random House, 1986).

Chapter 9/ Posture

1. Cailliet, R., and Gross, L. *The Rejuvenation Strategy* (Garden City, NY: Doubleday, 1987): 52.
2. Grandjean, E. *Fitting the Task to the Man,* 4th ed. (London: Taylor and Francis, 1989): 11.
3. Cailliet and Gross. *Rejuvenation*: 54.
4. Bhatnager, V., et al. "Posture, Postural Discomfort, and Performance." *Human Factors* 27(2) (Apr. 1985): 189–99; "Remedies for a Painful Case of Terminal-itis." *U.S. News & World Report* (Jan. 9, 1989): 60–61.
5. Cailliet and Gross. *Rejuvenation*; Cailliet, R., quoted in "Good Posture: An Antidote for Aging." *Shape* (Jul. 1987): 24.
6. Migdow, J. A., and Loehr, J. E. *Take a Deep Breath* (New York: Villard, 1986): 97.

7. Cailliet and Gross. *Rejuvenation*: 53.
8. Kraus, H. *Backache, Stress and Tension* (New York: Pocket Books, 1969): 40; Imrie, D., with Dimson, C. *Good Bye to Backache* (New York: Fawcett, 1983): 128–29.
9. Åstrand, P.-O., and Rodahl, K. *Textbook of Work Physiology: Physiological Bases of Exercise* (New York: McGraw-Hill, 1986): 112; Hanna, T. *The Body of Life* (New York: Knopf, 1980).
10. Riskind, J. H., and Gotay, C. C. "Physical Posture: Could It Have Regulatory or Biofeedback Effects on Motivation and Emotion?" *Motivation and Emotion* 6(3) (1982): 273–98; Weisfeld, G. E., and Beresford, J. M. "Erectness of Posture as an Indicator of Dominance or Success in Humans." *Motivation and Emotion* 6(2) (1982): 113–31; Wilson, E., and Schneider, C. "Static and Dynamic Feedback in the Treatment of Chronic Muscle Pain." Paper presented at the Biofeedback Society of America meeting, New Orleans (Apr. 16, 1985); Winter, A., and Winter, R. *Build Your Brain Power* (New York: St. Martin's, 1986); *The Neuropsychology of Achievement* (Sybervision Systems, Inc., Fountain Square, 6066 Civic Terrace Ave., Newark, CA 94560; 1985).
11. Barlow, W. Quoted in *Somatics* (Spring–Summer, 1987): 11.
12. Barlow, W. *The Alexander Technique* (New York: Knopf, 1972): 8.
13. Imrie. *Good Bye*: 128–29.
14. Riskind and Gotay. "Physical Posture."
15. Bhatnager, V., et al. "Posture, Posture Discomfort, and Performance." *Human Factors* 27(2) (Apr. 1985): 189–99.
16. Ekman, P., et al. "Autonomic Nervous System Activity Distinguishes Among Emotions." *Science* (Sep. 16, 1983): 1208–10; Greden, J., et al. *Archives of General Psychiatry* 43 (1987): 269–74; Zajonc, R. B. "Emotions and Facial Difference: A Theory Reclaimed." *Science* (Apr. 5, 1985); Duclos, S. E., et al. "Emotion-Specific Effects of Facial Expressions and Postures of Emotional Experience." *Journal of Personality and Social Psychology* 57(1) (1989): 100–108.
17. Cooper, M. *Change Your Voice, Change Your Life* (New York: Macmillan, 1984): 5; Rubin, L. S. *Voice Handbook* (Professionally Speaking, 119 W. 57th St., Suite 911, New York, NY 10019; 1986); Blumenthal, D. "Taking a Sounding." *New York Times Magazine* (Aug. 15, 1982): 51.
18. Cailliet and Gross. *Rejuvenation*: 56.
19. Heller, J., and Henkin, W. A. *Bodywise* (Los Angeles: Tarcher, 1986): 92; Cailliet and Gross. *Rejuvenation*: 56.
20. Cailliet and Gross. *Rejuvenation*: 56–57.
21. Cailliet and Gross. *Rejuvenation*: 64–65.
22. Barker, S. *The Alexander Technique* (New York: Bantam, 1978): 24.
23. Langan, L. M., and Watkins, S. M. "Pressure of Menswear on the Neck in Relation to Visual Performance." *Human Factors* 29(1) (1987): 67–71.
24. Stellman, J., and Henifin, M. S. *Office Work Can Be Dangerous to Your Health* (New York: Fawcett, 1989): 88.
25. Travell, J. G. *Office Hours: Day and Night* (New York: World Publishing, 1968): 270, 284, 285, 301, 302. Cited in Travell, J. G., and Simons, D. G. *Myofascial Pain and Dysfunction* (Baltimore: Williams and Wilkins, 1983): 112.
26. Stellman and Henifin. *Office Work*: 84.
27. Stellman and Henifin. *Office Work*: 85.
28. Cailliet and Gross. *Rejuvenation*: 127.

29. Roach, M. "Do You Fit into Your Office?" *Hippocrates/In Health* (Jul.–Aug. 1989): 44.
30. "Don't Be Slack About Good Posture." *University of California, Berkeley Wellness Letter* (Oct. 1986): 6.
31. Cailliet and Gross. *Rejuvenation*: 127.
32. Gould, N. "Back-Pocket Sciatica." *New England Journal of Medicine* 290 (1974): 633.
33. Lettvin, M. *Maggie's Back Book* (Boston: Houghton Mifflin, 1976): 131; Cailliet and Gross. *Rejuvenation*: 127.
34. Sweigard, L. *Human Movement Potential: Its Ideokinetic Function* (New York: Harper and Row, 1977): 272.
35. Cailliet and Gross. *Rejuvenation*: 129.
36. *Medical Tribune* 27 (1986): 31.

Chapter 10/ Exercise

1. Rippe, J. M. *Fit for Success* (Englewood Cliffs, NJ: Prentice Hall, 1989): 30.
2. Chen, M. S. "Wellness in the Workplace: Beyond the Point of No Return." *Health Values* 12(1) (1988): 16–22; Schwartz, D. C. "Career Wellness." *Fitness in Business* (Feb. 1989): 138–39; "Worksite Wellness Key to Productive Workforce." *Worksite Wellness Works* (May 1989): 2; Rosen, R. "Healthy People, Healthy Companies: Striking the Critical Balance." *Advances* 6(1) (1989): 8–11; Frecknall, P. "How Much Can Mind-Body Techniques Save by Reducing Absenteeism?" *Advances* 6(1) (1989): 63–65.
3. Bennis, W., and Nanus, B. *Leaders: The Strategies for Taking Charge* (New York: Harper and Row, 1985): 116.
4. Rippe. *Fit for Success*: 155.
5. "Health Benefits of Exercise in an Aging Society." *Archives of Internal Medicine* 147 (1987): 353–56; Powell, K. E., et al. "Physical Activity and the Incidence of Coronary Heart Disease." *Annual Review of Public Health* 8 (1987): 253–87; Proceedings of the American Heart Association 59th Scientific Sessions, 1988.
6. "The Health Benefits of Exercise (Part 1 of 2)." *The Physician and Sports Medicine* 15(10) (Oct. 1987): 115–32; "The Health Benefits of Exercise (Part 2 of 2)." *The Physician and Sports Medicine* 15(11) (Nov. 1987): 121–31.
7. Frymoyer, J. W., et al. "Epidemiologic Studies of Low Back Pain." *Spine* 5 (1980): 419–22; Kraus, H. *Backache, Stress and Tension* (New York: Fawcett, 1969).
8. Jensen, J., et al. *New England Journal of Medicine* (Oct. 17, 1985): 973–75; Lane, N. E., et al. "Long-Distance Running, Bone Density, and Osteoarthritis." *Journal of the American Medical Association* (Mar. 7, 1986): 1147–52; Block, J. E., et al. "Does Exercise Prevent Osteoporosis?" *Journal of the American Medical Association* 257(22) (Jun. 1987): 3115–17.
9. Åstrand, P.-O. *Health and Fitness* (New York: Barron's, 1977): 28–30.
10. Sime, W. E. "Psychological Benefits of Exercise." *Advances* (Journal of the Institute for the Advancement of Health, New York) 1(4) (Fall 1984): 15–29. 90 references cited; Roth, D. L., and Holmes, D. S. "Influence of Aerobic Exercise Training and Relaxation Training on Physical and Psychological Health Following Stressful Life Events." *Psychosomatic Medicine* (Jul.–Aug. 1987); Morgan, W. P., and Goldston, S. E. *Exercise and Mental Health* (Washington, DC: Hemisphere Publishing, 1987).

11. Simon, H. B. "The Immunology of Exercise." *Journal of the American Medical Association* 252(19) (Nov. 16, 1984); "Health Benefits of Exercise in an Aging Society"; Paffenbarger, R. S., et al. *Journal of the American Medical Association* (Jul. 27, 1984); Paffenbarger, R. S., et al. *New England Journal of Medicine* (Mar. 5, 1986).

12. Blair, S. N., et al. "Physical Fitness and All-Cause Mortality: A Prospective Study of Healthy Men and Women." *Journal of the American Medical Association* 262(17) (Nov. 3, 1989): 2395–2401.

13. Sinyor, D., et al. "Aerobic Fitness Level and Reactivity to Psychosocial Stress." *Psychosomatic Medicine* 45 (1983): 205–17; Keller, S., and Seraganian, P. "Physical Fitness Level and Autonomic Reactivity to Psychosocial Stress." *Journal of Psychosomatic Research* 28(4) (1984): 279–87.

14. Dienstbier, R. A. "Arousal and Physiological Toughness: Implications for Mental and Physical Health." *Psychological Review* 96(1) (1989): 84–100.

15. Eliot, R. S., and Breo, D. L. *Is It Worth Dying For?* Rev. ed. (New York: Bantam, 1989): 138.

16. Gondoloa, J., and Tuckman, B. *Journal of Social Behavior and Personality* 1(1) (1986); Backer, T. E. "How Health Promotion Programs Can Enhance Workplace Creativity," in Klarreich, S. H. (Ed.). *Health and Fitness in the Workplace* (New York: Praeger, 1987): 325–37.

17. Backer. "How Health Promotion."

18. U.S. Department of Health and Human Services, Public Health Service, National Institutes of Health. *Exercise and Your Heart* (1981). NIH Publication No. 83-1677 (Superintendent of Documents, U.S. Government Printing Office, Washington, DC 20402).

19. Hage, P. "Exercise Guidelines: Which to Believe?" *Physician and Sports Medicine* 10 (1982): 23.

20. American College of Sports Medicine. *Guidelines for Graded Exercise Testing Prescription*, 3rd ed. (Philadelphia: Lea & Febiger, 1986).

21. Åstrand. *Health*: 12.

22. Olsen, E. "Exercise, More or Less." *Hippocrates* (Jan.–Feb. 1988): 65-72; Åstrand. *Health*: 12; Stamford, B. A., and Shimer, P. *Fitness Without Exercise* (New York: Warner, 1990); *Journal of the American Medical Association* 262 (1989): 2395–2401.

23. Winter, A., and Winter, R. *Build Your Brain Power* (New York: St. Martin's, 1986): 70.

24. Funk, E. "Avoiding Altitude Sickness." *Summit County Journal* (Brekenridge, CO: Jan. 12, 1978): 7.

25. Asimov, I. *Isaac Asimov on the Human Body and the Human Brain* (New York: Bonanza, 1984): 211.

26. Lynch, J. J. Study published in *Psychosomatic Medicine*, quoted in Lynch, J. *Language of the Heart* (New York: Basic Books, 1985).

27. Sharkey, B. J. *Physiology of Exercise* (Champaign, IL: Human Kinetics, 1984): 336; Cailliet, R. *Understand Your Backache* (Philadelphia: F. A. Davis, 1984): 122–24; Cailliet, R., and Gross, L. *The Rejuvenation Strategy* (New York: Doubleday, 1987); Dickinson, A., and Bennet, K. "Do It Right: The Sit-up." *Shape* (Jul. 1983): 28.

28. Daniels, L., and Worthingham, C. *Therapeutic Exercise for Body Alignment and Function* (Philadelphia: Saunders, 1977): 77; Yessis, M. "Kinesiology." *Muscle & Fitness* (Feb. 1985): 18–19, 142.

29. Shyne, K., and Dominquez, R. H. "To Stretch or Not to Stretch?" *The Physician and Sports Medicine* 10 (1982): 137–40; Mirkin, G. *Dr. Gabe Mir-*

kin's Fitness Clinic (Chicago: Contemporary Books, 1986): 16–19; Yessis, M., and Trubo, R. *Secrets of Soviet Sports Fitness and Training* (New York: Arbor House, 1988): 78.

30. McArdle, W. D., Katch, F. I., and Katch, V. I. *Exercise Physiology: Energy, Nutrition, and Human Performance* (Philadelphia: Lea and Febiger, 1986).

31. Shellock, F. G. "Physiological Benefits of Warm-up." *The Physician and Sports Medicine* 11 (1983): 134–39; Shellock, F. G. "Physiological, Psychological, and Injury Prevention Aspects of Warm-Up." *NSCA Journal* 8 (5) (1986): 24–27; Shellock, F. G., and Prentice, W. E. "Warming-Up and Stretching for Improved Physical Performance and Prevention of Sports-Related Injuries." *Sports Medicine* 2 (1985): 267–78.

32. Shyne and Dominquez. "To Stretch"; Mirkin. *Mirkin's Fitness Clinic*: 16–19; Yessis and Trubo. *Soviet Sports*: 78.

33. France, K. "Competitive vs. Non-Competitive Thinking During Exercise: Effects on Norepinephrine Levels." Paper presented at the annual meeting of the American Psychological Association, Toronto, Canada (Aug. 1984).

34. Buchalew, M. W., University of North Carolina at Asheville. Study reported in Stamford and Shimer. *Fitness Without Exercise*: 48.

35. Nieman, D. C. *The Sports Medicine Fitness Course* (Palo Alto: Bull Publishing, 1986): 156.

Chapter 11/ Nutrition

1. *Heart Facts 1990*. American Heart Association (7320 Greenville Ave., Dallas, TX 75231); Doll, R., and Peto, R. "The Causes of Cancer: Quantitative Estimates of Avoidable Risks of Cancer in the United States." *Journal of the National Cancer Institute* 66 (1981): 1192. Higginson, J. In *Proceedings of the Eighth Canadian Cancer Research Conference* (Oxford: Pergamon, 1969): 40–75; Reddy, B., et al. "Nutrition and Its Relationship to Cancer." *Advances in Cancer Research* 32 (1980): 237–345; "How to Cut the Risk of Cancer." *FDA Consumer* (Apr. 1988): 22–29; Wynder, E. L., and Gori, G. B. "Contribution of the Environment to Cancer Incidence: An Epidemiologic Exercise." *Journal of the National Cancer Institute* 58 (1977): 825–32.

2. For highlights, refer to Klarreich, S. H. (Ed.). *Health and Fitness in the Workplace* (New York: Praeger, 1987); Blanchard, M., and Tager, M. J. *Working Well* (New York: Simon and Schuster, 1985); and *Fit for Success: Proven Strategies for Executive Health* (Englewood Cliffs, NJ: Prentice Hall, 1989); Wurtman, J. J. *Managing Your Mind and Mood Through Food* (New York: Harper and Row, 1987).

3. Snowdon, D. A., and Phillips, R. L. "Does a Vegetarian Diet Reduce the Occurrence of Diabetes?" *American Journal of Public Health* 75(5) (May 1985): 507–12; "Position of the American Dietetic Association: Vegetarian Diets." *Journal of the American Dietetic Association* 88(3) (Mar. 1988): 351; *Australian and New Zealand Journal of Medicine* (Aug. 1984); Ballentine, R. *Transition to Vegetarianism* (Honesdale, PA: Himalayan Institute, 1987); Liebman, B. "Are Vegetarians Healthier Than the Rest of Us?" *Nutrition Action* (Jun. 1983): 8; *British Medical Journal* 291 (Jul. 6, 1985); *Journal of the Royal Society of Medicine* 79 (Jun. 1986); Burr, M. L., and Sweetnam, P. M. "Vegetarianism, Dietary Fiber, and Mortality." *American Journal of Clinical Nutrition* 36(5) (Nov. 1982): 873–77; Dwyer, J., director, Frances

Stern Nutrition Center, Tufts–New England Medical Center, quoted in *Environmental Nutrition* (May 1987); *Environmental Nutrition* (May 1987); "A.D.A. Report: Position Paper on the Vegetarian Approach to Eating." *Journal of the American Dietetic Association* 77(1) (1980): 61–69; *Journal of the American Dietetic Association* 88(3) (Mar. 1988): 351.

4. "No Fast Fix for a Bad Diet." Gallup Poll for the American Dietetic Association reported in *USA Today* (Feb. 21, 1990).

5. Jenkins, D. A., et al. "Nibbling Versus Gorging: Metabolic Advantages of Increased Meal Frequency." *New England Journal of Medicine* (Oct. 5, 1989): 929–34.

6. Brody, J. E. *Jane Brody's Good Food Book* (New York: Norton, 1985): 187.

7. Wurtman, J. J. *Managing Your Mind*.

8. Kostas, G., and Rojohn, K. "Nutrition Tips: Eating on the Run — The Cooper Clinic Positive Eating Program." (Aerobics Center, Dallas, TX, 1986).

9. Leveille, T. "Adipose Tissue Metabolism: Influence of Eating and Diet Composition." *Federation Proceedings* 29 (1970): 1294–1301; Lukert, B. "Biology of Obesity." In Wolman, B. (Ed.). *Psychological Aspects of Obesity: A Handbook* (New York: Van Nostrand Reinhold, 1982): 1–14; Szepsi, B. "A Model of Nutritionally Induced Overweight: Weight 'Rebound' Following Caloric Restriction." In Bray, G. (Ed.). *Recent Advances in Obesity Research* (London: Newman, 1978).

10. Vash, P. D. "Outsmarting the Fat Cell." *Shape* (Mar. 1987): 72–74.

11. Willett, W., and MacMahon, B. "Diet and Cancer: An Overview." *New England Journal of Medicine* 310 (1984): 633–38; Alabaster, O. *The Power of Prevention: Reduce Your Risk of Cancer Through Diet and Nutrition* (New York: Simon and Schuster, 1985); *Journal of the National Cancer Institute* 77(1) (1986): 33–42.

12. Brody. *Good Food*: 12.

13. Berenson, G. *American Journal of Diseases of Children* 133 (1979): 1049; *Atherosclerosis* 5 (1985): 404; Report of the American Heart Association Nutrition Committee. *Atherosclerosis* 4 (1982): 177–91; Puska, P., et al. "Controlled Randomized Trial of the Effect of Dietary Fat on Blood Pressure." *Lancet* (1) (1983): 1; *Journal of Hypertension* 4(4) (1986): 407–12.

14. Williams, H. *Kidney International* 13 (1978): 410; Kromhout, D., et al. *New England Journal of Medicine* 312 (May 9, 1985): 1205.

15. Danforth, E. "Calories: A Scientific Breakthrough." *Shape* (Mar. 1986): 47; Danforth, E. "Diet and Obesity." *American Journal of Clinical Nutrition* 41 (May 1985): 1132–45.

16. Hallfrisch, J., et al. "Modification of the United States' Diet to Effect Changes in Blood Lipids and Lipoprotein Distribution." *Atherosclerosis* 57(2–3) (Nov. 1985): 179–88; Connor, S. L., and Connor, W. E. *The New American Diet* (New York: Simon and Schuster, 1986); Walford, R. *The 120-Year Diet* (New York: Simon and Schuster, 1986): 116; Alabaster. *Prevention*: 87–88 and 107.

17. *Tufts University Diet & Nutrition Letter* 5(3) (May 1987): 1–2.

18. Schaefer, E. J., et al. "The Effects of Low Cholesterol, High Polyunsaturated Fat, and Low Fat Diets on Plasma Lipid and Lipoprotein Cholesterol Levels in Normal and Hypercholesterolemic Subjects." *American Journal of Clinical Nutrition* 34 (1981): 1158–63.

19. *Tufts University Diet & Nutrition Letter* 5(1) (Mar. 1987): 2.

20. Cooper, K. H. *Controlling Cholesterol* (New York: Bantam, 1988): 42, 44.

21. Tornberg, S. A., et al. "Risks of Cancer of the Colon and Rectum in Relation to Serum Cholesterol and Beta-Lipoprotein." *New England Journal of Medicine* 315(26) (Dec. 25, 1986): 1629–34; Mannes, G. A., et al. "Relation Between the Frequency of Colorectal Adenoma and the Serum Cholesterol Level." *New England Journal of Medicine* (Dec. 25, 1986): 1634–38.
22. Montgomery, A. "Cholesterol Tests: How Accurate Are They?" *Nutrition Action* (May 1988): 1–7.
23. Stanford University Center for Research in Disease Prevention. "Stanford Heart Disease Prevention Program." *Prevention* (Feb. 1986): 38.
24. Hoeg, J. M., et al. "An Approach to the Management of Hyperlipoproteinemia." *Journal of the American Medical Association* 255(4) (Jan. 24–31, 1986): 512–21; Anderson, J. W., and Chen, W. L. "Plant Fiber: Carbohydrate and Lipid Metabolism." *American Journal of Clinical Nutrition* 32 (1979): 346–63; Anderson, J. W., et al. "Hypocholesterolemic Effects of Oatbran or Bean Intake for Hypercholesterolemic Men." *American Journal of Clinical Nutrition* 40 (1984): 1146–55; Kirby, R. W., et al. "Oat-Bran Intake Selectively Lowers Serum Low-Density Lipoprotein Cholesterol Concentrations of Hypercholesterolemic Men." *American Journal of Clinical Nutrition* 34 (1981): 824–28.
25. *Tufts University Diet & Nutrition Letter* 5(1) (Mar. 1987): 2; Cooper. *Controlling Cholesterol*: 80–83.
26. Migdow, J. A., and Loehr, J. E. *Take a Deep Breath* (New York: Villard, 1986): 97.
27. Hanson, P. G. *The Joy of Stress* (Kansas City: Andrews, McMeel & Parker, 1986): 27.
28. Leathwood, P., and Pollet, P. "Diet-Induced Mood Changes in Normal Populations." *Journal of Psychiatric Research* 17 (1983): 147–50; Lieberman, H., et al. "The Behavioral Effects of Food Constituents: Strategies Used in Studies of Amino Acids, Protein, Carbohydrates and Caffeine." *Nutrition Reviews* (Suppl. May, 1986): 61–69; Lieberman, H., et al. "Mood, Performance and Sensitivity: Changes Induced by Food Constituents." *Journal of Psychiatric Research* 17 (1984): 135–45; Spring, B. "Effects of Foods and Nutrients on the Behavior of Normal Individuals," in Wurtman, J. J., and Wurtman, R. J. (Eds.). *Nutrition and the Brain*, vol. 7 (New York: Raven Press, 1986): 1–47; Christensen, L. "Impact of Dietary Change on Emotional Distress." *Journal of Abnormal Psychology* 94 (1985): 565–79.
29. Wurtman. *Managing Your Mind*.
30. Wurtman, J. J. Personal communication. (Dec. 15, 1987); Spring, B., et al. "Carbohydrates, Tryptophan, and Behavior: A Methodological Review." *Psychological Bulletin* 102 (1987): 234–56; Benton. *Biological Psychiatry* 24 (1988): 95–100; Lieberman, H. R., et al. "Aging, Nutrient Choice, Activity, and Behavioral Responses to Nutrients." *Annals of the New York Academy of Science* 561 (1989): 196–208; Wurtman, R. J., and Wurtman, J. J. "Do Carbohydrates Affect Food Intake via Neurotransmitter Activity?" *Appetite* 11(Supp. 1) (1988): 42–47; Wurtman, J. "Recent Evidence from Human Studies Linking Central Serotoninergic Function with Carbohydrate Intake." *Appetite* 8(3) (1987): 211–13; Wurtman, R. J. "Dietary Treatments That Affect Brain Neurotransmitters." *Annals of the New York Academy of Science* 499 (1987): 179–90; Leathwood, P. "Food-Composition, Changes in Brain Serotonin Synthesis and Appetite for Protein and Carbohydrate." *Appetite* 8(3) (1987): 202–5; Spring, B., et al. "Psychobiological Effects of Car-

bohydrates." *Journal of Clinical Psychiatry* 50(Suppl.) (May 1989): 27–34; Wurtman, J. J. "Carbohydrate Craving, Mood Changes, and Obesity." *Journal of Clinical Psychiatry* 49(Suppl.) (Aug. 1989): 37–39; Okuyama, H. "Does Food Affect Brain Function?" *Tanpakushitsu Kakusan Koso* 35(3) (Mar. 1990): 275–79; Wurtman, R. J., and Wurtman, J. J. "Carbohydrates and Depression." *Scientific American* 260(1) (Jan. 1989): 68–75.

31. Wurtman, J. Quoted in "Peak Performance Brain Food." *Omni Longevity* 2(6) (Apr. 1988): 67.
32. Spring. "Carbohydrates."
33. Wurtman. *Managing Your Mind*: 27.

Chapter 12/ Healthy Environments

1. Hoffer, W. "Errors on the Job Can Be Reduced." *Nation's Business* 76(4) (Apr. 1988): 62–64.
2. Backer, T. E. "How Health Promotion Programs Can Enhance Workplace Creativity," in Klarreich, S. H. (Ed.). *Health and Fitness in the Workplace* (New York: Praeger, 1987): 333.
3. Robertson, A. S., et al. "Comparison of Health Problems Related to Work and Environmental Measurements in Two Office Buildings with Different Ventilation Systems." *British Medical Journal* 291(6492) (Aug. 10, 1985): 373–75; Taylor, C. W. "Promoting Health, Strengthening, and Wellness Through Environmental Variables," in Matarazzo, J. D., et al. (Eds.). *Behavioral Health: A Handbook of Health Enhancement and Disease Prevention* (New York: Wiley, 1984): 130–48.
4. Rice, F. "Do You Work in a Sick Building?" *Fortune* (Jul. 2, 1990): 86–88; "EPA: Pollution Higher Indoors." *USA Today* (Sep. 11, 1986).
5. *Science News* (Sep. 28, 1985).
6. "New CPSC Study Report: Indoor Air Worse Than Outdoor." *Human Ecologist* 26 (Summer 1984): 9–10.
7. "Got That Stuffy, Run-Down Feeling?" *Time* (Jun. 6, 1988): 76.
8. "Surgeon General, Citing Risks, Urges Smoke-Free Workplace." *New York Times* (Dec. 17, 1986).
9. "Cigarette Smoking: The Bottom Line." *American Cancer Society* (Nov. 1986).
10. "Smokers Make Poor Drivers." *USA Today* (Sep. 22, 1986).
11. *Western Journal of Medicine* 146 (1986): 1.
12. "Formaldehyde: Assessment of Health Effects." National Academy of Sciences Commission on Toxicology (Mar. 1980): vi; Fawcett, S. "Formaldehyde: If It Smells, Watch Out!" *Medical Self-Care* (Summer 1984): 21–23.
13. *The Cancer Prevention Letter* 1(4) (1986): 1–3; "Spider Plant Meets the Foam Monster." *Harrowsmith* (Apr.–May 1986): 124.
14. "Reduce Your Pollutants." *Women's Sports & Fitness* 12(1) (Mar. 1990): 11.
15. Stellman, J., and Henifin, M. S. *Office Work Can Be Dangerous to Your Health* (New York: Fawcett, 1989): 93.
16. Marks, J. G. "Allergic Contact Dermatitis from Carbonless Paper." *Journal of the American Medical Association* (Jun. 12, 1981): 2331.
17. LaMarke, F. P., et al. "Acute Systematic Reaction to Carbonless Copy Paper Associated with Histamine Release." *Journal of the American Medical Association* (Jul. 8, 1988): 242.

18. McCormick, E. J., and Sanders, M. *Human Factors in Engineering,* 5th ed. (New York: McGraw-Hill, 1987).
19. Stellman and Henifin. *Office Work:* 106.
20. Wineman, J. Quoted in Meer, J. "The Light Touch." *Psychology Today* (Sep. 1985): 60–67.
21. Taylor. "Promoting Health."
22. Grandjean, E. *Fitting the Task to the Man: A Textbook of Occupational Ergonomics,* 4th ed. (London: Taylor and Francis, 1989): 253.
23. Hoffer. "Errors on the Job": 62.
24. Gilbert, S. "Noise Pollution." *Science Digest* (Mar. 1985): 28; Stellman and Henifin. *Office Work:* 142–43.
25. Stellman, J., et al. "Air Quality and Ergonomics in the Office: Survey Results and Methodological Issues." *American Industrial Hygiene Association Journal* 46(5) (1985): 286–93; Stellman, J., et al. "Work Environment and the Well-Being of Clerical and VDT Workers." *Journal of Occupational Behavior* 8 (1987): 95–114; Klitzman, S., and Stellman, J. "The Impact of the Physical and Psychosocial Environment on Office Workers." *Social Science and Medicine* 29(6) (1989): 733–42.
26. Safranek, M. D. "Effect of Auditory Rhythm on Muscle Reactivity." *Physical Therapy* (Feb. 1982): 161–88.
27. Shabecoff, P. "Issue of Radon Peril: New National Focus on Ecology." *New York Times* (Sep. 10, 1986); Eckholm, E. "Radon: Threat is Real." *New York Times* (Sep. 2, 1986).
28. Shabecoff. "Radiation Peril"; Eckholm. "Radon."
29. Baranski, S., and Czerski, P. *Biological Effects of Microwaves* (Stroudsburg, PA: Dowden, Hutchinson, and Ross, 1976); Samuels, M., and Bennett, H. Z. *Well Body, Well Earth* (San Francisco: Sierra Club, 1984): 122.
30. Samuels and Bennett. *Well Body:* 122.
31. "Researchers See More Danger in Microwave Radiation." *Business Week* (Dec. 7, 1987): 127.
32. Stellman and Henifin. *Office Work:* 52.
33. Baranski and Czerski. *Biological Effects*; Shute, N. "The Other Kind of Radiation." *American Health* (Jul.–Aug. 1986): 54–58.
34. "Are Electric Blankets Safe?" *Consumer Reports* (Nov. 1989): 715–16.
35. Adey, W. R. "Tissue Interactions with Nonionizing Electromagnetic Fields." *Physiological Review* 61 (1981): 435–514; Singer, S. J., and Nicholson, G. L. "The Fluid Mosaic Model of the Structure of Cell Membranes." *Science* 175 (1972): 720–31; Marron, M. T., et al. "Mytotic Delay in Heterokaryons and Decreased Respiration." *Experientia* 24 (1978): 589–90; Marron, M. T., et al. "Cell Surface Effects of 60-Hz Electromagnetic Fields." *Radiation Research* 94 (1983): 217–20; Hansson, H. A. "Lamellar Bodies in Purkinje Nerve Cells Experimentally Induced by Electric Field." *Brain Research* 216 (1981): 187–91. Bawin, S., and Adey, W. "Sensitivity of Calcium Binding in Cerebral Tissue to Weak Environmental Electrical Fields Oscillating at Low Frequency." *Proceedings of the National Academy of Sciences* 73 (1976): 1999; Wiltschko, W., and Wiltschko, R. "Magnetic Compass of European Robins." *Science* 176 (1972): 62; Larkin, R. P., and Southerland, P. J. "Migrating Birds Respond to Project Seafarer's Electromagnetic Field." *Science* 195 (1977): 777; Samuels and Bennett. *Well Body:* 125.
36. Phillips, J. L., et al. "Transferrin Binding to Two Human Carcinoma Cell Lines: Characterization and Effect of 60-Hz Electromagnetic Fields." *Cancer*

Research 46 (1986): 239–44; Winters, W. D. "Biological Functions of Immunologically Reactive Human and Canine Cells Influenced by *in vitro* Exposure to 60-Hz Electric and Magnetic Fields" (1986). Cited in Ahlbom, A., et al. "Panel's Final Report: Biological Effects of Power Line Fields, New York State Power Lines Project Scientific Advisory Panel Final Report." State of New York Department of Health (Jul. 1, 1987).

37. Konig, H., et al. *Biological Effects of Environmental Electromagnetism* (New York: Springer-Verlag, 1981): 218.

38. "Are Electric Blankets Safe?"

39. "Danger from a Glowing Screen." *U.S. News & World Report* (Jun. 18, 1990): 76; Special Report. *Macworld* (Jul. 1990); Poch, D. I. *Radiation Alert* (Garden City, NY: Doubleday, 1985); DeMatteo, P. *Terminal Shock: The Health Hazards of Video Display Terminals* (Toronto: NC Press, 1985).

40. "Fit to Drink?" *Consumer Reports* (Jan., 1990): 27–43.

41. Kilpatrick, D. "Environmentalism: The New Crusade." *Fortune* (Feb. 12, 1990): 44–55.

Chapter 13/ Sleep and Rest

1. Lamberg, L. *The American Medical Association Guide to Better Sleep* (New York: Random House, 1984).

2. Dotto, L. *Asleep in the Fast Lane* (New York: Morrow, 1990): 179.

3. Horne, J. A. "Sleep Loss and 'Divergent' Thinking Ability." *Sleep* 11(6) (1988): 528–36; Arnot, R. B. *CBS News* (Feb. 25, 1986).

4. *Psychology Today* (Dec. 1988): 18.

5. Dotto. *Asleep in the Fast Lane*; Horne, J. A. *Why We Sleep* (Oxford: Oxford University Press, 1988); Adam, K., and Oswald, I. "Sleep Helps Healing." *British Medical Journal* (Nov. 24, 1984): 1400-1401.

6. Horne. *Why We Sleep*.

7. Horne. *Why We Sleep*; Horne. "Sleep Loss."

8. Horne. *Why We Sleep*.

9. Hauri, P. "Behavioral Treatment of Insomnia." *Medical Times* 107(6) (1986): 36–47; Regestein, Q. R. "Practical Ways to Manage Insomnia." *Medical Times* 107(6) (1986): 19–23.

10. Broughton, R. "Performance and Evoked Potential Measures of Various States of Daytime Sleepiness." *Sleep* 5(Suppl. 2) (1982); Dotto. *Asleep in the Fast Lane*: 138; Hauri. "Behavioral Treatment"; Regestein. "Practical Ways."

11. Quoted in Hopson, J. "The Unraveling of Insomnia." *Psychology Today* (Jun. 1986): 44.

12. Naitoh, P. *Napping and Human Performance During Irregular or Prolonged Work* (San Diego: Naval Health Research Center, 1988).

13. Dinges, D. F., et al. "The Benefits of a Nap During Prolonged Work and Wakefulness." *Work and Stress* 2(2) (1988): 139–53.

14. Shapiro, C. M., et al. "Fitness Facilitates Sleep." *European Journal of Applied Physiology* 53 (1984): 1–4; Baekland, F., Downstate Medical Center, NY, 1966 study, and Shapiro, C., and Zloty, R. B., University of Manitoba studies, both reported in Mirkin, G., *Dr. Gabe Mirkin's Fitness Clinic* (Chicago: Contemporary Books, 1986).

15. Kales, A., and Kales, J. D. *Evaluation and Treatment of Insomnia* (New York: Oxford University Press, 1984).

16. Lamberg, L. "White Noise on FM: Twisted Sister vs. the Sandman." *American Health* (May 1986): 20.
17. Hauri. "Behavioral Treatment"; Regestein. "Practical Ways."
18. *Medical Journal of Australia* (Jan. 21, 1984).
19. Cailliet, R., and Gross, L. *The Rejuvenation Strategy* (New York: Doubleday, 1987): 136; Dunkell, S. *Sleep Positions* (New York: Signet, 1977): 79–80.
20. Williams, G. III. "Early Morning Dangers: Why Your Body Hates to Wake Up." *American Health* (Dec. 1986): 56–59; Arnot, R. B. *CBS News* (Jan. 13, 1987).
21. Moore-Ede, M., et al. *The Clocks That Time Us* (Cambridge: Harvard University Press, 1982).

Chapter 14/ Self-Renewal and Social Support

1. O'Reilly, B. "Is Your Company Asking Too Much?" *Fortune* (Mar. 12, 1990): 39–46.
2. Dumaine, B. "Cool Cures for Burnout." *Fortune* (Jun. 20, 1988): 78–84; Klarreich, S. H. "Burnout," in Klarreich, S. H. (Ed.). *Health and Fitness in the Workplace* (New York: Praeger, 1987): 183–99.
3. Dumaine. "Cool Cures": 78.
4. Jaffe, D. T., and Scott, C. D. *From Burnout to Balance* (New York: McGraw-Hill, 1984): 127.
5. Stamp, D. Quoted in Kiechel, W. III. "12 Reasons for Leaving at Five." *Fortune* (Jul. 16, 1990): 117–18.
6. Ornstein, R., and Sobel, D. *Healthy Pleasures* (Reading, MA: Addison-Wesley, 1989). More than 1,000 scientific and medical references cited.
7. Kiechel. "12 Reasons."
8. Ornstein and Sobel. *Healthy Pleasures*: 131, 200–201.
9. Jaffe and Scott. *From Burnout to Balance*: 142; Ljungdahl, L. "Laugh If This Is a Joke." *New England Journal of Medicine* 261 (1989): 558; Dillon, K. M., et al. "Positive Emotional States and Enhancement of the Immune System." *International Journal of Psychiatry in Medicine* 15(1) (1985–1986): 13–18; "The Mind Fights Back: Scientists Study How Smiles and Laughter Boost the Immune System." *Washington Post* (Jan. 9, 1985); Brody, J. E. "Increasingly, Laughter as Potential Therapy for Patients Is Being Taken Seriously." *New York Times* (Apr. 7, 1988); Eckman, P., et al. "Autonomic Nervous System Activity Distinguishes Among Emotions." *Science* 221 (1983): 1208–10; Berk, A. L. S., et al. *Clinical Research* 36 (1988): 121, 435A; Berk, A. L. S., et al. *The Federation of American Societies for Experimental Biology (FASEB) Journal* 2 (1988): A1570.
10. Isen, A. M. "Toward Understanding the Influence of Positive Affect on Social Behavior, Decision Making, and Problem Solving: The Role of Cognitive Organization." Paper presented at the annual meeting of the American Association for the Advancement of Science, Boston (Feb. 11–15, 1988); Isen, A. M., et al. "The Influence of Positive Affect on the Unusualness of Word Associations." *Journal of Personality and Social Psychology* 48 (1985): 1413–26; Isen, A. M., et al. "Positive Affect Facilitates Creative Problem Solving." *Journal of Personality and Social Psychology* 52 (1987): 1122–31; Isen, A. M. "Positive Affect, Cognitive Processes, and Social Behavior." *Advances in Experimental Social Psychology* 20 (1987): 203–53.

11. "Humor and Productivity: Laughing Matters — At Work." *American Health* (Sep. 1988): 46.
12. Williams, R. *The Trusting Heart* (New York: Times Books, 1989).
13. House, J. S., et al. "Association of Social Relationships and Activities with Mortality: Prospective Evidence from the Tecumseh Community Health Study." *American Journal of Epidemiology* 116(1) (1982): 123–40; Berkman, L. F., and Syme, L. O. "Social Networks, Host Resistance, and Mortality: A Nine-Year Follow-Up of Alameda County Residents." *American Journal of Epidemiology* 102(2) (1979): 186–204; Eisenberg, L. "A Friend, Not an Apple, a Day Will Keep the Doctor Away." *Journal of the American Medical Association* 66 (1979): 551–53; Syme, L. "People Need People." *American Health* (Jul.–Aug. 1982): 49–51; Cohen, S., and Wils, T. "Stress, Social Support, and Buffering Hypothesis." *Psychological Bulletin* 98 (1985): 310–57; Caplan, G. "Mastery of Stress: Psychological Aspects." *American Journal of Psychiatry* 138 (1981): 413–20; Lynch, J. J. *The Broken Heart: Medical Consequences of Loneliness* (New York: Basic Books, 1977); Ornstein, R., and Sobel, D. *The Healing Brain* (New York: Simon and Schuster, 1987).
14. Jaffe, D. T., and Scott, C. D. *Take This Job and Love It* (New York: Simon and Schuster, 1988): 185.
15. Research by Princeton University psychologist John B. Jemmott III. Cited in Elias, M. "Friends May Help Keep Disease Away." *USA Today* (Oct. 11, 1989).
16. Segal, J. *Winning Life's Toughest Battles: Roots of Human Resilience* (New York: McGraw-Hill, 1986): 18.
17. Fisher, R., and Brown, S. *Getting Together: Building a Relationship That Gets to Yes* (Boston: Houghton Mifflin, 1988).
18. Ferguson, T. "Social Support Systems as Self-Care." *Medical Self-Care* (Winter 1979–1980): 3.
19. Work/Family Directions, Inc. Research cited in *Achieving Balance* (Great Performance, Inc., Portland, OR, 1990).
20. Kanter, R. M. *Work and Family in the United States* (New York: Russell Sage Foundation, 1977).
21. Bolger, N., et al. "The Contagion of Stress Across Multiple Roles." *Journal of Marriage and the Family* 51 (Feb. 1989): 175–83; Bolger, N., et al. "Marital Problems Affect Job." American Psychological Study, reported in *USA Today* (Nov. 8, 1989).
22. Yankelovich, D., and Harman, S. *Starting with the People* (Boston: Houghton Mifflin, 1988); Ludeman, K. *The Worth Ethic* (New York: Dutton, 1989); Covey, S. R. *The Seven Habits of Highly Effective People* (New York: Simon and Schuster, 1989); Kiechel, W. III "The Workaholic Generation." *Fortune* (Apr. 10, 1989): 50–62; O'Reilly, B. "Why Grade 'A' Executives Get an 'F' as Parents." *Fortune* (Jan. 1, 1990): 36–46; O'Reilly, B. "Is Your Company."
23. Curran, D. *Stress and the Healthy Family* (Minneapolis: Winston Press, 1985): 158.
24. Greiff, B. S. "The Executive Family," in *The American Family: Current Perspectives*, Harvard Seminar Series (Cambridge: Harvard University Press, 1979); Greiff, B. S., and Munter, P. *Tradeoffs: Executive, Family, and Organizational Life* (New York: New American Library, 1980).
25. Kanter, R. M. *When Giants Learn to Dance: Mastering the Challenges of Strategy, Management, and Careers in the 1990s* (New York: Simon and Schuster, 1989).

26. Pierce, J. L., et al. *Alternative Work Schedules* (Newton, MA: Allyn and Bacon, 1988); Christensen, K. *A Look at Flexible Staffing and Scheduling* (New York: Conference Board, 1989).
27. Elias, M. "Flextime Workers Win Praise." *USA Today* (Jan. 8, 1990).
28. Elias, M. "'Flex-Time' Gives Employees Muscle." *USA Today* (Oct. 11, 1989).
29. O'Reilly, B. "Is Your Company."
30. Covey, S. R. *The Seven Habits of Highly Effective People* (New York: Simon and Schuster, 1989): 188.
31. Kiechel. "12 Reasons."
32. Rodgers, F. S., and Rodgers, C. "Business and the Facts of Family Life." *Harvard Business Review* (Nov.–Dec. 1989): 121–29. From research conducted by Ellen Galinsky at Merck and Company, Rahway, NJ, 1983, 1984, and 1986.
33. Bond, Terry. *Employer Supports for Child Care*. Report for the National Council of Jewish Women, Center for the Child, New York (Aug. 1988).
34. Rodgers and Rodgers. "Business and Family": 123.
35. Rodgers and Rodgers. "Business and Family": 123–24.
36. The most insightful report to date on corporate actions is "Business and the Facts of Family Life" by Fran Sussner Rodgers and Charles Rodgers, mentioned earlier in this chapter.
37. Rodgers and Rodgers. "Business and Family": 125.
38. Burden, D., and Googins, B. *Boston University Balancing Job and Homelife Study* (Boston University School of Social Work, 1986).
39. "A Killer of Women, Too." *U.S. News & World Report* (Dec. 18, 1989): 75–76.
40. Rodgers and Rodgers. "Business and Family": 128.

Chapter 15/ High-Stress Business Travel

1. Hyatt Travel Futures Project Report on Business Travelers (1988).
2. Dumaine, B. "How Managers Can Succeed Through Speed." *Fortune* (Feb. 13, 1989): 54–59; Stalk, G., and Hout, T. M. *Competing Against Time: How Time-Based Competition Is Reshaping Global Markets* (New York: Free Press, 1990).
3. Trunzo, J. Quoted in "How America Has Run Out of Time." *Time* (Apr. 24, 1989): 59–67; Hoffman, E. "Have Office, Will Travel." *Psychology Today* (Sep. 1988): 43–46.
4. "Going Global." *Business Week* (Oct. 20, 1989): 9–18; Tully, S. "The Hunt for the Global Manager." *Fortune* (May 21, 1990): 140–44.
5. Dumaine, B. "Cool Cures for Burnout." *Fortune* (Jun. 20, 1988): 78–84.
6. Levine, R. "Waiting Is a Power Game." *Psychology Today* (Apr. 1987): 24–33.
7. Buffington, P. W. "The Waiting Game." *Sky* (Apr. 1988): 78–84.
8. "Special Report: The Portable Executive." *Business Week* (Oct. 10, 1988): 102–12; Hoffman. "Have Office."
9. Quick, J. C. Quoted in *Psychology Today* (Sep. 1988): 46.
10. Dientsbier, R. A. "Arousal and Physiological Toughness: Implications for Mental and Physical Health." *Psychological Review* 96(1) (1989): 84–100; Keller, S., and Seraganian, P. "Physical Fitness Level and Autonomic Reactivity to Psychosocial Stress." *Journal of Psychosomatic Research* 28(4) (1984): 279–87.

11. Mautz, W., et al. "Enhancement of Ozone-Induced Lung Injury by Exercise." *Journal of Toxicology and Environmental Health* 16(6) (1985); Carey, B. "A Jog in the Smog." *Hippocrates* (May–Jun. 1989): 94–96.

12. Wurtman, J. J. *Managing Your Mind and Mood Through Food* (New York: Harper and Row, 1988); Leathwood, P., and Pollet, P. "Diet-Induced Mood Changes in Normal Populations." *Journal of Psychiatric Research* 17 (1983): 147–50; Lieberman, H., et al. "The Behavioral Effects of Food Constituents: Strategies Used in Studies of Amino Acids, Protein, Carbohydrates, and Caffeine." *Nutrition Reviews*, Suppl. (May 1986): 61–69; Lieberman, H., et al. "Mood, Performance and Sensitivity: Changes Induced by Food Constituents." *Journal of Psychiatric Research* 17 (1984): 135–45; Spring, B. "Effects of Foods and Nutrients on the Behavior of Normal Individuals," in Wurtman, J. J., and Wurtman, R. J. (Eds.). *Nutrition and the Brain*, vol. 7 (New York: Raven Press, 1986): 1–47; Christensen, L. "Impact of Dietary Change on Emotional Distress." *Journal of Abnormal Psychology* 94 (1985): 565–79.

13. McArdle, W. D., Katch, F. I., and Katch, V. L. *Exercise Physiology: Energy, Nutrition, and Human Performance* (Philadelphia: Lea and Febiger, 1986): 451; Miller, P. M. *Hilton Head Executive Stamina Program* (New York: Rawson, 1986): 26; Swarth, J. *Stress and Nutrition* (San Diego: Health Media of America, 1986): 23; Brooks, G. A., and Fahey, T. D. *Exercise Physiology: Human Bioenergetics and Its Applications* (New York: Macmillan, 1985): 462.

14. Miller. *Hilton Head*: 26.

15. Slonim, N. B., et al. *Respiratory Physiology*, 3rd ed. (St. Louis: Mosby, 1976); Browne, L., et al. "The Nine Stresses of Flight." *Journal of Emergency Nursing* 13(4) (Jul.–Aug. 1987): 232–34.

16. "Beware of Unfriendly Air on Lengthy Flights." *USA Today* (Oct. 30, 1989): 6D; Hendley, J. O. "Risk of Acquiring Respiratory Tract Infections During Air Travel." *Journal of the American Medical Association* (Nov. 20, 1987): 2764.

17. Marth, E., et al. "Aircraft Noise: Changes of Biochemical Parameters." *Zentralblatt Für Bakteriologie, Mikrobiologie und Hygiene* 185(Serie B) (1988): 498–508; Browne et al. "Nine Stresses of Flight."

18. Langan, L. M., and Watkins, S. M. "Pressure of Menswear on the Neck in Relation to Visual Performance." *Human Factors* 29(10) (1987): 67–71.

19. "Health: Don't Let Flying Strain Your Back." *Business Week* (Dec. 15, 1986): 113.

20. Cruickshank, J. M., et al. "Air Travel and Thrombotic Episodes: The Economy Class Syndrome." *The Lancet* (Aug. 27, 1988): 497–98.

21. Perkins, E. Quoted in "Finding Comfort in the Friendly Skies." *Successful Meetings* (Dec. 1988): 117–18.

22. *Management Review* 77 (Oct. 1988): 7–8; Upjohn Company Study on Business Travel. Quoted in *USA Today* (Mar. 20, 1989).

23. Preston, F. S. "Travel and Performance." *Medicine and Science in Law* 24(4) (1984): 249–55.

24. Czeisler, C. H., et al. "Bright Light Induction of Strong (Type O) Resetting of the Human Circadian Pacemaker." *Science* (Jun. 16, 1989): 1328–33; Czeisler, C. H., et al. "Human Sleep: Its Duration and Organization Depend on Its Circadian Phase." *Science* (Dec. 12, 1980); Kronauer, R., and Czeisler, C. Quoted in "Jet Lag Breakthrough." *Condé Naste's Traveler* (Sep. 1989): 35–36.

25. Beyond a long list of recent research articles, one noteworthy report is from Argonne National Laboratory, #1984-754-904 (9700 South Cass Ave., Argonne, IL 60439; 1984), and one of the best books on this subject is *Overcoming Jet Lag* by Dr. Charles F. Ehret and Lynne Waller Scanlon (New York: Berkley, 1983).
26. Ehret and Scanlon. *Overcoming Jet Lag*: 98–99.
27. Ehret and Scanlon. *Overcoming Jet Lag*: 81.
28. Mrosovsky, N., and Salmon, P. A. "A Behavioral Method for Accelerating Re-Entrainment of Rhythms to New Light-Dark Cycles." *Nature* (Nov. 26, 1987): 372–73; Van Reeth, O., and Turek, F. W., *Nature* (May 9, 1989); Klein, K. E., and Wegmann, D. H., in Scheving, L. E., et al. (Eds.). *Chronobiology* (Tokyo: Igaku Shoin, 1974): 564–70.

Chapter 16/ The Further Reaches of the Mind

1. Salk, J. Quoted in Helvarg, D. "A Conversation with the Old Master." *San Diego* 5 (1984): 194–200.
2. Kra, S. *Aging Myths* (New York: McGraw-Hill, 1986); "Building a Better Brain." *Omni Longevity* 1(1) (Nov. 1986): 1–2; Schaie, K. W. (Ed.). *Longitudinal Studies of Adult Psychological Development* (New York: Guildford Press, 1983); "Senility Reconsidered: Treatment Possibilities for Mental Impairment in the Elderly." Task force sponsored by the National Institute on Aging, Bethesda, MD. *Journal of the American Medical Association* (Jul. 18, 1980): 259–60; Duara, R., et al. "Cerebral Glucose Utilization as Measured with Positron Emission Tomography in 21 Resting Healthy Men Between the Ages of 21 and 83 Years." *Brain* 106 (1983): 761–75; Diamond, M. C., et al. "Differences in Occipital Cortical Synapses from Environmentally Enriched, Impoverished, and Standard Colony Rats." *Journal of Neuroscience Research* 1 (1987): 109–19; Rosenzweig, M. R. "Experience, Memory, and the Brain." *American Psychologist* (Apr. 1984).
3. Rosenzweig, M. R., and Bennett, E. "The Physiological Imprint of Aging." U.S. Department of Health Research Grant Report, National Institutes of Health (May 1966) (University of California's Lawrence Berkeley Laboratory (Jun. 24, 1980); Goleman, D. "The Aging Mind Proves Capable of Lifelong Growth." *New York Times* (Feb. 21, 1984); Diamond, M. C., et al. "Differences."
4. Diamond, M. C. Quoted in "Building a Better Brain"; Diamond, M. C. *Enriching Heredity: The Impact of the Environment on the Anatomy of the Brain* (New York: Free Press, 1989).
5. Kandel, E. R., and Schwartz, J. H. "Molecular Biology of Learning: Modulation of Transmitter Release." *Science* 218(4571) (1982): 433–43; Clark, G. "Cell Biological Analysis of Associative and Non-Associative Learning." Paper presented at the annual meeting of the American Association for the Advancement of Science, New York (May 26, 1984); News feature, University of Illinois at Urbana (May 26, 1984).
6. *Special Report on Aging.* U.S. Department of Health, National Institutes of Health Publication No. 80-1907 (Feb. 1980).
7. Coleman, P. Quoted in "Building a Better Brain."
8. Sandman, C. Quoted in *Psychology Today* (Nov. 1987): 20.

9. Colarelli, S. Quoted in Roberts, M. "Eight Ways to Rethink Your Workstyle." *Psychology Today* (Mar. 1989): 44.
10. Isen, A. M., et al. "The Influence of Positive Affect on the Unusualness of Word Associations." *Journal of Personality and Social Psychology* 48 (1985): 1413–26; Isen, A. M., et al. "Positive Affect Facilitates Creative Problem Solving." *Journal of Personality and Social Psychology* 52 (1987): 1122–31; Isen, A. M. "Positive Affect, Cognitive Processes, and Social Behavior." *Advances in Experimental Social Psychology* 20 (1987): 203–53.
11. Csikszentmihalyi, M. *Flow: The Psychology of Optimal Experience* (New York: Harper and Row, 1990): 117–42.
12. Schank, R. C. *The Creative Attitude* (New York: Macmillan, 1988): 348.
13. Langer, E. J. *Mindfulness* (Reading, Mass.: Addison-Wesley, 1989): 145.
14. Schank. *Creative Attitude*: 348.
15. Goldberg, P. *The Intuitive Edge* (Los Angeles: Tarcher, 1984): 168–69.
16. Storr, A. *Solitude: A Return to the Self* (New York: Free Press, 1989).
17. Ruggiero, V. R. *The Art of Thinking* (New York: Harper and Row, 1984).
18. Shaw, M. E. *Group Dynamics*, 3rd ed. (New York: McGraw-Hill, 1981).
19. Miner, F. C., Jr. "Group Versus Individual Decision Making: An Investigation of Performance Measures, Decision Strategies, and Process Losses/Gains." *Organizational Behavior and Human Performance* (Feb. 1984): 112–24.
20. Nelson, R. J., et al. "Variations in the Proportional Representations of the Hand in Somatosensory Cortex of Primates." Paper presented at the Society for Neuroscience meeting, Boston (Nov. 13, 1980); Jenkins, W. M., et al. Coleman Memorial Laboratories, University of California at San Francisco. Paper presented at the Society for Neuroscience meeting, Anaheim (Oct. 13, 1984).
21. Gondola, J., and Tuckman, B. *Journal of Social Behavior and Personality* 1(1) (1986).
22. Backer, T. E. "How Health Promotion Programs Can Enhance Workplace Creativity." In Klarreich, S. H. (Ed.). *Health and Fitness in the Workplace* (New York: Praeger, 1987): 325–37.
23. Winter, A., and Winter, R. *Build Your Brain Power* (New York: St. Martin's, 1986): 17–43.
24. Cattell, R. B. *Abilities: Their Structure, Growth and Action* (Boston: Houghton Mifflin, 1971).
25. Elsayad, M., et al. "Intellectual Differences of Adult Men Related to Age and Physical Fitness Before and After an Exercise Program." *Journal of Gerontology* 35 (May 1980): 383–87.
26. Waterman, R. H., Jr. *The Renewal Factor* (New York: Bantam, 1987).
27. Borysenko, J. *Minding the Body, Mending the Mind* (Reading, MA: Addison-Wesley, 1987): 91–93.
28. Raiport, G. *Red Gold: Peak Performance Techniques of the Russian and East German Olympic Victors* (Los Angeles: Tarcher, 1989): 39–46.
29. *Journal of Physiology* (London) 160 (1962): 106–54; *Journal of Physiology* (London) 165 (1962–1963): 559–68.
30. Raiport. *Red Gold*; Winter and Winter. *Build Your Brain Power*.
31. Bloomfield, H. H., and Felder, L. *The Achilles Syndrome* (New York: Ballantine, 1985).
32. Sheikh, A. A. (Ed.). *Imagery: Current Theory, Research, and Application* (New York: Wiley Interscience, 1984); Marks, D. F. (Ed.). *Theories of Image Formation* (New York: Brandon House, 1986); Sheikh, A. A. (Ed.). *Imagi-*

nation and Healing (Farmingdale, NY: Baywood, 1984); Sheikh, A. A., and Sheikh, K. S. (Eds.). *Imagery in Education* (Farmingdale, NY: Baywood, 1985); Sheikh, A. A. (Ed.). *Imagery in Sports* (Farmingdale, NY: Baywood, 1988); Suinn, R. M. *Seven Steps to Peak Performance* (Lewiston, NY: Hans Huber, 1986).

33. Miller, E. E. *Power Vision: Mastering Life Through Mental Image Rehearsal.* Audiotape program and manual (Chicago: Nightingale-Conant, 1987).

34. Kosslyn, S. *Visual Cognition* (Cambridge: MIT Press, 1986).

35. Miller, E. E. *Software for the Mind* (Berkeley: Celestial Arts, 1987): 49.

36. Miller. *Power Vision.*

37. Zilbergeld, B., and Lazarus, A. A. *Mind Power: Getting What You Want Through Mental Training* (Boston: Little, Brown, 1987): 19.

Index

About the Author

Robert K. Cooper is chairman and CEO of Advanced Excellence Systems (AES), a management development and corporate consulting firm. He earned his Ph.D. in health sciences and psychology at the Union Graduate School in Cincinnati, has taken graduate work in psychology from the University of Michigan, and has directed university and corporate research projects.

Dr. Cooper has lectured at leading business schools, including the Stanford University Graduate School of Business, and works with a number of *Fortune 500* and *Fortune Global 500* companies. He is regularly featured on national television and radio programs and is a professional member of the American Management Association and National Speakers Association. He presents lectures and seminars for executive conferences, strategic leadership sessions, and management development programs worldwide.

In addition to his corporate expertise, Dr. Cooper is a certified instructor for national preventive medicine organizations and is the author of *Health & Fitness Excellence: The Comprehensive Action Plan.*

Advanced Excellence Systems (AES) is a management development and consulting firm specializing in performance-based programs to establish and sustain the competitive advantage — in innovation, speed, work quality, customer service, productivity, decision making under stress, and work-family balance.

Robert K. Cooper and his associates offer a variety of company-specific programs, including keynote addresses, lectures, executive seminars, and management development workshops. AES also designs scientifically based assessments to pinpoint performance capabilities and vulnerabilities, and provides a variety of in-depth consulting services and training programs — custom-tailored for applications in management, sales, service, and manufacturing.

For further information, contact:

ADVANCED EXCELLENCE SYSTEMS (AES)

5620 SMETANA DRIVE

SUITE 270

MINNEAPOLIS, MN 55343

Telephone: 612-938-0445